Physicians at War

The Dual-Loyalties Challenge

INTERNATIONAL LIBRARY OF ETHICS, LAW, AND THE NEW MEDICINE

VOLUME 41

The titles published in this series are listed at the end of this volume.

Fritz Allhoff
Editor

Physicians at War

The Dual-Loyalties Challenge

Springer

Dr. Fritz Allhoff
Western Michigan University
Kalamazoo, MI
USA
fritz.allhoff@wmich.edu

ISBN: 978-1-4020-6911-6 e-ISBN: 978-1-4020-6912-3

Library of Congress Control Number: 2008922459

Printed on acid-free paper

9 8 7 6 5 4 3 2 1

springer.com

To military physicians, for your humanity, compassion, and service

Contents

in Johannesburg, South Africa. His research focuses on ethical issues associated with, and the history of, infectious disease and genetics. He recently co-edited *Ethics and Infectious Disease* (Blackwell, 2006); and he has published articles in the *American Journal of Bioethics, Bioethics, Developing World Bioethics*, the *Hastings Center Report*, and the *Journal of Medical Ethics*, among other places.

Introduction

Physicians at War: The Dual-Loyalties Challenge[†]

Fritz Allhoff[‡]

1 Introduction

This project began during the 2004–2005 academic year, when I was on a research fellowship at the Institute for Ethics of the American Medical Association (AMA). Just after I began the fellowship, two articles were published in *The Lancet* by Steve Miles in which he discussed alleged violations of military medical ethics that may have transpired through physician involvement in hostile interrogations.[1,2] Then, right before the holiday break, we received notice that the *New England Journal of Medicine* would be publishing a similar essay by Gregg Bloche and Jonathan Marks, in its first issue of 2005.[3] The American Medical Association in general, and the Institute for Ethics in particular, was extremely concerned about Miles's papers and the forthcoming one by Bloche and Marks. Not only were these extremely visible publications, but many thought that the allegations they contained were of grave ethical concern. The AMA, which publishes *The Code of Medical Ethics*, takes very seriously the moral status of the medical profession and therefore was very interested in these articles. (Recently, the AMA's Council on Ethical and Judicial Affairs published an opinion on physician involvement in interrogation,[4] which represents the culmination of its thinking on these topics.)

† I thank Marcus Adams for comments on the penultimate draft of this paper.

‡ Department of Philosophy, Western Michigan University and Centre for Applied Philosophy and Public Ethics, The Australian National University. Please direct correspondence to fritz.allhoff@wmich.edu.

[1] Steven H. Miles, "Abu Ghraib: Its Legacy for Military Medicine," *The Lancet* 364.9435 (2004): 725–729.

[2] Steve H. Miles, "Military Medicine and Human Rights," *The Lancet* 364.9448 (2004): 1851–1852.

[3] M. Gregg Bloche and Jonathan H. Marks, "When Doctors Go to War," *New England Journal of Medicine* 352.1 (January 6, 2005): 3–6.

[4] The Council on Ethical and Judicial Affairs, CEJA Report 10, A-06, "Physician Participation in Interrogation" (American Medical Association, 2006). Reprinted in this volume, pp. 261–271.

F. Allhoff (ed.), *Physicians at War: The Dual-Loyalties Challenge.*

Having already had a background in some elements of military ethics, and the torture debate in particular,[5] my fellowship year quickly evolved to explore physician involvement in interrogations. One element of this project was to research some of the underlying moral issues, though another was to talk to those responsible for military ethics (including military medical ethics) education. This research led me to speak with those teaching military ethics at the US Military Academy at West Point, the US Naval Academy, and the US Air Force Academy, as well as those teaching military medical ethics at US Army Medical Department Center & School (Fort Sam Houston) and the Uniformed Services University of the Health Sciences (Bethesda, Maryland). After I left the AMA, I was also able to spend some time at the Australian Defence Force Academy (Canberra, Australia). In all cases, I was extremely impressed with the professionalism and commitment to ethics that was displayed at each of these training academies.

When starting the research, however, one of the first things that I noticed was how little academic work had been done in military medical ethics. The Borden Institute, an agency of the US Army Medical Department Center & School, had produced two outstanding books which were meant to be used as textbooks for the teaching of military medical ethics.[6] Steve Miles[7] and Michael Gross[8] have each written books about these topics, though these emerged, at least in part, from the previously mentioned journal articles of 2004. Finally, a symposium was held in a prestigious bioethics journal, *Cambridge Quarterly of Healthcare Ethics* (2006).[9] The point, though, is that few discussions regarding military medical ethics have been held until the past few years. As a final programmatic note, the topic of physician involvement in interrogations was afforded the plenary session at the largest biomedical ethics conference of the year, the American Society of Bioethics and the Humanities (2005). This session was somewhat unbalanced, however, insofar as all three speakers argued for exactly the same conclusion (i.e., there was no conservative or dissenting voice), though a response panel aimed to remediate this shortcoming. It was at this meeting that I met Fritz Schmuhl of Springer, who encouraged the production of this volume, particularly given the interest in the two sessions at that meeting.

In the remainder of this introduction, I would like to provide a discussion of some of the frameworks and issues that appear in this volume (§2) and then to provide a

---

[5]See, for example, Fritz Allhoff, "Terrorism and Torture," *International Journal of Applied Philosophy* 17.1 (2003): 105–18. See also Fritz Allhoff, "A Defense of Torture: Separation of Cases, Ticking Time-Bombs, and Moral Justification," *International Journal of Applied Philosophy* 19.2 (2006): 243–64.

[6]Office of the Surgeon General, Department of the Army, United States of America, *Military Medical Ethics*, 2 vols. (Bethesda, MD: Department of Defense, Office of the Surgeon General, US Army, Borden Institute, 2003).

[7]Steven H. Miles, *Oath Betrayed: Torture, Medical Complicity, and the War on Terror* (New York: Random House, 2006).

[8]Michael L. Gross, *Bioethics and Armed Conflict* (Cambridge, MA: MIT Press, 2006).

[9]I authored an essay in this symposium; see Fritz Allhoff, "Physician Involvement in Hostile Interrogations," *Cambridge Quarterly of Healthcare Ethics* 15 (2006): 392–402. Reprinted in this volume, pp. 91–104.

discussion of how some of these issues might be resolved (§3); the essays in the volume explore these frameworks, issues, and resolutions in greater detail.

2 The Dual-Loyalties Challenge

The motivating premise behind this volume is that, in times of armed conflict, physicians can arguably be subject to dual-loyalties. This concept has been explored in greater detail elsewhere[10] but, for present purposes, we might understand it as the existence of simultaneous obligations which might come into conflict with each other. While dual-loyalties can generalize to all sorts of contexts, our present concern is with the ones that apply to physicians during armed conflict. In these scenarios, physicians have medical obligations to those in medical need. We could ground such obligations in various ways, but the most straightforward way is to acknowledge the medical duties of beneficence and non-malfeasance, both of which have been traditional foundations of medical ethics. According to these duties, physicians are morally bound to render aid insofar as they can and not to (intentionally) make anyone medically worse off.

Such medical duties, however, might come into conflict with non-medical duties, and there are such non-medical duties that we would expect to be expressly manifest during times of war. For example, military physicians are subject to the chain of command and therefore have an obligation to obey their orders. To be sure, it might not *always* be the case that following orders from the chain of command is morally obligatory, but we can presumably suppose that, at least in the cases of just war, there is a (defeasible) reason—which we could cache out in terms of military efficiency, for example—for obeying commands and that, therefore, such commands have some sort of positive moral status. Second, the physician, in virtue of medical training, might be able to promote national security or, more nebulously, the greater good, and therefore absorb the associative moral obligations.

Of course, these non-medical obligations could precisely oppose the medical obligations previously mentioned. Consider, for example, physician participation in weapons development, which is covered in Part III of this volume. We can easily imagine cases wherein physicians are operating on the just side in a conflict against an evil regime and that their expertise could be applied to chemical or biological weapons; we could further imagine that such weapons would be effective against the enemy and lead to a quicker dissolution of the conflict. With such weapons, it could be the case that there would be fewer casualties overall—perhaps by shortening the war—or even that the existence of such weapons would be psychologically debilitating enough to the enemy that the conflict could rapidly come to an end. If this is a terrorist regime, then national security could legitimize the development of

[10]See, for example, Physicians for Human Rights and the School of Public Health and Primary Health Care, University of Cape Town, Health Sciences Faculty, *Dual-loyalty Human Rights in Health Professional Practice: Proposed Guidelines & Institutional Mechanisms*. Excerpts reprinted in this volume, pp. 15–38. See also the other essays in Unit I.

the weapons or, regardless, such weapons might serve the greater good—including the citizenry, present and future, which falls under the dissolved evil regime—and therefore be morally justified. But, despite the moral considerations that would count in favor of such weapons development, there are contrary considerations that would inveigh against it. In particular, the development of weapons could violate the physician obligation of non-malfeasance since those weapons would be used to harm some individuals.[11] What, then, should physicians do? Are they morally permitted to participate in weapons development?

Before moving on to a more general discussion of these challenges, let me point out some other specific contexts in which such challenges arise. Many of these are covered in this volume, but I will briefly mention them in this section. In particular, we could see the above frameworks also applying in the following: physician involvement in torture (Part II) and battlefield triage/medical neutrality (Part IV). Starting with torturous interrogations, it could easily be the case that such interrogations serve important military objectives, and that medical knowledge could make the interrogations more expedient, perhaps by conducting them in ways that invoke physical or psychological vulnerabilities of the interrogatee. Again, though, any application of medical knowledge that makes the interrogatee worse off than he/she otherwise would have been could be viewed as problematic when viewed through the lens of medical ethics.[12] Therefore, this is another instance of the dual-loyalties conundrum.

Finally, consider some of the issues that physicians might face on the battlefield. In particular, I have battlefield triage and medical neutrality in mind. The scenario in these cases is that there are some number of individuals in need of medical attention such that the demand for such attention exceeds the supply. Some decision, then, must be made about how those resources should be allocated. Medical obligations would suggest that these decisions should be made on medical grounds alone: resources should be invested in ways to optimize (medical) outcomes. Just to take an example, imagine that there are two wounded soldiers, one of ours and one of the enemy and that there are only resources to tend to one of them. Imagine, further, that the enemy is slightly worse off, though both are very much in need. Medically, it could easily be the case that treatment should be provided to the enemy, since he is less likely to survive absent medical care. The other soldier, however, is on *our side*. Should the physician tend to the enemy, despite the fact that this could lead to the death of an allied comrade? Or, more generally, should physicians exercise (political) *neutrality* when making medical decisions? What if the injured enemy were a high-ranking officer who could be an important strategic asset? It could be the case that resuscitating such an offer could, ultimately, lead to the realization of various

[11] In my own view, this conclusion does not follow since I think that non-malfeasance should be understood in an aggregative mode: if physicians harm a few people such that more people are not harmed later—through, let's say, continued military conflict—it seems to me that such an act is not just licensed, but rather required by an appeal to non-malfeasance. This is an unpopular view that I will not develop here, but see Allhoff (2003) for related discussion.

[12] In fact, this is precisely the view taken by the AMA in its report. See pp. 261–271, this volume. For a dissent, see my essay, pp. 91–104.

military objectives; we could further stipulate that such objectives had moral significance. If the physician chooses to save the enemy officer over our private, is this *fair*? If such an officer were *less* in medical need then, despite the military advantages, then it would seem medical virtues would mandate the treatment of the private, though this could have adverse consequences for key military objectives. These questions can become even murkier when we abstract away from "micro" decisions (e.g., save this person or that one) and try to achieve some clarity about the general triage practices that should be endorsed; in any case, such situations can clearly manifest the dual-loyalties concern.

3 Addressing the Challenge

In the previous section, I introduced the notion of the dual-loyalties challenge and showed how it could be instantiated in various contexts: weapons development, torture, and battlefield triage/medical neutrality. In this section, I want to consider various ways to remediate the challenge, and I take it that there are, conceptually, four different options here. First, we could hold that medical and non-medical values are *commensurable* and that, in any given case, we just have to make adjudications about which pull more strongly. Second and third, we could hold that these values are *incommensurable*, but that one or the other set of values does not apply. One option is that non-medical obligations are patently irrelevant to medical decision making; the other is that medical obligations are inappropriate in these contexts. Fourth, we might say that the values are incommensurable, yet all apply. It is not clear to me how this fourth option is a *solution* to the challenge as it merely posits intractability. And I think, therefore, that it is simply implausible: we all believe that there are right and wrong courses of action in the scenarios mentioned in §2, and I want to suggest that we all believe this because one of the first three options listed must be correct.

The first option is the one that might seem the most straightforward: we acknowledge the existence of conflicting obligations, and then we just have to figure out which set carries more weight (while accepting the countervailing force of the contrary). So we could say, for example, that it is *prima facie* bad for physicians to develop weapons while, at the same time, allowing that complicity in weapons programs could nevertheless be justified if the stakes were high enough. As more lives hung in the balance, as the enemy regime were more evil, or as all other options had been exhausted, we might postulate increasing moral merit in physicians developing these weapons. Absent such features, though, perhaps there would not be sufficient countervailing moral weight for physician involvement in such a program given their medical obligations.

This line is not without problems, both epistemic and metaphysical. Regarding the epistemic ones, we simply do now *know* how many lives might be at stake, or what the consequences will be of us having (or not having) chemical or biological weapons. Metaphysically, we might meaningfully ask how many lives are *worth* a single transgression against non-malfeasance, and thence beckons the specter of incommensurability. The epistemic worries, though, are just that, epistemic: whether we *know* the relevant stakes, it hardly follows that there does not *exist* some proper course of action, and we then have to do the best we can to determine what it is. The commensurability problem is a difficult one as well, and people choosing this approach to resolving the challenge will surely owe us an account of their thinking in this regard.

Let me also point out another answer that might present itself here, which is more empirical than conceptual. In setting up the above challenges (in §2), I made various suppositions, and people might simply deny that any of these is reasonable. For example, in the torturous interrogation case, I asked that we consider an interrogation that advanced the greater good, despite its transgression of medical virtues. It is certainly an open possibility here to deny that such an interrogation is *possible*, perhaps by denying the plausibility of any sort of utility forecast that would justify the interrogation. In the torture debate more generally, this is a common line,[13] though I think that there are responses.[14] This approach, then, admits of the commensurability of the conflicting obligations while, at the same time, denying that there will ever be much pull coming from one of the directions; a quick look at the literature would suggest that the non-medical obligations are more commonly thought to be the impotent ones. Regardless, I think that this is the approach that it most intuitive, though there is some work to be done regarding how the commensurability would be understood.

Second, we could resolve the challenge by saying that one of the two directions (necessarily, as opposed to contingently) exerts no pull. The more common direction that this would take is to deny that extra-medical considerations can have any import on medical considerations. This strategy is one that we might appropriate, in a different context, to Michael Walzer.[15] Walzer has postulated "spheres of justice" exist such that we can only make distributions of resources within some sphere based on considerations internal to it, rather than to some distributive logic that would be motivated from some other sphere. In applying that structure to our context, it would therefore be inappropriate to make decisions regarding *medicine* by appeal to *extra-medical* considerations: medicine occupies its own sphere of justice and, therefore, medical decisions must be based on medical considerations alone. Note, then, that this view is patently is one of incommensurability: it does not *matter*, for example, whether there are tremendous extra-medical benefits to be gained through some action that violates tenets of medical justice since the former are inadmissible regarding considerations of the latter. On this view, there is no dual-loyalties challenge since there are no *dual* loyalties in the first place: physicians must make medical decisions based *solely* on medical considerations and chains of command, national security,

[13] See, for example, Jean Maria Arrigo, **"A** Utilitarian Argument against Torture," *Science and Engineering Ethics* 10.3 (2004):1–30. See also Matthew Wynia, "Consequentialism and Harsh Interrogations," *American Journal of Bioethics* 5. I (2005): 4–6.

[14] See, for example, Fritz Allhoff, "A Defense of Torture: Separation of Cases, Ticking Time-Bombs, and Moral Justification," *International Journal of Applied Philosophy* 19.2 (2006): 243–64.

[15] Michael Walzer, *Spheres of Justice* (New York: Basic Books, 1983).

and the greater good are impotent against such considerations. While Walzer did not explicitly apply his framework to this present context, such an application is nevertheless fairly straightforward.

This view is not without problems, though many people will nevertheless find it compelling. As far as I can tell, the most pressing objection would have to do with how we individuate different spheres. As I laid it out in the previous paragraph, the medical sphere was conveniently insulated from the non-medical realm, and this insulation provided a solution to the dual-loyalties challenge. However, this structure could receive pressure in either of two directions. First, we might wonder whether this medical sphere is *too small*. In fact, the reason it offers a solution to the dual-loyalties challenge is that it is precisely of the scope that would do so and, therefore, might be thought to be idiosyncratic or *ad hoc*. What is so special about medicine such that it gets its own sphere of justice? The postulation of such a sphere almost seems to be question-begging against "greater good" considerations, since it eliminates those considerations out of hand (e.g., by asserting a sphere which they cannot penetrate). We could certainly carve up the spheres differently, and maybe "greater good" could be some such sphere, of which medicine were a proper part. Regardless, it would seem that the postulation of some sphere needs to be *motivated* in some way, and it is not clear to me what the motivation for a medical sphere would be.[16] Conversely, maybe the medical sphere is *too big* (as opposed to too small). If there is a medical sphere, there could very well be sub-medical spheres: just as some features set off the medical sphere from others, features within it might be used to set off facets of it from itself. The problem would then be that this conception of spheres could lead to a sufficiently high number of them such that they would not be useful in particular cases. Regardless, the proponents of spheres will have to say something about *why* there is a sphere of medicine and why it does not either get subsumed under a bigger sphere or fracture into multiple smaller ones; only such a compelling story here would preserve the merits of this answer.

Finally, we could resolve the dual-loyalties challenge in the third way, which is again to deny that there are dual loyalties at all. While the spheres of justice approach negates the relevance of extra-medical obligations, a converse approach holds that *only* extra-medical obligations are admissible and that medical obligations do not apply. Again, this line would deny that there is a dual-loyalties *challenge* since there would not be competing obligations at all. This is undoubtedly the least popular of all the options and, as far as I can tell, I am the only person who defends it.[17] The idea here is that medical obligations apply only to *physicians* and that there is conceptual space for medically-trained military functionaries who are nonetheless not physicians.[18] Physicians are members of the medical *profession*, and this carries with it various moral features. For example, they have taken an oath

[16] In the book (and in subsequent literature), this topic is explored, though I take it to continue to be one that assails the position.

[17] See Allhoff(2006), pp. 395–400. Reprinted in this volume, pp. 96–104 [section entitled "Are Medically Trained Interrogators *Physicians*?"].

[18] I acknowledge that, despite this contention, the title of this volume nevertheless invokes 'physicians'. I do this most proximately for ease of use, but also in recognition of the consensus view on this issue.

to abide by various features of that profession, including providing care for those in need. But we could easily imagine medically trained personnel who are not members of this profession: they may never have taken the oath nor ever planned to provide positive medical services. Rather, they could use their medical training in an adversarial way, such as through the development of weapons or through participation in hostile interrogations.

I want to suggest that medical obligations do not apply to these people, whom I take to be something other than physicians. The contrary view would have to hold that, *regardless* of these people's non-participation in the medical profession, the obligations nevertheless attach to them. I think that this line is problematic for various reasons, and provide those arguments later in this volume. A second critique of this position—which came out as a response to my paper and is therefore not considered within it—is that the people that I would otherwise exempt from medical obligations are, *in fact*, physicians: they *have* taken the associative oaths and *are* members of the medical profession. I do not disagree with this claim, but it does nothing to erode the conceptual space that I aim to delimit. Rather, it seems completely possible to me that military physicians could *opt out* of the profession, and that some of their obligations would thereafter dissolve. (Some, however, would not, such as the obligation to preserve confidences obtained through participation in the profession.) Furthermore, there is no reason that these personnel had to take whatever oaths would ground medical obligations: we could easily imagine a medically-trained force that completely rejects these values altogether.

In this introduction, I have discussed briefly the issues that motivate and constitute the volume. In §2, I introduced the notion of the dual-loyalties challenge, which is further discussed in Part I. I also introduced some particular issues in which this challenge is manifest: physicians and torture (Part II); physicians and weapons development (Part III); and physicians on the battlefield (Part IV). Each of these parts comprises papers which explore the associative dimensions in greater detail, and display a range of different perspectives thereof. In §3, I discussed various options to resolve the dual-loyalties challenge; these are also variously considered throughout the following essays. At the end of the volume, I have included three appendices, which are statements published by the World Health Organization and the American Medical Association regarding physician involvement in armed conflict.

Thank you for your interest in this project; I hope that you find the following essays engaging and provocative!

References

Allhoff, Fritz. 2003. Terrorism and Torture. *International Journal of Applied Philosophy* 17.1: 105–118.

Allhoff, Fritz. 2006. Physician Involvement in Hostile Interrogations. *Cambridge Quarterly of Healthcare Ethics* 15: 392–402. Reprinted in this volume, pp. 91–104.

Allhoff, Fritz. 2006. A Defense of Torture: Separation of Cases, Ticking Time-Bombs, and Moral Justification. *International Journal of Applied Philosophy* 19.2: 243–264.

Arrigo, Jean Maria. 2004. A Utilitarian Argument Against Torture. *Science and Engineering Ethics* 10.3: 1–30.

Bloche, M. Gregg and Jonathan H. Marks. 2005. When Doctors Go to War. *New England Journal of Medicine* 352.1 (January 6): 3–6.

Gross, Michael L. 2006. *Bioethics and Armed Conflict*. Cambridge, MA: MIT.

Miles, Steve H. 2004. Military Medicine and Human Rights. *The Lancet* 364.9448: 1851–1852.

Miles, Steven H. 2004. Abu Ghraib: Its Legacy for Military Medicine. *The Lancet* 364.9435: 725–729.

Miles, Steven H. 2006. *Oath Betrayed: Torture, Medical Complicity, and the War on Terror*. New York: Random House.

Office of the Surgeon General, Department of the Army, United States of America. 2003. *Military Medical Ethics*, 2 vols. Bethesda, MD: Department of Defense, Office of the Surgeon General, US Army, Borden Institute.

Physicians for Human Rights and the School of Public Health and Primary Health Care. *Dual-loyalty & Human Rights in Health Professional Practice: Proposed Guidelines & Institutional Mechanisms*. Cape Town, South Africa: University of Cape Town, Health Sciences Faculty. Excerpts reprinted in this volume, pp. 15–38.

Walzer, Michael. 1983. *Spheres of Justice*. New York: Basic Books.

Wynia, Matthew. 2005. Consequentialism and Harsh Interrogations. *American Journal of Bioethics* 5.1: 4–6.

Part I
Physicians and Dual-Loyalties

Dual-Loyalty and Human Rights in Health Professional Practice: Proposed Guidelines and Institutional Mechanisms[1]

International Dual-Loyalty Working Group[2]

1 Introduction

1.1 The Problem of Dual-Loyalty and Human Rights

The problem of dual-loyalty—simultaneous obligations, express or implied, to a patient and to a third party, often the state—continues to challenge health professionals. Health professional ethics have long stressed the need for loyalty to people in their care. In the modern world, however, health professionals are increasingly asked to weigh their devotion to patients against service to the objectives of government or other third parties. Dual-loyalty poses particular challenges for health professionals throughout the world when the subordination of the patient's interests to state or other purposes risks violating the patient's human rights. Efforts to bolster ethical codes to address these challenges have only marginally succeeded, as will be discussed in Chapter 2 (not herein included).

The goals of this project are to identify the dimensions of dual-loyalty and to propose guidelines and mechanisms for the prevention of complicity by health professionals in human rights violations. This introductory chapter defines what dual-loyalty is, explains how professional ethics and human rights relate in solving dual-loyalty problems, and explores the obligations of health professionals

[1] The following selection has been excerpted from a complete report (of the same title) published by and copyrighted by Physicians for Human Rights and the School of Public Health and Primary Health Care, University of Cape Town, Health Sciences Faculty. Used with permission. I have left references to parts of the report not included in this selection in case the interested reader wishes to further pursue them. The entire report is available at http://physiciansforhumanrights.org/library/documents/reports/report-2002-duelloyalty.pdf. Note that §1 discusses general theoretical issues in the dual-loyalty context, whereas §4.5 considers proposed guidelines for military settings. This has been reformatted for consistency with the other essays in this volume.

[2] This workgroup is a collaborative initiative of Physicians for Human Rights and the School of Public Health and Primary Health Care, University of Cape Town, Health Sciences Faculty. Leonard S. Rubenstein, Leslie London, and Laurel Baldwin-Ragaven directed the project, and Adrian van Es led the military sub-group.

F. Allhoff (ed.), *Physicians at War: The Dual-Loyalties Challenge.*

to respect human rights. These introductory comments provide the background for a description of the motivation for and scope of this project.

1.2 The Concept of Dual-Loyalty

Since ancient times, many societies have held healthcare professionals to an ethic of undivided loyalty to the welfare of the patient. Current international codes of ethics generally mandate complete loyalty to patients.[3] The World Medical Association (WMA) Declaration of Geneva, the modern equivalent of the Hippocratic Oath, asks physicians to pledge that "the health of my patient shall be my first consideration" and to provide medical services in "full technical and moral independence."[4] The WMA International Code of Medical Ethics states that "a physician shall owe his patients complete loyalty and all the resources of his science."[5]

In practice, however, health professionals often have obligations to other parties besides their patients—such as family members, employers, insurance companies and governments—that may conflict with undivided devotion to the patient. This phenomenon is dual-loyalty, which may be defined as clinical role conflict between professional duties to a patient and obligations, express or implied, real or perceived, to the interests of a third party such as an employer, an insurer or the state.[6]

---

[3] These refer to ethical codes promulgated by international and national bodies of health professionals such as the World Medical Association and intergovernmental organs like the United Nations.

[4] World Medical Association, *Declaration of Geneva*. This and other ethical codes adopted by international bodies applicable to health professions can be found in Amnesty International, Ethical Codes and Declarations Relevant to the Health Professions. See Appendix 1 for full citations.

[5] World Medical Association, *International Code of Medical Ethics*.

[6] For an overview of dual-loyalty, see M. Gregg Bloche, "Clinical Loyalties and the Social Purposes of Medicine," *Journal of the American Medical Association* 281.3 (1999): 268–274. For a discussion of dual-loyalty concerns in everyday practice, see British Medical Association, *Medical Ethics Today: Its Practice and Philosophy*. It should be noted that not every conflict or ethical dilemma presents a dual-loyalty problem. Questions of transactions by health professionals with an entity in which they have a financial interest, for example, represent a direct conflict between the health professional and a patient rather than a problem of allegiance or submission by the health professional to an external agency or authority. In medical triage of ill and injured patients, health professionals may face conflicts between the medical needs of some patients at the expense of others; however, there is inherently no dual loyalty problem as the term is defined here since making these often difficult decisions means balancing the medical needs of patients rather than considering non-medical interests of a third party. Dual-loyalty can arise in triage situations if, however, the decision is influenced by social objectives, such as gender or racial preferences. By contrast, where the reimbursement policies of a third party are such as to influence the health professional's judgment in ways that are detrimental to the patient's best interest, a dual-loyalty conflict may be said to exist. This project concerns dual-loyalty conflicts that have the potential to violate human rights.

The dual-loyalty problem is usually understood in the context of a relationship with an individual patient. In many parts of the world, however, clinicians have responsibilities to communities of patients, for prevention, health education and clinical care. Dual-loyalty conflicts can and do arise in these settings as well.

In cases where dual-loyalty exists, elevating state over individual interests may nevertheless serve social purposes often accepted as justifiable.[7] Evaluations for adjudicative purposes are a common example. A medical evaluation of an individual's condition that is relevant to resolution of a lawsuit or a claim for disability benefits requires the health professional to express opinions about individuals that may result in their exclusion from desired benefits or their being deprived of a desired outcome. Such an evaluation is generally accepted as a justifiable departure from complete loyalty to the individual because of the overriding need for objective medical evidence to resolve the claim in a fair and just manner.

Such socially and legally accepted departures from undivided loyalty to the patient are not restricted to evaluations. For example, a health professional may be required to breach confidentiality in a relationship with a patient in order to protect third parties from harm or to notify a health authority of communicable diseases for health surveillance purposes. However, in all circumstances where departure from undivided loyalty takes place, what is critical to the moral acceptability of such departures is the fairness and transparency of the balancing of conflicting interests, and the way in which such balancing is, or is not, consistent with human rights.

1.3 Dual-Loyalty and Human Rights

Dual-loyalty becomes especially problematic when the health professional acts to support the interests of the state or other entity instead of those of the individual in a manner that violates the human rights of the individual. The most insidious human rights violations stemming from dual-loyalty arise in health practice under a repressive government, where pervasive human rights abuses, combined with restrictions on freedom of expression, render it difficult both to resist state demands and to report abuses. In addition, closed institutions, such as jails, prisons, psychiatric facilities and the military, impose high demands for allegiance on health professionals even in the face of often-common human rights violations against individuals held there. But violations of human rights at the behest of the state by health professionals also take place in open societies, for example, in cases of institutionalized bias or discrimination against women, members of a particular ethnic or religious group, refugees and immigrants, or patients who are politically or socially stigmatized. Violations of people's rights of access to health care may also arise from policies imposed by governments, or in health systems, including privately managed health systems, in which health professionals are called upon to withhold treatment from certain groups of people in discriminatory ways.

[7] See Bloche, "Clinical Loyalties and the Social Purposes of Medicine."

The problem is compounded when the health professional's conduct is constrained by pressure to yield to other powerful interests, especially those of the state. The pressure may be a product of legal requirements, threats of professional or personal harm for non-compliance, the culture of the institution or society where the professional practices, or even the professional's own sense of duty to the state.[8] In repressive political regimes or in closed institutions like prisons and jails, the personal consequences can be quite severe.

1.4 Human Rights, Bioethics and the Resolution of Dual-Loyalty Conflicts

Many health professionals are generally familiar with bioethical frameworks to assist in resolving difficult clinical dilemmas, typically arising in end-of-life situations or in the context of limited resources. Less familiar to health professionals is analysis of the human rights dimensions to healthcare practice.[9] This project seeks to extend the ambit of health professionals' decision making to include the protection of patients' human rights in cases of dual-loyalty. The frameworks of bioethics and human rights each present approaches to resolving competing claims in principled ways. Where dual-loyalty conflicts are associated with human rights violations, it is essential for health professionals to recognize the contributions human rights approaches can make. The following sections outline the respective approaches: one based on human rights and another on bioethics, and how their complementarities can be used to resolve dual-loyalty conflicts that threaten violations of human rights.

1.4.1 Human Rights

Human rights have best been described as "rights of individuals in society" that take the form of "… legitimate, valid, justified claims—upon his or her society—to various 'goods' and 'benefits' deemed essential for dignity and well-being."[10] These claims are not abstractions or based on natural law, social contract, or political theory but stem from international governmental consensus around moral principles considered universal. In the modern era, they were first embodied in the Universal Declaration of Human Rights (UDHR), adopted in the aftermath of World War II,

---

[8] Some commentators have suggested that health professionals are at times unaware or even unconscious of the connections between clinical practices and the furtherance of social norms that may not be in the patient's interest. See M. Gregg Bloche, "Caretakers and Collaborators," *Cambridge Quarterly of Healthcare Ethics* 10.3 (2001): 275–284.

[9] British Medical Association, *The Medical Profession and Human Rights: A Handbook for a Changing Agenda* (London: Zed Books, 2001), 478–502.

[10] Louis Henkin, *The Age of Rights* (New York: Columbia University Press, 1990), 4.

and then extended through international treaties. Grounded on the premise that "all human beings are born free and equal in dignity and rights,"[11] the UDHR enumerates specific rights, many of which have been adopted in international and regional treaties that bind states that have ratified the treaties.[12] Once a treaty is ratified by a state, it becomes law in the state and binds its conduct.

Human rights obligations generally impose duties upon the state rather than private individuals and entities. But the state/private distinction does not fully do justice to the scope of human rights obligations. In certain circumstances, the state has a duty to assure that the conduct of private actors is consistent with human rights. Thus, for example, states have obligations not merely to refrain from racial discrimination but to "prohibit and bring to an end" to discrimination, including racial discrimination, by "any person, group or organization"[13] that interferes with "the right to public health, medical care, social security and social services."[14] Similarly, states have obligations to protect the rights of workers in relations with employers.

Operationalizing the UDHR, principally an aspirational document, are two foundational human rights treaties: the International Covenant on Civil and Political Rights and the International Covenant on Economic, Social and Cultural Rights.[15] The former recognizes principally the rights to life, liberty, security of the person, freedom from torture and cruel, degrading and inhuman treatment, freedom from unjust discrimination, due process of law, and free expression and association. These rights are not subject to balancing against other state interests and none may be "derogated," or suspended, unless the state officially proclaims the existence of a national emergency and only to the extent "strictly necessary" to meet the exigencies of the situation; and, any derogation cannot involve discrimination on the basis of race, color, sex, language, birth, property,[16] religion or social origin.[17]

Moreover, certain rights, including the right to be free from torture and cruel, inhuman, or degrading treatment can never be subject to derogation. The obligations not to engage in discrimination on the basis of race and gender have been elaborated with more specificity in the Convention on the Elimination of all forms of Racial Discrimination and the Convention for the Elimination of all forms of

---

[11] United Nations, *Universal Declaration of Human Rights*, art. 1.

[12] Not all states have ratified all human rights treaties, but so many states have agreed to them and the norms have become universal such that the state's obligations can be considered binding under customary international law. See Henry Steiner and Philip Alston, *International Human Rights Law in Context* (Oxford: Oxford University Press, 2000).

[13] United Nations, *Convention on the Elimination of All Forms of Racial Discrimination*, art. 2, sec. 1(d).

[14] Id., art. 5(e).

[15] Human rights instruments, treaties and declarations are all available at the web site of the UN High Commissioner for Human Rights, www.unhchr.ch. These covenants, moreover, are supplemented by regional instruments such as the *Inter-American Convention on Human Rights* and the *European Convention on Human Rights*. Also, see Appendix 2.

[16] Property and birth can be understood to encompass caste and class.

[17] United Nations, *International Covenant on Civil and Political Rights*, art. 4.

Discrimination against Women. Under these conventions, states are bound not to engage in discrimination themselves and also to take affirmative steps to eliminate discrimination in society. Moreover, the conventions prohibit discriminatory effects of policies and practices as well as intentional discrimination.

Nations have also adopted a treaty specific to the problem of torture, the Convention Against Torture and Other Cruel, Inhuman and Degrading Treatment and Punishment, which sets out both standards of conduct for states and monitoring mechanisms by UN bodies. Other treaties also bear on health and indirectly on the conduct of health professionals. The Convention on the Rights of the Child systematically sets out states' obligations to children. Another convention, dating from 1951, sets out the requirements of states in the treatment of refugees. In addition, the United Nations General Assembly has promulgated standards and guidelines designed to protect human rights of prisoners, people with mental illness and mental retardation, and other vulnerable groups.

The International Covenant on Economic, Social and Cultural Rights (1966) sets forth obligations states have to meet people's basic material needs, to protect the family as an institution, and to establish rights to work, health, social security and housing, among others. For health professionals, the most important provision is Article 12, which provides that "Every human being is entitled to the enjoyment of the highest attainable standard of health conducive to living a life in dignity." In 2000, the UN Committee responsible for interpretation of this Covenant issued a General Comment, or explanation of Article 12 that, while not binding, does serve as a useful guide for monitoring.[18]

The Committee interpreted Article 12 consistent with past interpretations of the Covenant on Economic, Social and Cultural Rights as imposing three types of duties on governments. The first core obligation is to respect, requiring states to refrain from interfering directly or indirectly with the enjoyment of the right to the highest attainable standard of health, for example, by denying or limiting equal access to health care for all persons, engaging in state-sponsored discrimination in health services, marketing unsafe drugs, or limiting access to family planning and reproductive health services. The second is the obligation to protect, requiring states to prevent third parties from interfering in the right to the highest attainable standard of health, for example, by permitting providers to discriminate or by failing to control marketing of medicines and harmful products like tobacco. The third is the obligation to fulfill, requiring states to adopt appropriate legislative, administrative, budgetary and other steps toward the full realization of the right to the highest attainable standard of health.[19] This obligation requires states to have a national

[18] United Nations, Committee on Economic, Social and Cultural Rights, *The Right to the Highest Attainable Standard of Health*, "General Comment 14."

[19] Id., para. 33. The Committee makes clear that Article 12 does not articulate a right to "be healthy," but rather demands action by states to provide the underlying conditions, health policies and services that enable individuals to obtain the highest attainable standard of health for themselves. See also Audrey R. Chapman and Sage Russell, eds., *Core Obligations: Building a Framework for Economic, Social and Cultural Rights* (Antwerpen, The Netherlands: Intersentia, 2002).

strategy for enabling all members of society to achieve the highest attainable standard of health, to assure that marginalized groups have access to clean water, education and essential health services, to immunize its population against communicable diseases, to provide information to prevent the spread of disease, and to take other steps the Committee sets out.[20]

Although fulfillment of the right to the highest attainable standard of health is subject to resource limitations and of course does not require that every health service (e.g., cosmetic surgery) be made available to all, the Committee makes clear that the Covenant obliges "each State party to take the necessary steps to the maximum of its available resources and failure to do so constitutes a violation." Moreover, the Committee sets out "core" obligations that exist irrespective of resource constraints. These include, among others, non-discriminatory and equitable access to health care services "especially for marginalized groups," maternal and child health care services, availability of immunizations against infectious diseases, a public health strategy for the society, essential drugs and access to information about the main health problems in the community.[21]

The rights described in the two foundational covenants are mutually reinforcing and are commonly said to be indivisible. A person cannot enjoy political freedoms unless he or she has the education to be able to exercise those freedoms. Similarly, a person who has access to health care is nonetheless denied health and well-being if forced to live in a repressive society. The connections are evident, too, on a macro scale: as Amartya Sen has explained, no substantial famine has occurred in a democratic country.[22] In Chapter 2 [not herein included], greater detail about how these human rights apply to specific problems of dual-loyalty is provided.

In sum, the most basic and fundamental purpose of human rights is to respect and protect individual persons. For health professionals, a human rights framework provides a steady moral compass, a blueprint of a just and humane social order that at its core articulates the principles of the dignity and equality of every human being. Decisions made to respect, protect, and fulfill human rights therefore seek to ensure that a rights analysis informs how such conflicts can be resolved. Put another way, a human rights analysis enables the health professional to resolve these conflicts by reference to an agreed-upon, universally applicable set of moral principles. In health care settings, consideration of human rights concerns, as elaborated through the various instruments, conventions and treaties discussed above, should be a requisite for resolving dual-loyalty conflicts.

---

[20] Rights related to the highest attainable standard of health are also reflected in other treaties, particularly the *UN Convention on the Rights of the Child* and the *UN Convention on the Elimination of all forms of Discrimination against Women.*

[21] United Nations, Committee on Economic, Social and Cultural Rights, *The Right to the Highest Attainable Standard of Health*, "General Comment 14," para. 43.

[22] Amartya Sen, *Development as Freedom* (Oxford: Oxford University Press, 1999), 51.

1.4.2 Bioethics

Bioethics is a discipline that enables clinicians to engage in analyses that will determine their courses of action in particularly compelling and morally complex clinical situations. Bioethical analysis can help health professionals address the difficult dilemmas that arise in everyday clinical work and provide guidance for identifying rational arguments to substantiate their moral choices in ways that aim to be reasoned and constant.

There are at least two aspects to such a bioethics paradigm: one is ethics formulated as professional codes of conduct that seek to provide guidance to clinicians facing ethical dilemmas[23] and the other is the process of resolving clinical dilemmas through philosophical reasoning. A widely recognized framework for resolving morally difficult situations in health care identifies four ethical principles and addresses their scope of application.[24] It has been argued that these four principles together with concern for their scope or coverage "encompass most if not all of the moral issues in health care" and reflect the range of moral commitments or options available to support the resolution of competing choices.[25] These have been laid out as:

- Respect for the decision-making ability of autonomous persons (autonomy or self-determination)
- The duty to maximize benefit to the person or people in care (beneficence); often taken together with
- The mandate to avoid the causation of harm (non-maleficence)
- Fairness in deciding competing claims, often to resources, but also to human rights and laws or social policy (justice)

Within this framework, bioethical reasoning invokes the application of these principles in a thoughtful and systematic way to provide guidance for appropriate decisions when faced with a clinical or patient-management dilemma. By balancing these principles, and taking into account the contextual factors in which the dilemma occurs as well as the evidentiary support data, clinicians will more often than not make decisions about what they ought to do.

More recent developments have sought to expand the scope of bioethics to include its application beyond the individual clinical encounter to considerations of the health of an entire population.[26] It is now widely recognized that societal factors,

---

[23] See footnotes 4–6, for example.

[24] Tom L. Beauchamp and James F. Childress, *Principles of Biomedical Ethics* (Oxford: Oxford University Press, 2001).

[25] Raanan Gillon, "Preface: Medical Ethics and the Four Principles," in *Principles of Health Care Ethics*, eds. Raanan Gillon and Lloyd (Chichester: Wiley, 1994) xxi.

[26] Jonathan M. Mann et al., "Health and Human Rights," *Health and Human Rights: An International Journal* 1.1 (1994): 7–23; Nancy E. Kass, "An Ethics Framework for Public Health," *American Journal of Public Health* 91.11 (2001): 1776–1782; Marc J. Roberts and Michael Reich, "Ethical Analysis in Public Health," *Lancet*. 359.9311 (2002): 1055–1059; Dan E. Beauchamp and Bonnie Steinbock, *New Ethics for the Public's Health* (Oxford: Oxford University Press, 1999); Anthony Kessel, "Public Health Ethics: Teaching Survey and Critical Review." *Social Science and Medicine* (in press).

such as socioeconomic inequalities, discrimination and a lack of respect for dignity have profound effects on health status and life expectancy,[27] and that health disparities are increasingly a matter of ethical concern.[28] This provides a compelling reason for the health sector to identify the moral basis for policies and programs that affect the interests and well-being of groups and populations. However, there is no dominant or presently coherent body of ethical theory, much less one that commands international consensus, on society's obligations in the public health domain[29]—though reliance on the principle of justice to resolve ethical dilemmas in public health in the most fair manner remains attractive.[30] While each of the four principles may have possible application, depending on the specific nature of violations, human rights offers a societal level framework for identifying, understanding, and responding to the social determinants of health.[31]

1.4.3 Human Rights and Bioethics

In many ways, human rights and bioethics complement each other. The four principles speak strongly to key human rights concepts. The interdiction against participation by health professionals in torture, a key human rights prohibition,[32] is grounded in non-maleficence, the duty to do no harm. Respecting women's autonomy on reproduction promotes health and the right of access to reproductive health care while combating gender discrimination. Acting in accord with the principle of justice, clinicians who promote fairness in their management of patient—for example, by eschewing racial and gender bias—also uphold human dignity. The four principles are, in general, consistent with human rights tenets. Yet the principles do not focus on compliance with human rights standards.

---

[27] Institute of Medicine, *Unequal Treatment: Confronting Racial and Ethnic Disparities in Health Care*; David B. Evans et al., "Comparative Efficiency of National Health Systems: Cross National Econometric Analysis," *British Medical Journal* 323 (2001): 307–310; David B. Evans et al., "Measuring Quality: From the System to the Provider," *International Journal for Quality in Health Care* 13.6 (2001): 439–446.

[28] Fabienne Peter and Timothy Evans, "Ethical Dimensions of Health Equity," in *Challenging Inequalities in Health. From Ethics to Action*, Timothy Evans, Margaret Whitehead, Finn Diderichsen, Abbas Bhuyia, and Meg Wirth, eds. (New York: Oxford University Press, 2001) 25–33.

[29] Roberts and Reich, "Ethical Analysis in Public Health"; Jonathan M. Mann, "Medicine and Public Health, Ethics and Human Rights," in *Health and Human Rights: A Reader*, Jonathan M. Mann, Sofia Gruskin, Michael A. Grodin, and George J. Annas (New York: Routledge, 1999), 439–452.

[30] Norman Daniels, *Just Health Care* (New York: Cambridge University Press, 1985).

[31] Mann, "Medicine and Public Health, Ethics and Human Rights."

[32] See the UN *Convention Against Torture and Other Cruel, Inhuman and Degrading Treatment and Punishment* and the WMA *Declaration of Tokyo: Guidelines for Medical Doctors Concerning Torture and Other Cruel, Inhuman or Degrading Treatment or Punishment in Relation to Detention and Imprisonment.*

Indeed, bioethics often treats human rights compliance as just one of many competing obligations to be considered.[33] Moreover, the four principles do not provide a method for arriving at concrete decisions—particularly decisions about how to prioritize competing principles. Historical traditions in North America tend, in practice, to privilege individual autonomy over other principles,[34] but even there none of the principles has inherent primacy. Various moral theories and philosophical traditions may be invoked to give relative weights to the four principles in particular circumstances.[35]

As a result, there is space for enormous variability in moral decision-making. Moral disagreements per se are not a bad thing and should not make us skeptical about bioethical reasoning. But such disagreements become problematic when human rights are at stake. Therefore, as stated earlier, in health care settings, consideration of human rights concerns, as elaborated through the various international human rights instruments, conventions and treaties should be a pre-requisite for resolving dual-loyalty conflicts.

Although not usually the case, it is possible in theory for the process of ethical reasoning to arrive at decisions that are inconsistent with human rights. Two examples illustrate the potential disassociation between bioethical reasoning and the human rights approach.

1. Not everyone who needs dialysis and renal transplant can receive such treatments. In clinical practice, decisions about eligibility for renal dialysis involve some form of explicit rationing, usually in the form of agreed-upon criteria for entry into and/or maintenance on the program. Bioethical reasoning is usually critical to informing the development of such criteria, which typically balance beneficence and respect for patient autonomy with considerations of likely capacity to benefit, based on the medical utility of treating any given patient. Typically, patients with other risk factors who have lower likelihood of success on a transplant program are excluded at the outset, so that resources are allocated to those who can "most benefit" from the program. Although some lose out while others gain, ethical reasoning can justify the decision on the basis that all patients are subjected to the same criteria. Unfairness would only be demonstrable if an individual was unfairly treated in the process. Bioethical reasoning, even in its application of the principle of justice, is weaker where criteria for program eligibility discriminate against whole groups of people, usually those for whom social stratification and disadvantage have created social patterning of the risk factors that lead to the

---

[33] For example, see Raanan Gillon, "Medical Ethics: Four Principles Plus Attention to Scope," *British Medical Journal* 309 (1994): 184–188; and World Health Organization, "25 Questions and Answers on Health and Human Rights," 22.

[34] See for example, Ezekiel Emanuel, Amitai Etzioni, Martha Nussbaum, Margaret Walker.

[35] There are multiple schools and philosophical traditions that bioethicists draw upon. To cite a few examples: utilitarianism, contractarianism, communitarianism, virtue based and relationship ethics.

individual's disqualification.[36] As a result, group disadvantage may be weakly addressed in a bioethics framework, and the effects of discrimination against whole groups receive less emphasis in the balancing of bioethical principles. In contrast, human rights standards would view the problem through the prism of discrimination. Analysis would focus on whether clinical protocols were directly or indirectly resulting in unfair treatment, not only of individuals but also of groups subjected to social inequalities.[37] Less emphasis would be placed on the capacity for individual benefit or on questions of autonomy or beneficence. As a result, application of a human rights framework may result in somewhat different decisions about what is fair and just in renal dialysis, particularly because of its capacity to discern group patterning and consider the implications of racial or other prohibited forms of discrimination in decisions about the fairness of a policy.[38]

2. A second example further illustrates the potential for divergence between human rights and bioethics approaches. In 1997, the provincial health department asked a teaching hospital in Cape Town, South Africa to implement a policy of non-treatment for illegal immigrants, and to report all such immigrants to the Department of Home Affairs.[39] In deliberating whether to implement this policy, the ethics committee of the institution concluded that while containing costs in health care was a legitimate objective for public policy and that the health services were entitled to protect scarce resources for citizens or legitimate immigrants, it was not the health professional's role to be part of such gate-keeping. As a result, the hospital issued an order that placed the onus onto hospital clerical staff to identify and report illegal immigrants seeking health care, sparing the clinicians from such a responsibility. The inherent discriminatory context in which such gatekeeping was to take place, and the potential violations of human rights that may result from mandatory reporting, did not enter sufficiently into the ethical reasoning process. Indeed, in many ways, the policy mimicked earlier policies

[36] M. Lowe et al., "These Sorts of People Don't Do Very Well: Race and Allocation of Health Care Resources," *Journal of Medical Ethics* 21.6 (1995): 356–360; Arnold M. Epstein et al. "Racial Disparities in Access to Renal Transplantation—Clinically Appropriate or Due to Underuse or Overuse?" *New England Journal of Medicine* 343.21 (2000): 1537–1544; Kevin A. Schulman et al., "The Effect of Race and Sex on Physicians' Recommendations for Cardiac Catheterization," *New England Journal of Medicine*. 340.8 (1999): 618–626.

[37] See, for example, Sofia Gruskin and Daniel Tarantola, "Health and Human Rights," in *Oxford Textbook of Public Health*, Roger Detels et al., eds. (Oxford: Oxford University Press, 2004); Ichiro Kawachi and Bruce P. Kennedy, *The Health of Nations: Why Inequality is Harmful to Your Health* (New York: New Press, 2002).

[38] Charles Ngwena, "The Recognition of Access to Health Care as a Human Right in South Africa: Is it Enough?" *Health and Human Rights: An International Journal* 5.1 (2000): 26–44; Craig Scott and Philip Alston, "Adjudicating Constitutional Priorities in a Transnational Context: A Comment on the Soobramoney's Legacy and Grootboom's Promise," *South African Journal on Human Rights* 16 (2000): 206–268.

[39] Groote Schuur Hospital Notice #12/97, cited in the Health and Human Rights Project, *Final Submission to the Truth and Reconciliation Commission*.

implemented by the apartheid government in its attempts to arrest anti-apartheid activists seeking medical care at state hospitals for injuries sustained in civil disobedience protests.[40]

In contrast, a human rights approach starts and concludes with the issues of discrimination and access to health care, irrespective of who conducts the gate-keeping. Any policy that results in significant violations of human rights that cannot be adequately justified by public health criteria[41] would be deemed unacceptable.

In sum, both the human rights and bioethics approaches generally attempt to promote morally desirable outcomes. Just as bioethics reasoning seeks to balance contrasting principles, human rights approaches sometimes have to balance competing rights.[42] Yet, even though in recent years many professional bodies have adopted human rights principles in their ethical codes,[43] there has been insufficient attention paid to bringing these two paradigms or discourses together conceptually.

It is possible to operate within an ethics framework in ways that focus only on the dyadic relationship of the clinician and patient without considering the context in which that relationship is constructed. Likewise, there is little uniformity on how to weigh conflicting principles of bioethics or how far to extend their scope. In the case of dual-loyalty, respect for human rights (insofar as this connotes respect for human dignity and the inviolability of personhood) is a pre-condition to engaging in ethical decision-making. Where human rights are at stake in a dual-loyalty conflict, it is necessary to look to human rights norms to guide the resolution of these conflicts.

1.5 The Obligation of Health Professionals to Respect Human Rights

As discussed earlier, human rights obligations generally fall to governments, not to individuals. But the power and legal standing of human rights norms have enormous implications for the behavior of health professionals. Most generally, the

---

[40] Laurel Baldwin-Ragaven et al., *An Ambulance of the Wrong Colour* (Cape Town, South Africa: University of Cape Town Press), 69.

[41] Gruskin and Tarantola ("Health and Human Rights") citing the UNECOSOC 1985, list the conditions under which restrictions of rights could be considered as being 'necessary' and carried out in accordance with the law: the restriction is in the interest of a legitimate objective of general interest; the restriction is strictly necessary in a democratic society to achieve the objective; there are no less intrusive and restrictive means available to reach the same goal; and the restriction is not imposed arbitrarily, i.e., in an unreasonable or otherwise discriminatory manner.

[42] Note that in some situations, balancing rights may not be permitted. These are situations that threaten non-derogable rights, such as freedom from torture.

[43] See, for example, the compilation of *International Instruments, Resolutions, Declarations and Statements on Torture* compiled by the International Rehabilitation Council for Torture Victims; World Medical Association, *Resolution on Human Rights*; International Council of Nurses, *Nurses and Human Rights*; International Council of Nurses, *Ethical Concepts Applied to Nursing*.

International Covenant on Civil and Political Rights declares that all people have "a responsibility to strive for the promotion and observance of the rights recognized" in the Covenant.[44]

Beyond this general obligation, applicable to the health professional as citizen,[45] are specific obligations imposed by the nature of professionalism, reinforced by the authority given through licensing. Professionalism entails a social pact in which society and its institutions accord the health professional status, power and prestige in exchange for a guarantee that he or she will meet certain standards of practice. It is these expectations that bestow upon health professionals a particular obligation to respect their patients' human rights.

How might a health professional become complicit in a human rights violation? First, when employed by or acting on behalf of the state, health professionals may become agents through which the state commits a violation, for example, by participating in torture of an individual at the behest of state interrogators.

Second, even in private doctor-patient encounters, health professionals can become complicit in violations by adhering to—and thus furthering—state health policies and practices that unjustly discriminate on the basis of race, sex, class, or other prohibited grounds, or that deny equitable access to health care. Where the state has failed to take necessary steps to establish a health system that affords equitable access to health services, the health professional participating in that system has an obligation to press for alternative policies designed to end the violations.

Third, even where no explicit state policy is involved, in circumstances where the health professional engages in cultural or social practices that violate human rights, for example, "virginity examinations" or genital mutilation of women, he or she becomes the vehicle by which the violation is accomplished. Most human rights treaties require states to take affirmative steps to end social or cultural practices that discriminate or otherwise violate the human rights of individuals in private relationships, thereby making it clear that tolerance of the underlying conduct is impermissible.

For example, the Convention on the Elimination of all forms of Discrimination against Women (CEDAW) provides that states parties "shall take all appropriate measures ... to modify the social and cultural patterns of conduct of men and women, with a view to achieving the elimination of prejudices and customary and all other practices which are based on the idea of the inferiority or the superiority of either of the sexes or on stereotyped roles for men and women."[46] The Convention on the Elimination of all forms of Racial Discrimination contains similar language.

---

[44] United Nations, *International Covenant on Civil and Political Rights*, preamble.

[45] For a discussion on the imperative for ordinary citizens to act against injustice, see Judith Shklar, *The Faces of Injustice* (New Haven, CT: Yale University Press, 1990).

[46] United Nations, *Convention on the Elimination of all forms of Discrimination Against Women*, art. 5(b).

The commitment to eliminating discrimination in the sphere of civil life thus creates a norm that should govern the conduct of a private health professional as much as it does the state and its citizenry.

The language of ethical codes guiding medical and nursing practice increasingly reinforces values that derive from international human rights law.[47] Indeed, many professional associations have explicitly adopted human rights language in their own ethical principles.[48] Numerous ethical codes and declarations hold that protecting the human rights of patients is considered within the scope of professional duty. Both the World Medical Association and the International Council of Nurses have affirmed the centrality of human rights in health practice.[49] The WMA Declaration of Tokyo focuses on avoiding complicity of health professionals in torture, linking a human rights obligation to fundamental ethical norms: "a doctor must have complete clinical independence in deciding upon the care of a person for whom he or she is medically responsible. The doctor's fundamental role is to alleviate the distress of his or her fellow men, and no motive, whether personal, collective or political, shall prevail against this higher purpose."[50] The International Council of Nurses' Ethical Concepts Applied to Nursing Code emphasizes that "inherent in nursing is respect for life, dignity, and the rights of man."[51] The Code goes on to elaborate that the care provided by nurses must not be restrained by "considerations of nationality, race, creed, color, age, sex, politics or social status."[52]

1.6 Loyalty and Human Rights: The Need for This Project

As noted above, subordinating loyalty to the patient to the interests of the state is only permissible to serve a higher social purpose. Violations of human rights cannot constitute permissible social purposes. Professional conduct that abets human rights abuse is thus illegitimate. In recent years there has been increasing attention by health professionals and professional associations to promoting, and even leading, efforts to promote human rights. They have done this through promulgation of standards and, even more importantly, through actions to protect the human rights of patients. However, four sets of problems remain.

---

[47] See, for example, the compilation of International Instruments, Resolutions, Declarations and Statements on Torture compiled by the International Rehabilitation Council for Torture Victims.

[48] See note 40.

[49] World Medical Association, *Resolution on Human Rights*; ICN, *Nurses and Human Rights*.

[50] World Medical Association, *Declaration of Tokyo: Guidelines for Medical Doctors Concerning Torture and Other Cruel, Inhuman or Degrading Treatment or Punishment in Relation to Detention and Imprisonment*, sec. 4.

[51] International Council of Nurses, *Ethical Concepts Applied to Nursing*.

[52] Id.

1.6.1 Extent of Dual-Loyalty Problems

In a wide variety of contexts, settings and clinical roles, health professionals are subjected to demands by governments (and in certain circumstances by other powerful third parties) to subordinate their patients' human rights to third party interests, usually those of the state. The structure of employment relationships, including sources of compensation, supervision and legal authority; expectations to defer to embedded social practices even if they violate human rights; and the state's ability to apply pressure to secure compliance with its demands, all render it difficult for health professionals to maintain fidelity to patients' human rights. As a result, dual-loyalty conflicts resulting in human rights violations are common. The variety of circumstances and settings in which violations of human rights take place on account of dual-loyalty are described in the next chapter [not herein included].

1.6.2 The Lack of Education and Training

In some parts of the world, awareness of the relevance of human rights to clinical and community practice is increasing. Nevertheless, health professionals do not usually receive training and guidance to identify situations where dual-loyalty violates a person's human rights and even less so on how to formulate and implement appropriate responses. Existing guidelines and ethical codes for health professionals do not provide a firm foundation for assessment of the state's demands. Health professionals lack clear guidance concerning the evaluation of state and other third party demands for subordination of patients' interests. In many cases, the state claims that subordinating patients' interests serves the common good, for example, by enhancing prison security or compelling drug-abusing mothers to receive treatment. But existing guidelines and ethical codes do not advise health professionals how to evaluate these claims—and how to determine when protecting the human rights of patients requires that health professionals turn state interests aside.[53]

Guidance is especially murky in cases where state complicity consists only of health professionals doing nothing, passively accepting situations that contribute to violations of human rights. In these cases, the protection of human rights requires an affirmative stance by the health professional in favor of the patient or larger community. Ethical guidance provided to health professionals is largely silent on questions of advocacy, providing space for the state to encourage health professionals to conceptualize their function narrowly so as not to interfere with its priorities.

Similar gaps in guidance and training, together with pressures to conform, exist in circumstances where health professionals confront often-embedded cultural

[53] The UN Principles of Medical Ethics explicitly prohibit any such distinctions: "There may be no derogation from the foregoing provisions on any grounds whatsoever, including public emergency." *UN Principles of Medical Ethics*, principle 6.

prejudices that, when applied to health care, interfere with human rights. Examples include denial of reproductive health services to women and institutionalized discrimination in health services. Yielding to these policies and attitudes makes health professionals complicit in human rights violations, but they have few places to turn to develop appropriate responses. To break established patterns of care requires attention not only to general, overarching statements about health professionals' human rights obligations, but guidance about responses in particular circumstances, so that health professionals can assume the responsibilities a human rights-respecting posture asks of them.

1.6.3 Systemic Flaws and Limitations

Institutional structures often inhibit health professionals from meeting their human rights obligations. These structures include: the nature of employment relationships with the state; administrative mechanisms that lack procedures for contesting state demands; disincentives to promote human rights; and licensing and professional organizations that play no part in providing support to health professionals when they are challenged in meeting their human rights obligations. Especially in highly politicized or repressive environments, institutional structures to support responses consistent with the human rights of patients are non-existent or ineffective, forcing the individual health professional to have to make wrenching choices that may require him or her to risk personal safety.

To address the problem of dual-loyalty and human rights, the relationship of the health professional to the state (particularly where the health professional is an employee of the state) must be restructured. This relationship should protect the independence of the health professional from state pressures, minimizing the compulsion to succumb to the state's demands and expectations. Administrative mechanisms to protect whistle blowers must be established. In addition, licensing boards and professional associations need mechanisms to support health professionals who seek to comply with their ethical and human rights obligations in the face of state demands to the contrary. Collective action by colleagues in the professions may be required to enable individual health professionals to fulfill their obligations. For this reason, medical, nursing and other organizations should protect and advocate for colleagues who are at risk of becoming engaged in human rights abuses.

1.6.4 The Larger Social Context in Which Dual-Loyalty Occurs

Lack of guidance and support for health professionals is especially poignant in an environment where the health system itself violates human rights because it fails to meet basic health needs, because distribution of existing resources is inequitable, or because of racial, gender or ethnic discrimination. Practicing in such an environment can lead the health professional to become complicit in human rights violations despite the professional's personal commitment to human rights. For example, in some societies systematic racial or ethnic discrimination pervades health policy. A primary care physician who denies or limits care in the service of discriminatory policies elevates conformance to state policies over loyalty to patient needs. In the same vein, social policies that reduce women's ability to protect their reproductive health may lead health professionals to deny women the means to protect their health. The more the health professional "adjusts" his or her conduct to the constraints and inequities built into the system, the more the professional participates in the violation.[54]

The systemic nature of role conflict may constrain the power of the individual practitioner to fulfill the human rights of individual patients and communities of patients for whom the practitioner has responsibilities. These communities may include diverse patient populations as well as groups of people often marginalized and neglected, many of whom do not seek care but are in serious need of care. The health professional will often have obligations to all members of the community beyond those seen as patients in clinical settings that raise challenging ethical questions, requiring them to affirm human rights.

Professional organizations and codes of conduct have begun to acknowledge the systemic dimensions of dual-loyalty problems. The Turkish Medical Association, for example, has been active both in seeking to end torture and to protect physicians who are pressured not to report it. The British Medical Association is addressing the roles of physicians who practice in prisons and other difficult settings. Nevertheless, a great deal more needs to be done. Indeed, in most countries there is typically no connection made between institutionalized or structural discrimination, inequity, and the ethical requirements of practice. Moreover, the codes and associations of health professionals by and large address only the behavior of individual clinicians, giving little attention to the obligations of the profession as a whole.

[...]

4.5 *Guidelines for Military Health Professionals*

4.5.1 Preamble

Health professionals working in institutions that serve state interests, where human rights are easily at risk, are most likely to be confronted with dual-loyalty conflicts. Among these, military health professionals face unique conflicts. They must navigate their way between very different and sometimes antagonistic or even irreconcilable goals: on the one hand, to preserve life, attend to the sick, and reduce suffering

[54] This phenomenon is well documented in South Africa under apartheid. See American Association for the Advancement of Science, *Human Rights and Health: The Legacy of Apartheid* (New York: AAAS, 1998), 111–113.

(the obligation of the health professional), and on the other, to support killing and inflicting harm on the enemy (the obligation of the military officer or soldier).

As long as the interests of the patient and the military organization are in line with each other, dual-loyalty conflicts can be avoided. As one military physician put it: "What's good for the patient is good for the military, and you want a fit, happy troop." But even in peacetime the two objectives may conflict. The military health professional is a member of civil society's health professions subject to ethical and human rights standards and goals. As such, the military health professional attends to the soldier who is sick, wounded, or in need of other medical attention and who, like any other patient, seeks the expertise, counseling, and support of his doctor or nurse in privacy and confidentiality. Indeed, this medical function is protected by international humanitarian law, which forbids warring parties from interfering or obstructing efforts by medical personnel to care for the sick and wounded, regardless of affiliation.

From the military's point of view, however, even treatment goals can be subordinated or reinterpreted to reinforce military objectives. For example, usual principles of triage demand that in medical emergencies health professionals attend to the most seriously injured first. But in battle the commander may compel the physician to attend first to soldiers with less severe wounds as a means to return them to battle quickly and maximize force strength; meanwhile the most seriously injured suffer or may die. Similarly, treatment of sick or traumatized soldiers in both physical and mental health may differ from standard civilian protocols in order to serve military purposes, for example, preparing the soldier as soon as possible for new battle engagements rather than seeking the best long term outcome for the patient. Soldiers are often not entitled to exercise informed consent regarding medication and vaccines. Indeed, even interventions to promote the health and well-being of soldiers are designed to further the fitness of troops for battle or other military tasks.

In more extreme circumstances, the ethical medical role can be even more severely compromised. A military health professional may be requested to declare troops fit for engagement even when they are not. The health professional may be called upon to participate or advise in interrogation of suspects of terrorism, insurgency, or espionage to an extent that may amount to torture or cruel and inhuman treatment, to prepare (and be present at) executions, or to administer pharmaceutical substances or vaccines to soldiers (own or enemy) without medical justification. He or she may be called on to participate in biological, chemical or pharmaceutical research and experimentation where civilian protocols, regulations and supervision are reduced or absent. When such research takes place in secrecy—often for legitimate reasons of national security—the military health professional may be required or asked to yield to security interests and forego medical ethical principles and professional codes of conduct.

These dual-loyalty conflicts place the health professional in an untenable position. In some of the above examples the practitioner is put in a situation where the underlying conduct violates human rights. In other cases the health professional may be called upon to support a violation of the laws of war, such as supporting acts of violence against a civilian population. Further, during engagements and missions, military health professionals are likely to witness human rights violations on the battle field or in peace-enforcing actions. Yet their duty to report these violations may be inconsistent with the perceived needs of the combat unit.

A complex dual-loyalty problem may arise in jurisdictions where military service is voluntary and members of the armed forces are generally held to have voluntarily waived some of their rights by choosing to join the armed services. As patients, they take some responsibility in advance for deciding the extent to which they are willing to "give up" their rights, including, for example, the right to doctor-patient confidentiality. However, this agreement does not mean all of a military patient's rights are necessarily waived and health care providers should therefore not exceed what is "necessary" in any disclosure. Indeed, it is debatable whether the waiving of rights by conscripts could be reasonably accepted as voluntary.

Health professionals engaged in peacekeeping face other dual-loyalty conflicts. In such operations, military health professionals confront the medical needs of civilian populations in the area of their assignment; yet they may be subject to rules and regulations preventing them from providing professional assistance to these civilians.

Military health professionals—being members of the troops and placed in the hierarchical chain of command[55]—thus face an extraordinary set of medical-ethical and human rights conflicts. The following Guidelines are meant to address these conflicts. The Guidelines follow the World Medical Association's Regulations in Time of Armed Conflict in insisting that the health professional in the military is bound by the same standards of practice as civilian health professionals.

4.5.2 Scope and Context

The following Guidelines apply to military doctors and other military health professionals, both in times of combat and in peacekeeping and peace-enforcing operations. These guidelines apply both to the individual health professional and to the military institutions and civil authorities and organizations related to the services of the military health professional.

4.5.3 Guidelines

1. **The military health professional's first and overruling identity and priority is that of a health professional**

Commentary: Although this guideline appears self-evident, many military organizations teach physicians that they are officers or soldiers first and physicians second. As such, they are supposed to make their medical skills available exclusively for

[55] In many armed forces, the military health professional, as a non-combatant, is not in the chain of command in the sense of having the power to give orders to combat soldiers. In addition, the health professional may not be subject to the same obligation to fight in order to avoid surrender.

military purposes. In some countries, such as France, the military physician is trained in a separate military medical school, rather than trained as a military doctor after graduating from civilian medical school. Even where such training takes place, the primacy of the medical function should always be reinforced, even if there exist circumstances where the needs of the military prevail over the needs of the soldiers.

2. **Civilian medical ethics apply to military health professionals as they do to civilian practitioners**

Commentary: The starting point for the conduct of military health professionals should be the ethical and human rights standards of civilian professionals, with exceptions only for absolutely essential military purposes. These exceptions should be reviewed on a regular basis. Where deviations from normative ("regular") medical ethics are proposed, such deviations should be subject to careful review and oversight by a suitable structure such as a medical ethical commission with membership that includes an adequate number of civilian health professionals skilled in ethical issues.

Upholding medical ethics includes the obligation to obtain informed consent for treatment. The health professional should consider his or her relationship to the individual under treatment or evaluation as comparable to a civilian health professional-patient relationship rather than as part of a military hierarchy. In considering modes of treatment, a health professional should engage in the same kinds of dialogue with a patient about medical procedures as he or she would in civilian practice. Adherence to civilian informed consent practice does not imply that there will never be circumstances where consent is not required, but rather that the same standards should apply as in civilian health practice. For example, compulsory vaccinations should only be administered without consent in the military to the extent that such vaccinations can be administered in the absence of consent in civilian practice. Even though joining the armed forces may imply "voluntary" waiving of some patient rights, this does not relieve the health professional of responsibility to apply general rules of obtaining informed consent.

3. **The military health professional should adhere to the principle of confidentiality in a manner consistent with practice in civil society**

Commentary: Many military organizations consider the health professional as part of the chain of command who must thus disclose information concerning patients to his or her commanding officer, whether that officer is a health professional or not. This blanket abrogation of the confidentiality principle is not always necessary to achieve military objectives, however. Information about a person's medical condition may be needed to make a determination for fitness to serve, but this function is no different from fitness to work determinations in the civilian employment context (except that soldiers are not permitted to withhold consent and leave the position). Military health professionals can provide their opinions and disclose their medical judgments about fitness for duty, extent of disability (and projected length of disability), or required restrictions in a soldier's scope of responsibilities without providing detailed medical information and without sharing the information with personnel not directly involved in the assignment decision. The information disclosed should be made known to the soldier.

Divulging confidential information simply on the basis of command interests should, as in civilian society, be regarded as unethical behavior. Exceptions to this general rule should be reviewed by a mechanism similar to that applicable in civilian life as described in General Guidelines 7 and 8 [not herein included].

4. The military health professional is a member of the national and international health professionals' community

Commentary: In many, if not most, countries the military medical community identifies itself with the military rather than with the larger medical community. This identification may be due in part to training and organization, but it is also psychological. Military health professionals sometimes feel that they are not an accepted part of the civilian medical society. In other circumstances they do not separate their role from that of the military generally. The supremacy and priority of the military health professional's identity as a professional can be promoted by this Guideline as well as by the membership of military health professionals in national and international associations.

5. The military health professional should treat the sick and wounded according to the rules of medical needs and triage

Commentary: The Geneva Conventions require medical attention according to usual medical practice for persons outside of combat, whether civilians or wounded enemy soldiers. Thus, a guideline requiring adherence to the usual rules of triage should not be controversial. Because this principle is so often breached, it warrants repetition. Existing international human rights and humanitarian law and international professional codes of conduct support the responsibility to follow the rules of triage. The military health professional should ensure on the basis of a pre-engagement agreement that he or she will be able to treat civilians of his or her "own side" and civilians and military (POW and otherwise) of the "enemy side" or those caught in between, with the understanding that medical need and triage be the exclusive criteria for selection. A similar guideline should apply in peacekeeping operations where emergency medical care is needed.[56]

Finally, the usual rules of triage should apply with respect to soldiers within a health professional's own unit. As indicated above, the military's goal in returning the maximum number of wounded soldiers to battle as quickly as possibly often results in different rules of triage than those applied in civilian life. In the military context, the least wounded may receive treatment first, while treatment for the most seriously wounded is delayed. The delay in treatment increases the risk of death to the more severely wounded. This practice should be considered unacceptable.

6. Health professionals should not participate in research or development of chemical or biological weapons (CBW) that could be used for purposes of killing, disabling, torturing or in any way harming human life

Commentary: Military health professionals may be called upon to apply their specific expertise for offensive chemical and biological weapons research. Such

[56] The question to what extent the military health professional is required to serve the health needs of the civilian population of the area assigned should be explicit.

projects to develop weapons of mass destruction against civilian populations are often shielded by formal or informal secrecy and immunity. Military health professionals have participated in horrific chemical and biological weapons experimentation[57] on human beings, hidden behind a wall of secrecy and immunity. This guideline prohibits such participation because it is fundamentally inconsistent with human rights.

Any research involving methods to protect human beings from the effects of CBW weapons, or with materials that could directly or indirectly contribute to CBW weapons, must be subject to systems of ethical review and scrutiny. Such systems of ethical review and scrutiny, even when conducted in secrecy due to national security concerns, should have built into them mechanisms for civilian participation in the oversight of research.

7. **The military health professional should refrain from direct, indirect and administrative forms of cooperation in torture and cruel, inhuman and degrading treatment and punishment at all times, including in wartime and during interrogation of prisoners**

Commentary: The Guideline prohibiting civilian health professionals from participating in cruel and unusual treatment and punishment applies to military health professionals as well. Military health professionals have been called upon to assist in interrogation of prisoners and, in some cases, domestic dissidents. Despite their military status, however, these professionals are bound by existing prohibitions on medical participation in torture and cruel and inhuman treatment. Special attention should be given to practices such as certifying fitness of individuals to undergo intensive forms of interrogation, to be punished for non-cooperation, or to be subjected to medical and/or pharmaceutical "treatment" after such interrogations or punishments.

8. **The military health professional should refrain from direct, indirect, preparatory and administrative participation in capital punishment, both within the military court martial system and elsewhere**

Commentary: Many countries that have abandoned capital punishment for criminal offenses permit its use in military courts. In such cases the military health professional is likely to be involved when he or she is requested to declare the sentenced prisoner fit for execution. International codes prohibiting the participation of medical personnel in capital punishment and contain no exceptions for the military setting. It is never justified for health professionals to participate, directly or indirectly, in capital punishment.

9. **Military health professionals should report violations of human rights that interfere with their ability to comply with their duty of loyalty to patients to appropriate authorities and report human rights violations perpetrated by their own troops as well as by others**

Commentary: Military health professionals should maintain their independence and report human rights violations as civilian health professionals do (see General

[57] South Africa's Chemical and Biological Weapons Programme, Special Investigation into Project Coast. *Truth and Reconciliation Commission Final Report*, Vol. II, Chapter 6, 29 October 1998.

Guideline 12 [not herein included]). The military health professional should especially take steps to report violations of the Geneva Conventions.

10. The health professional should not engage or participate in any form of human experimentation among members of military services unless the research will provide significant health and other benefits for military personnel and facilitate promotion of their human rights

Commentary: It is the view of the Working Group that true "voluntary informed consent" is extremely difficult to obtain in the military setting, because of the various overt and covert factors which govern the relationship between military personnel, their chain of command and the health professional. There may however, be some particular circumstances when research with military personnel may provide Significant health and other benefits and facilitate promotion of their human rights. The Working Group acknowledges, moreover, that research issues are not strictly part of its mandate; we would thus welcome further discussion with and guidance from those directly involved in the ethics of research.

References

American Association for the Advancement of Science. 1998. *Human Rights and Health: The Legacy of Apartheid.* New York: AAAS.

Baldwin-Ragaven, Laurel et al. 1999. *An Ambulance of the Wrong Colour.* Cape Town, South Africa: University of Cape Town Press.

Beauchamp, Dan E. and Bonnie Steinbock. 1999. *New Ethics for the Public's Health.* Oxford: Oxford University Press.

Beauchamp, Tom L. and James F. Childress. 2001. *Principles of Biomedical Ethics.* Oxford: Oxford University Press.

Bloche, Gregg. 1999. Clinical Loyalties and the Social Purposes of Medicine. *Journal of the American Medical Association* 281.3: 268–274.

Bloche, M. Gregg. 2001. Caretakers and Collaborators. *Cambridge Quarterly of Healthcare Ethics* 10.3: 275–284.

British Medical Association. 2001. *The Medical Profession and Human Rights: A Handbook for a Changing Agenda.* London: Zed Books.

Chapman, Audrey R. and Sage Russell, eds. 2002. *Core Obligations: Building a Framework for Economic, Social and Cultural Rights.* Antwerpen, The Netherlands: Intersentia.

Daniels, Norman. 1985. *Just Health Care.* New York: Cambridge University Press.

Epstein, Arnold M. et al. 2000. Racial Disparities in Access to Renal Transplantation—Clinically Appropriate or Due to Underuse or Overuse? *New England Journal of Medicine* 343.21: 1537–1544.

Evans, David B. et al. 2001. Comparative Efficiency of National Health Systems: Cross National Econometric Analysis. *British Medical Journal* 323: 307–310.

Evans, David B. et al. 2001. Measuring Quality: From the System to the Provider. *International Journal for Quality in Health Care* 13.6: 439–446.

Gillon, Raanan. 1994. Preface: Medical Ethics and the Four Principles. In *Principles of Health Care Ethics*, eds. Raanan Gillon and Lloyd, xxi. Chichester: Wiley.

Gillon, Raanan. 1994. Medical Ethics: Four Principles Plus Attention to Scope. *British Medical Journal* 309: 184–188.

Groote Schuur Hospital Notice #12/97, cited in the Health and Human Rights Project, *Final Submission to the Truth and Reconciliation Commission.*

Gruskin, Sofia and Daniel Tarantola. 2004. Health and Human Rights. In *Oxford Textbook of Public Health*, eds. Roger Detels et al. Oxford: Oxford University Press.

Henkin, Louis. 1990. *The Age of Rights*. New York: Columbia University Press.

Kass, Nancy E. 2001. An Ethics Framework for Public Health. *American Journal of Public Health* 91.11: 1776–1182.

Kawachi, Ihiro and Bruce P. Kennedy. 2002. *The Health of Nations: Why Inequality is Harmful to Your Health*. New York: New Press.

Kessel, Anthony. Forthcoming. Public Health Ethics: Teaching Survey and Critical Review. *Social Science and Medicine*.

Lowe, M. et al. 1995. These Sorts of People Don't Do Very Well: Race and Allocation of Health Care Resources. *Journal of Medical Ethics* 21.6: 356–360.

Mann, Jonathan M. 1999. Medicine and Public Health, Ethics and Human Rights. In *Health and Human Rights: A Reader*, eds. Jonathan M. Mann et al., 439–452. New York: Routledge.

Mann, Jonathan M. et al. 1994. Health and Human Rights. *Health and Human Rights: An International Journal* 1.1: 7–23.

Ngwena, Charles. 2000. The Recognition of Access to Health Care as a Human Right in South Africa: Is it Enough? *Health and Human Rights: An International Journal* 5.1: 26–44.

Peter, Fabienne and Timothy Evans. 2001. Ethical Dimensions of Health Equity. In *Challenging Inequalities in Health. From Ethics to Action*, eds. Timothy Evans et al., 25–33. New York: Oxford University Press.

Roberts, Marc J. and Michael Reich. 2002. Ethical Analysis in Public Health. *Lancet*. 359.9311: 1055–1059.

Scott, Craig and Philip Alston. 2000. Adjudicating Constitutional Priorities in a Transnational Context: A Comment on the Soobramoney's Legacy and Grootboom's Promise. *South African Journal on Human Rights* 16: 206–268.

Schulman, Kevin A. et al. 1999. The Effect of Race and Sex on Physicians' Recommendations for Cardiac Catheterization. *New England Journal of Medicine* 340.8: 618–626.

Sen, Amartya. 1999. *Development as Freedom*. Oxford: Oxford University Press.

Shklar, Judith. 1990. *The Faces of Injustice*. New Haven, CT: Yale University Press.

Smedley, Brian D. et al. *Unequal Treatment: Confronting Racial and Ethnic Disparities in Health Care*. Washington, DC: The National Academies Press, 2002.

South Africa's Chemical and Biological Weapons Programme. 1998. Special Investigation into Project Coast. *Truth and Reconciliation Commission Final Report*, Vol. II, Chapter 6, 29 October 1998.

Steiner, Henry and Philip Alston. 2000. *International Human Rights Law in Context*. Oxford: Oxford University Press.

United Nations. *Convention on the Elimination of All Forms of Discrimination Against Women*, art. 5(b).

United Nations. *Convention on the Elimination of All Forms of Racial Discrimination*. art. 2, sec. 1(d); art. 5(e).

United Nations. *International Covenant on Civil and Political Rights*. Preamble, art. 4.

United Nations. Committee on Economic, Social and Cultural Rights. *The Right to the Highest Attainable Standard of Health*. General comment 14.

United Nations. *Universal Declaration of Human Rights*, art. 1.

World Health Organization. *25 Questions and Answers on Health and Human Rights*, 22. Geneva: WHO, 2002.

World Medical Association. *Declaration of Geneva*.

World Medical Association. *International Code of Medical Ethics*.

World Medical Association. *Declaration of Tokyo: Guidelines for Medical Doctors Concerning Torture and Other Cruel, Inhuman or Degrading Treatment or Punishment in Relation to Detention and Imprisonment*.

World Medical Association. *Resolution on Human Rights*.

Guidelines to Prevent the Malevolent Use of Physicians in War[1]

Michael E. Frisina

1 Introduction

The question of how to prevent the malevolent use of physicians in war is not new. Historically the lines were far more distinct than they are today. When physicians were clearly noncombatants in a civilian culture tending to the sick and wounded of belligerent, armed combatants, regardless of country of origin, protecting and preserving the integrity of the healing arts was less complicated. Today physicians wear the uniform of their countries, travel imbedded with the fighting forces to intervene and to provide care and treatment to the sick or wounded soldier as quickly as possible with the best expectation of survival. Military physicians participate in medical research and development with suspicion regarding the benevolent nature of the research as to the outcomes and use for improving the means of healing as opposed to improving the means of killing and inflicting harm. The use of medical knowledge and those who apply this knowledge in a war scenario continually face the ethical burden to preserve the caring and compassionate nature of the healing arts.

The subject of military medical ethics is a microcosm of the subject of medical ethics as a body of knowledge and ethics as a whole. The mixture of military ethics and medical ethics makes for problematic bedfellows. The Borden Institute published *Military Medical Ethics*, Volumes 1and 2 in its series Textbooks of Military Medicine, devoting a unique body of scholarship on the merging of medical ethics and military ethics.[2] This publication serves as a reference tool in seeking understanding in the tension and dynamics of melding of these two professions in a phrase termed as mixed or dual agency of military physicians—serving two masters within the persona of both the profession of medicine and the profession of arms. That this tension is acknowledged is a good thing. That this tension exists is also a good thing for by its very nature, military medicine is an amalgam of both professions

[1] The views in this essay are strictly those of the author and do not reflect any official policy of the United States Army or the Government of the United States.

[2] Dave E. Lounsbury, *Military Medical Ethics*, vols. 1 and 2 (Textbooks of Military Medicine Series; Washington, DC: Borden Institute, 2003).

F. Allhoff (ed.), *Physicians at War: The Dual-Loyalties Challenge.*

revered by many and disdained by some as well. The American Medical Association is on record supporting the outstanding work of military physicians in treating sick and wounded soldiers while personally facing extreme circumstances to do so. Military medical personal are highly decorated for their courage and bravery in assisting their fallen comrades and list among the highest number of recipients of the Congressional Medal of Honor for their actions above and beyond the call of duty.[3]

The simple fact is that militaries do what they do to preserve the cultures and societies they are sworn to protect and to defend and military physicians perform a vital role not only in reducing pain and suffering and promoting healing, but also in conserving the fighting strength of the military. Society in general, and physicians in particular (whether civilian or military) have an obligation to fulfill that role on and off the battlefield as part of the universal commitment physicians have to uphold established and recognized codes and principles of medical ethics.[4]

2 Shifting Definitions

Presently, the fundamental discussion of preserving the nature of medical ethics within the military hinges on what medical ethics scholars call the patient-physician relationship.[5] This relationship, the healer-helper version of this relationship specifically, is the pivot point of the discussion of the ethical nature and conduct of physicians in war as it is in medicine in general. There are numerous models in the literature that suggest reasonable definitions for this relationship between patient and physician.[6] Though they vary in degree, these models all suggest that there is something unique and therapeutic in this relationship that has a distinct ethical component. A fundamental criterion relating these models is the element of time and relationship building between patient and physician that establishes the basis for the ethical as well as instrumental value of the relationship and inherent obligations. If the aspect of time and relationship building is a necessary and sufficient condition to creating an ethical obligation, clearly military physicians are challenged in this regard to the patients they may not know or spend very little time in the development of this relationship. Clearly on the battlefield there is very little relationship building between military physicians and those likely requiring their services. While some medical personnel are embedded and serve directly with their combatant

[3] The Congressional Medal of Honor Society, http://www.cmohs.org/society.htm, cited 4 June 2007.

[4] American Medical Association, *Code of Medical Ethics: Current Opinions with Annotations*, 2004–2005 ed. (Chicago, IL: AMA Press, 2004).

[5] P. Lain Entralgo, *Doctor and Patient*, Partridge F., trans. (New York: McGraw-Hill, 1969).

[6] Edmund Pelligrino, "The Moral Foundations of the Patient-Physician Relationship: The Essence of Medical Ethics," in *Military Medical Ethics*, vol. 1 (Washington, DC: Borden Institute, 2003).

cohorts, the majority of physicians are assigned to medical units and have no direct contact to soldiers they are likely to treat as patients especially those evacuated from the combat zone. This is not to say that absent of relationship building and adequate time in the midst of the treatment process that there is no clearly established ethical and legal patient-physician relationship only that this scenario pushes the limits of any of the suggested models currently recognized in the literature, civilian practice, or peacetime military healthcare practices.

The nature of patient-physician relationship is essential to preserving the ethical dimension of physician as healer and not some other role and application of medical knowledge. The physician as "helper and healer" model, perhaps the most traditional and ethically demanding upholds the ideal that the physician is a dedicated professional whose primary obligation is to the good of the patient served in a therapeutic role.[7] Without dispute, the Nuremberg Military Tribunals, that include the prosecution of so-called Nazi doctors, provides the basis for distinguishing between physicians and their use of medical knowledge to help and heal opposed to those who use such knowledge for the propagation of nontherapeutic measures that may include some areas of research and expanding medical science at large.[8] To separate and to desensitize oneself from the role of healer-helper and to denigrate the status of the patient to some nonpatient category of human being provides the means to disregard the tenets of fundamental human conduct and medical ethics. This process has been coined "shifting sands"[9] and refers to the convenience of shifting definitions to accommodate behavior that otherwise would be construed as unacceptable. Since the victims of the Nazi medical horrors were defined out of a class of human beings protected by codes of conduct, rule of law, and rudimentary elements of conventional decency, the behavior and conduct of these nefarious medical professionals was not construed in their minds as a violation of ethical duty and obligation. This distinction is central to a modern day casuistry pushing the limits of duty and obligation in the midst of unconventional warfare known as the "war on terror." National and international media sources have reported alleged misconduct of military and nonmilitary physicians to report the use of torture in prisoner interrogation and to allow the release of patient health information to interrogators to enhance their intelligence means by exploiting prisoners through the use of this health information.[10] Such conduct by medical physicians has

---

[7] Entralgo, *Doctor and Patient*.
[8] Robert Jay Lifton, *The Nazi Doctors* (New York: Basic Books, 1986)
[9] Ann Hornaday, "The war tapes: three soldiers on shifting sands," *Washington Post* (June 30, 2006).
[10] See, for example, Dana Priest and Barton Gellman, "U.S. decries abuse but defends interrogations: 'stress and duress' tactics used on terrorism suspects held in secret overseas facilities," *Washington Post* (26 December 2002); and M. Gregg Bloche and Jonathan H. Marks, "When doctors go to war," *N Engl J Med* 352.1 (2005): 3–6; Joe Stephens, "Army doctors implicated in abuse: medical workers helped tailor interrogations of detainees, article says," *Washington Post* (6 January 2005): A8.

clearly been recognized as a corruption of medical ethics in the past and under current guidelines, codes, and ethical constructs should be so today as well, current post 9/11 logic notwithstanding. This is to suggest that again by shifting definitions like, a terrorist is not a legal combatant, and hence not entitled to protective status of the Geneva Convention as prisoner or patient, suggest a slippery slope in the use of medical personnel in nontherapeutic roles. If we can argue by definition who counts or does not count as the patient then we can act toward that person then medical professionals can participate in nontherapeutic roles without a violation of ethical codes and principles generally governing the conduct of the use of their knowledge and skill.

Application of established standards, duties and obligation hinge ironically today on "the definition" as they did in the 1940s. Central to defending the use of physicians and health information for intelligence purposes is whether terrorists count as deserving protection under, say the constraints of the Geneva Conventions. Such discussion is eerily similar no doubt to whether Jews were considered worthy of similar established codes and practices of their day. Note the other similarity in this argument by analogy. It would seem that the strength of the patient-physician relationship to bind an ethical obligation stems from the one on one nature of relationship. One could argue that this obligation is less binding when applied to a group of people or community of people for example, al Qaeda terrorists. More vexing is the use of medical knowledge and physician skills for purposes that have no clear and distinct therapeutic basis. Mixing the pragmatic necessity for intelligence gathering from prisoners with well established and acceptable means pushes the proverbial envelope when doing so involves physicians and medical knowledge and health information for no therapeutic purpose. The use of physicians and the healing arts for means and purpose that is clearly intended to exploit and harm a human being regardless of wartime status, classification, or definition is simply unethical.

To be sure, only the "helper-healer" model of the patient-physician relationship preserves the ethical integrity of the military physician. This model derives its ethical basis in the specific role of the physician as healer and the externally derived "end" of medicine as a healing and helping profession. The other models of the patient-physician relationship imply a different theory of medicine and competing interests between the patient and physician. As such the physician may use medical knowledge for what we can construe as for both a good and bad purpose. While such purpose need not be inherently or intrinsically evil, the misuse of medicine causes such an act to no longer constitute medicine since by definition medicine must have a healing purpose. Hence in the examples relating to physician participation in interrogation, torture and other forms of application of medical knowledge outside the scope of a healing purpose is indicative of the unethical use of that knowledge. The highest good of medicine is grounded in our humanity and medicine advancing the highest good of each particular patient. This good is inherent in the patient-physician relationship most clearly in the "helper-healer" model. In this regard, military physicians are no different from their civilian counterparts in obligations to patients and that relationship. The moral obligation in this relationship, the good of the patient, is the genesis for the tension in the mixed or dual agency of the military physician but must carry a greater moral weight over military necessity and the exigencies of war. Shifting definitions do not apply only to the notion of who the patient is but also when a medical professional ceases to serve in the capacity of physician when the misuse of medical knowledge no longer serves the interest of the patient. This distinction will be developed in detail in the latter part this discussion.

3 The Problem

To provide explanation as to how the power of "shifting definition" adds clarity to otherwise unexplainable conduct and behavior of otherwise thoughtful and caring people, we shift to the notion of 'duress' and its likely applicability to our discussion of physician behavior in times of war. Simply stated, the essence of ethical behavior is voluntary ability to make choices regarding various courses of action. Presumably, as previously posited, the choice for physicians in relationship to patients, is to choose to serve the best interest of the patients. Even at times when the patient and physician disagree regarding what choices serve the best interest of the patient, reasonable accommodations are provided to the patient and it is usually expected that the physician act as the patient desires or defer and provide an alternate physician to serve the needs of the patient.

Building upon the obligation of physicians to protect their patients, an obligation explicit in the patient-physician relationship, we will use the concept of 'duress' to explain how physicians can lose perspective and perhaps violate this fundamental obligation during times of war and terror. These situations, not solely inherent to military physicians but existing in other models of patient-physician relationship, are best described by the term 'mixed agency'. Mixed agency is typically defined as a set of circumstances where the physician has competing obligations to the fundamental obligation to the patient.[11] In such circumstances the physician's ethical choice is complicated, more complex, and hence more difficult to make as the choice becomes one of competing obligations.

The unction of mixed agency, with many examples in the practice of civilian medicine, demonstrates the tension created by conditions of extreme pressure when the ability to reason critically about moral obligation measured against competing pragmatic demands is most likely to occur. Arguably the admitted tension existing in the nature of military medical ethics may be such to question the very morality of physicians serving in the armed forces. There exist published accounts of strongly held views in the literature on this very topic.[12] These include what are considered to be significant barriers to providing ethical military healthcare most

[11] Edmund G. Howe, "Ethical Issues regarding mixed agency of military physicians," *Soc Sci Med* 23.8 (1986): 803–815.

[12] Victor W. Sidel and Barry Levy, eds., *War and Public Health* (New York: Oxford University Press, 1997).

notably subordinating the best interest of the patient and overriding the patient's wishes without informed consent.[13] Given the alternative to physicians serving in the military, needless suffering and harm of sick and wounded soldiers, the merits of these arguments are left for the reader to study and engage in thoughtful analysis. In doing so, alternatives to uniformed physicians are necessary so as to fulfill the obligation to care for sick and wounded soldiers. If it is unethical or morally unacceptable and impracticable for that matter, for a physician to serve as both physician and soldier, what is the reasonable accommodation for providing medical services to those serving in a combat role? The most notable alternative acknowledged in the literature was suggested by Professor John Ryle, Cambridge University, in the 1930s and modified by more current thinkers today.[14] Essentially, Professor Ryle suggested that all medical personnel simply refuse, by form of conscientious objection, to withhold medical services to include inoculations, sanitary advice, clinical and surgical care so as to cripple the ability of armed belligerents from waging war in the first place.[15] The thesis appears quite simple, if there is no war there is no need for physicians to care for sick and wounded soldiers. The reader is left to debate the merits of such a proposition in a post 9/11 era.

One need not hang on either horn of this perceived irresolvable dilemma. While there may be a blurring of military physicians' role in combat, such blurring exists in other professions as well with equal burden of ethical challenges and within the practice of civilian medicine. For the remainder of this discussion, we will focus on upholding the obligation of physicians with excellent moral character to serve not only honorably but ethically in providing medical services with the awareness of the need to exert moral influence on the military command structure to preserve the integrity of the essence and legitimate end of military medicine and medical ethics.

4 The Nature of Duress

With the advent of modern media and embedded reporting in war, we as a people have been exposed to horrific images that in times past were only seen by those in the midst of the horror of war. Film footage and audio reporting that invades into the horror of civilian and military hospitals and its victims intended to sensationalize or inform, regardless of motive violates the fundamental right of privacy of the

---

[13] Victor W. Sidel and Barry Levy, "Physician-soldier: a moral dilemma? The essence of medical ethics," in *Military Medical Ethics*, vol. 1 (Washington, DC: Borden Institute, 2003).

[14] John A. Ryle, "Foreword," in *The Doctor's View of War*, Horace Joules, ed. (London: George Allen & Unwin, 1938), 7–10.

[15] Ibid.

patient.[16] Documentaries reporting on wartime casualties filmed in the midst of the screaming and terror of the wounded patient, no longer a combatant by definition but a wounded, injured, and suffering human being violates the fundamental aspect of physician obligation to protect the patient. Patients have a fundamental right to privacy in peacetime and there is no reasonable argument for the violation of this right in times of war.

Again the literature is replete with examples and essays that defend the fundamental right to privacy and we need not reexamine them here.[17] Established codes and practices like The World Medical Association declarations abound.[18] Fundamentally, when people place themselves in the care and trust of a physician, they are entitled to a legitimate expectation to confidentiality, privacy, dignity, autonomy, and informed consent. Exploitive in nature and free speech not withstanding, the graphic display of the treatment scenario of these patients in combat surgery hospitals without their consent is unethical and physicians have an obligation to protect these patients, be they civilian or military, from such exploitation and violation of established ethical principles.

This knowledge and awareness notwithstanding, the nature of war, its terror, horror, stress, and other behavioral dynamics challenge the best of us to the very core of our character and ethical conduct. All of which call more so for the need of public scrutiny and discussion of critical issues that place our ethical norms in doubt and severe challenge—especially our ethical norms of healthcare and biomedical research. Consequently this challenge now raises the issue of duress as a means to explain otherwise indefensible behavior and brings a cloud of doubt regarding one's moral accountability to act appropriately to codes of conduct and behavior when one is impaired and incapable of doing so.

Duress implies a sense of coercion. In a legal sense the word connotes an excuse rather than a defense of an illegal action. In our case, duress would imply an excuse and not a justification for failing as a physician to uphold fundamental patient rights in war particularly as a form of mitigation and extenuating circumstances. Though somewhat dated, Michael Walzer provides an excellent discussion of duress in his book, *Just and Unjust Wars*.[19] Though more dated in time, Aristotle's "principle of accountability" links to the notion of duress and the limits of accountability to one's intended or unintended action.[20] In a simplistic form, every human act is either

---

[16] Jerome A. Singh and T.L. DePellegrin, "Images of war and medical ethics," *BMJ* 326 (12 April 2003): 774–775.

[17] Catherine A. Hood et al., "Videos, photographs, and patient consent," *BMJ* 316 (1998): 1009–1011.

[18] World Medical Association Declaration of Helsinki, WMA General Assembly, Tokyo 2004, http://www.wma.net/e/policy/b3.htm, cited 4 June 2007.

[19] Michael Walzer, *Just and Unjust Wars*, 3rd ed. (New York: Basic Books, 2000).

[20] Susan D. Collins, *Aristotle and the Rediscovery of Citizenship* (New York: Cambridge University Press, 2006).

voluntary or involuntary. Praise, blame, and responsibility are attached to voluntary acts and to those in proportion to the voluntariness in the act. A voluntary act is not done under compulsion (duress) and is done with knowledge of the circumstances, and by choice (result of deliberation). Duress, ignorance, and absence of freedom constitute limits to the voluntary. So we have a sliding scale so to speak in what we call Aristotle's "principle of responsibility", namely, the greater the limits placed on me to act in a voluntary manner, the greater the duress and hence the less responsible I am for my conduct.

In the case of media exploitation of a patient, the physician might well argue the need to expose the horrors of war so as to bring social and political pressure to end the hostilities. One might view a typical utilitarian argument for maximizing the greater good. Unfortunately, inherent to the patient-physician relationship and fundamental obligations, physicians are not permitted to weigh the interests of their patients against competing interests. The World Medical Association declarations among others inherently uphold the fundamental right of the patient against other competing interests.[21] A loose Kantian version of the means-end principle would also suggest that to violate the fundamental right of the patient-physician relationship without consent would constitute an ethical harm to the patient.

It is reasonable to assume that in the very nature of war, ethical judgment will be impaired to the degree that the physician is close to or removed from the stress, fatigue, and other factors existing in combat. As such, duress is a likely explanation for conduct that appears inconsistent with established and known codes of ethics.[22] To the degree we would want to hold a physician morally accountable fits a sliding scale of judgment mitigated by the circumstances. One would likely be less willing to hold a combat surgeon culpable for moral misjudgment fighting to save the lives of seriously wounded soldiers in a daily routine exposed as well to harms way as opposed to a psychiatrist, acting in a role as "behavioral scientist," assisting in the interrogation of a prisoner for the purpose of extracting information and not providing treatment in the traditional patient-physician relationship. Another way of expressing the difficulties of these decisions reflects in a paraphrased version of the following quotation by former United States Army combat surgeon Colonel Basil Pruitt, "the certainty of ethical opinion is directly proportional to the square of the distance from the site of combat."[23]

---

[21] World Medical Association Declaration of Helsinki, WMA General Assembly, Tokyo 2004, http://www.wma.net/e/policy/b3.htm, cited 4 June 2007.

[22] Abbe L. Dienstag, "Fedorenko v. United States: war crimes, the defense of duress, and American Nationality Law," *Columbia Law Review* 82.1 (January 1982), 120–183.

[23] Basil A. Pruitt, Jr., "Trauma care in war and peace: the Army/ASST synergism: 1992 Fitts lecture," *J Trauma* 35.1 (1993): 78–87.

5 When Doctors Go to War

Resolving the matter of mixed agency draws us closer to a position of reasonable ethical accommodation for those who choose to serve both as medical professionals and soldiers. This very thought accepts a fundamental truth regarding the moral nature of military medicine. If the entire enterprise of military medicine has no moral basis then it would be impossible for one to engage in this activity as a voluntary moral agent. Since by its nature stealing horses is morally wrong, there can be no ethical horse thieves. Likewise, if military medicine is morally wrong, there can be no moral military physicians.

If one considers the ethos of both the military and medicine, we find that this melding of professions does not make for such strange bedfellows as one might naively assume. For example, both professions share in the ideals of protecting the innocent, caring for oppressed, and seek to nobly diminish human suffering. Fundamental moral principles that focus on shared values, legitimate moral obligation, and duty refute the arguments that military medicine and those who serve as both medical professionals and soldiers are immoral. So the question becomes how to serve morally within the confines of the competing obligations of mixed agency?

The most compelling argument against the ethical nature of military medicine is the perceived dilemma of mixed agency. As previously argued, this argument is not convincing since similar dilemmas occur in civilian healthcare as well, namely competing obligations from more than one morally acceptable choice. Civilian managed care and occupational health concerns are relevant civilian analogs to the mixed agency of military physicians, namely, obligations to conserve the fighting strength of the Army, the national security obligation, as opposed to the fundamental patient-physician relationship and the concomitant rights of the patient. Hence to suggest that situations may arise where a military physician might subordinate the best interest of the patient to the good of the fighting force and the completion of mission would require similar justification to managed care concerns regarding protecting the financial interest of insurance companies and subordinating the appropriate care and treatment of the patient. The problem is not in the mixed agency of nature of the melding of military and medicine but in how one is likely to choose in the context as a voluntary moral agent.

The argument of mixed agency assumes wrongly that military professionals serve in a blind allegiance to the chain of command. In fact, the nature of the roles of those serving as military medical professionals requires them to adhere to two sets of ethical codes and ethical principles, namely both as an officer and a physician. While obedience to the command structure is essential and necessary for order and discipline of the Army, this obligation, contained within the commissioning oath, explicitly applies only to lawful orders. "Absolute obedience" is not an overriding principle of the US military. On the contrary, blind obedience to unlawful orders has led to sanction and punishment for those who fail to distinguish properly their obligation to the command structure. The presence of ethical education in the development of the officer corps of the US military is evidence of the commitment to educate, develop, and promote an officer corps of the highest values, ethical principles and sound character. Future officers at the US Military Academy at West Point live and are developed in an honor system where one learns in early character development to "choose the harder right" and not to "lie, steal, or cheat or tolerate anyone who does."[24]

Sadly there are historical and current events and behaviors to suggest that what is taught is not always applied. Such is the fate of those who teach and students who fail to grasp the lessons of a character mentor and then must deal with the consequences of poor choices. As the noble knight tells us all in the Indiana Jones trilogy, "we must choose wisely." Poor choosing does not negate the ethical nature of a profession but exposes the flawed nature of human beings to conform behavior to ideals we posit in our ethical principles and constructs. A final illustration may serve best to support this distinction that the tension is not in mixed agency but in the final choosing of voluntary moral agents.

In summer of June 2005, authors of an article published by the *New England Journal of Medicine* share aspects of their interviews with doctors who helped devise and supervise the interrogation regimen at Guantánamo revealing that the program was explicitly designed to increase fear and distress among detainees as a means to obtaining intelligence.[25] "The accounts shed light on how interrogations were conducted and raise new questions about the boundaries of medical ethics in the nation's fight against terrorism."[26] Ethics experts outside the military raised serious questions regarding the conduct of medical professionals in activity outside of what we have termed the patient-physician relationship. In response to the NEJM article, a senior Pentagon spokesman declined to address the specifics in the accounts. But he suggested that the doctors advising interrogators were not covered by ethical requirements because they were not treating patients but rather were acting as behavioral scientists. He said that while some health care personnel are responsible for "humane treatment of detainees," what we have called the patient-physician relationship, some medical professionals "may have other roles," like serving as behavioral scientists assessing the character of interrogation subjects.[27] This is the mixed agency scenario that clearly sets the rub of the tension regarding military physicians. Note however, the subtle distinction in the official Pentagon response. Some medical professionals who "may have other roles" suggest that the

[24] The United States Military Academy Honor Code, http://www.usma.edu/Committees/Honor/Info/main.htm, cited 4 June 2007.

[25] Peter A. Clark, "Medical ethics at Guantanamo Bay and Abu Ghraib: the problem of dual loyalty," *J Law Med Ethics* 34.3 (2006): 570–581.

[26] D. Holmes and A. Perron, "Violating ethics: unlawful combatants, national security and health professionals," *J Med Ethics* 33 (2007): 143–145.

[27] Steven P. Cohen, M. Gregg Bloche, and Jonathan H. Marks, Doctors and interrogation,'' *N Engl J Med* 353 (2005): 1633–1634.

structure of medical ethics does not apply when a physician is not functioning in the role as helper-healer.[28] Specifically when a medical professional is using medical knowledge for some other purpose than to heal, as this Pentagon response indicates, the constructs of medical ethics do not apply. This thinking is unfortunately flawed and exposes a grave misunderstanding of the noncombatant nature of military medical personnel.

6 Noncombatant Status

Fundamental to the notion of a noncombatant status afforded to military medical personnel under the Hague and Geneva Conventions is that such personnel engage in only humane activities and do so for all parties engaged in war activity be they military or civilian, friendly or foe. This means a military physician is under obligation to treat civilians, wounded soldiers, friendly or enemy or in post 9/11 terminology, a "detainee," in need of care. Under this protective status military medical personnel only use a personal weapon in self-defense and in defense of themselves and their wounded patients. As such military medical personnel are not to participate and support direct combat operations as part of the fighting force but in a combat service support role providing medical and health services. By definition once a soldier is wounded, this human being ceases to be a belligerent hostile but simply a wounded soldier unable to properly defend against an attacker and afforded benevolent quarantine from attack or harm. Historically the reason for providing medical personnel protection under the uniformly recognized "red cross" was to protect them from inadvertent attack and preserve their capability to render aid and healing comfort to wounded soldiers. When medical personnel engage in non-medical activities, such as interrogation, they forfeit their protective status as noncombatants. Military commanders who willingly allow their medical personnel to jeopardize their protective status of noncombatant put them at personal risk and ultimately risk the mission of the medical department to "conserve the fighting strength."[29]

Unfortunately physicians have been involved with developing interrogation techniques and involved in outright torture for generations. This level of participation and involvement has many levels and of varying degrees and is not inclusive to the military. Unfortunately, when physicians accept this shifting role they cease to be physicians, *per se*, for they contradict the fundamental essence of their vocation, namely, the ethics of the healing relationship between patient and physician. Physicians in the military may be more susceptible to assisting in interrogation and

[28] Tom Koch, "Weaponising medicine: 'Tutti fratelli,' no more," *J Med Ethics* 32 (2006): 249–255.

[29] Geneva Convention (III) relative to the Treatment of Prisoners of War, Geneva (12 August 1949).

torture for many reasons including the predisposition to follow orders and reluctance to question the authority or legality of the order, the closed structure and hierarchy of the military system and the identification and assimilation of the physicians with the military unit to which they belong. Assimilation, which can take the form of subliminal duress and the affirmation of association, may be the most likely causes of behavior that can lead to an unethical choice. Shakespeare perhaps acknowledged this power of assimilation best in *Henry V*, "we few, we merry few, we band of brothers."[30] Identification with the military unit is a very powerful force in determining behavior as is the case in any "group think" phenomena. Consequently military physicians must be vigilant and constantly guard their status as noncombatants to preserve the integrity of medical ethics while serving in uniform and avoid too close an identification to the military unit and become complicit to unethical behavior or compromise their protective status as noncombatant. Department of Defense doctrine and Article 17 of the Geneva Conventions clearly proscribes physician involvement concerning treatment of prisoners and medical professional conduct. Arguments to suggest that physicians who assist interrogators or otherwise use their clinical skills for nontherapeutic purposes do not act as physicians are correct on that point; they are not acting as physicians. To suggest that in doing so these same physicians are therefore not subject to medical ethics is true in the sense of the role that they are no longer acting as physicians, by definition. The error in this argument is the failure to identify that fact that these individuals are only capable of serving in these nontherapeutic roles *because* they are by training physicians. It is the very idea and action of using this training and skill for nontherapeutic purposes, the perversion of the healing arts for nefarious purposes, that is unethical. Hence, while the participation of physicians in these nontherapeutic roles may be a pragmatic necessity, arguably legal, and politically justifiable in a post 9/11 era, there remains no sound argument for the ethical nature of this behavior.

7 Conclusion

The military physician, as physician, is constrained by a fundamental relationship inherent to the practice of medicine, the patient-physician relationship. While there are various models that define this relationship, the purest model in the sense that elicits the nature of medical ethics is the physician as helper and healer. When physicians choose to move outside this realm of role and function, they jeopardize their ethical standing within the structure defined by their knowledge and practice. This is not to say that physicians who participate in nontherapeutic activities are *de facto* unethical. The use of medical knowledge and those who apply this knowledge

[30] Alfred Harbage, ed., "The life of Henry the fifth" in *William Shakespeare: The Complete Works* (New York: Viking Penguin, 1969) 767, lines 20–69.

in a war scenario continually face the ethical burden to preserve the caring and compassionate nature of the healing arts.

Military physicians have an ethical obligation to fulfill the role of healing helper on and off the battlefield as part of the universal commitment physicians have to uphold established and recognized codes and principles of medical ethics. They share no similar obligation to use their training and knowledge for nontherapeutic practices whether those practices are judged good or bad in the context of medical ethics. Mixing the pragmatic necessity for intelligence gathering from prisoners with well established and acceptable principles of medical ethics pushes the proverbial envelope when doing so involves physicians and medical knowledge and health information for no therapeutic purpose. The use of physicians and the healing arts for means and purpose that is clearly intended to harm a human being regardless of wartime status, classification, or definition is simply unethical. All of us in healthcare share a common bond, "we few, we merry few," and universal obligation to our patients whether military or civilian, prisoner or terrorist. To allow for and continue in nontherapeutic practices by military medical personnel is a perversion of the fundamental nature of the medical profession and desensitizes the medical professional to tending to the basic needs of the patient–and anyone in need of healing and helping and compassion is the patient.

References

American Medical Association. 2004. *Code of Medical Ethics: Current Opinions with Annotations*, 2004–2005 ed. Chicago, IL: AMA.

Beam, Thomas E. and Linette R. Sparacino, eds. 2003. *Military Medical Ethics*, vols. 1–2 (*Textbooks of Military Medicine* series). Washington, DC: Office of the Surgeon General, Department of the Army, and Borden Institute.

Bloche, M. Gregg and Jonathan H. Marks. 2005. When doctors go to war. *N Engl J Med* 352.1: 3–6.

Clark, Peter A. 2006. Medical ethics at Guantanamo Bay and Abu Ghraib: the problem of dual loyalty. *J Law Med Ethics* 34.3: 570–581.

Cohen, Steven P., M. Gregg Bloche, and Jonathan H. Marks. 2005. Doctors and interrogation. *N Engl J Med* 353: 1633–1634.

Collins, Susan D. 2006. *Aristotle and the Rediscovery of Citizenship*. New York: Cambridge University Press.

Dienstag, Abbe L. 1982. Fedorenko v. United States: war crimes, the defense of duress, and American Nationality Law. *Columbia Law Rev* 82.1: 120–183.

Entralgo, P. Lain. 1969. *Doctor and Patient*. Partridge, F., trans. New York: McGraw-Hill.

Geneva Convention (III) relative to the Treatment of Prisoners of War. 1949. Geneva (12 August).

Harbage, Alfred, ed. 1969. The life of Henry the Fifth. In *William Shakespeare: The Complete Works*. New York: Viking Penguin. Page 767, lines 20–69.

Holmes, D. and A. Perron. 2007. Violating ethics: unlawful combatants, national security and health professionals. *J Med Ethics* 33: 143–145.

Hood, Catherine A. et al. 1998. Videos, photographs, and patient consent. *BMJ* 316: 1009–1011.

Hornaday, Ann. 2006. The war tapes: three soldiers on shifting sands. *Washington Post*, 30 June.

Howe, Edmund G. 1986. Ethical issues regarding mixed agency of military physicians. *Soc Sci Med* 23.8: 803–815.

Koch, Tom. 2006. Weaponising medicine: 'Tutti fratelli,' no more. *J Med Ethics* 32: 249–255
Lifton, Robert Jay. 1986. *The Nazi Doctors*. New York: Basic Books.
Priest, Dana and Barton Gellman. 2002. US decries abuse but defends interrogations: 'stress and duress' tactics used on terrorism suspects held in secret overseas facilities. *Washington Post*, 26 December.
Pruitt, Jr., Basil A. 1993. Trauma care in war and peace: the Army/ASST synergism: 1992 Fitts Lecture. *J Trauma* 35.1: 78–87s
Ryle, John A. 1938. Foreword. In *The Doctor's View of War*, ed. Horace Joules, 7–10. London: George Allen & Unwin.
Sidel, Victor W. and Barry Levy, eds. 1997. *War and Public Health*. New York: Oxford University Press.
Singh, Jerome A. and T.L. DePellegrin. 2003. Images of war and medical ethics. *BMJ* 326 (12 April): 774–775.
Stephens, Joe. 2005. Army doctors implicated in abuse: medical workers helped tailor interrogations of detainees, article says. *Washington Post*, 6 January 2005: A8.
The Congressional Medal of Honor Society. http://www.cmohs.org/society.htm. Cited 4 June 2007.
The United States Military Academy Honor Code. http://www.usma.edu/Committees/Honor/Info/main.htm. Cited 4 June 2007.
Walzer, Michael. 2000. *Just and Unjust Wars*, 3rd ed. New York: Basic Books.
World Medical Association Declaration of Helsinki. 2004. WMA General Assembly, Tokyo 2004. http://www.wma.net/e/policy/b3.htm. Cited 4 June 2007.

Dual Disloyalties: Law and Medical Ethics at Guantánamo Bay*,[1,2]

Jonathan H. Marks

1 Introduction

At a recent symposium held in Seton Hall Law School and simulcast to hundreds of academic institutions in the United States and abroad, I was asked to address the question: "Guantánamo Bay: How should we respond?" When I thought about this question, it occurred to me that we talk about "responding" in a number of ways. We respond in games, such as chess or bridge. But the detention policy of the Bush Administration (henceforth, the "Administration") is not a game—certainly not from the perspectives of those who are being (or have been) detained at Guantánamo Bay for prolonged periods since the "global war on terror" began. We also respond in conversation. However, we should not permit rhetoric to distract from action on the ground. Statements of interrogation and detention policy are one thing (especially when prepared for public consumption or in response to public criticism); interrogation and detention practices may be quite another. We respond in negotiation. That model, too, makes me uncomfortable. My intuition and my legal training tell me that some things should simply not be negotiable, among them certain absolute commitments to fundamental human rights: freedom from cruel, inhuman, and degrading (CID) treatment, as well as freedom from torture. This is, after all, the position adopted in two core human rights treaties: the International Covenant on Civil and Political Rights (ICCPR),[3] and the Convention against Torture and Other

*The citations for this essay have been rendered according to law journal conventions—as opposed to those exercised in the rest of the Volume—per the preferences of the author and his primary audience.

[1] This essay is a revised and expanded version of the essay, "Doctors as Pawns: Law and Medical Ethics at Guantánamo Bay," 37 Seton Hall Law Review 711–731 (2007).

[2] The author would like to thank Jean Maria Arrigo for providing access to the indispensable archive materials referred to in the body of this article, and M. Gregg Bloche for generous collaboration and support without which this essay could not have been written.

[3] G.A. Res. 2200A (XXI), 21 UN GAOR, Supp. No. 16, at 52, UN Doc. A/6316 (Dec. 16, 1966), *available at* http://www.unhchr.ch/html/menu3/b/a_ccpr.htm (stating in Article 4 that there can be no derogation from the prohibitions on either torture or cruel, inhuman, or degrading treatment even "[i]n time of public emergency which threatens the life of the nation").

F. Allhoff (ed.), *Physicians at War: The Dual-Loyalties Challenge.*

Cruel, Inhuman or Degrading Treatment or Punishment (henceforth, the "Torture Convention").[4] Finally, and perhaps most charitably, our "response" may be viewed as part of the political process—as deliberative democracy taking its natural course. But the political process seems to be taking far too long. There are detainees at Guantánamo who have been in United States custody for five years, and every additional day of detention deepens the profound psychological impact on them.[5] Three of the Guantánamo detainees have already taken their own lives.[6] Additionally, at least 25 detainees have failed in their suicide attempts (in some cases, multiple attempts),[7] while many more are clinically depressed.[8]

As I contemplated my own response to the Administration's counterterrorism policy for the symposium, I became preoccupied with three major concerns. First, despite my comments above, the treatment of detainees at Guantánamo and elsewhere does appear to have evolved into a kind of multi-party, multi-dimensional game of chess. The familiar array of players includes the three branches of government and the Fourth Estate—at times critical, but often stenographic[9]—as well as lawyers, academics, and members of human rights and civil liberties groups. However, health professionals at Guantánamo Bay—whether nominally serving in a care-giving capacity or as adjuncts to the interrogation mission—are also involved, as are their professional organizations.[10] A related concern, which I articulate further below, is that health professionals—whether physicians, psychologists, nurses, medics, or others—who have served or now serve at Guantánamo Bay, have become pawns in the mistreatment of detainees and in the debate over their treatment.

Second, a substantial part of the "game" of politico-legal move and countermove has involved the reinterpretation of the scope, meaning, and application of legal norms—particularly international legal norms. Three of the most conspicuous casualties in this process have been the definition of torture, the prohibition of cruel, inhuman, and degrading treatment and punishment, and the basic protections in Common Article Three of the Geneva Conventions.[11] When legal protections for

---

[4] G.A. Res. 39/46, annex, 39 UN GAOR, Supp. No. 51, at 197, UN Doc. A/39/51 (Dec. 10, 1984) (stating in Article 2(2) that "[n]o exceptional circumstances whatsoever, whether a state of war or a threat of war, internal political instability or any other public emergency, may be invoked as a justification of torture").

[5] *See generally* Physicians For Human Rights, Break Them Down: Systematic Use Of Psychological Torture By us Forces 48–71 (2005), *available at* http://www.physiciansforhumanrights.org/library/documents/reports/break-them-down-the.pdf (explaining the long-term psychological impact of prolonged isolation and aggressive interrogation procedures).

[6] Josh White, *Three Detainees Commit Suicide at Guantanamo*, Wash. Post, June 11, 2006, at A01.

[7] Id.

[8] It has been reported that one-fifth of Guantánamo detainees are on anti-depressants. *See, e.g.*, Editorial, *Inside Guantanamo: How We Survived Jail Hell*, Observer (London), Mar. 14, 2004, *available at* http://observer.guardian.co.uk/uk_news/story/0,6903,1168937,00.html.

[9] *See* Jonathan H. Marks, *Apology or Apologia: The Fourth Estate and the Case for War in Iraq, in* The Age of Apology: The West Faces its own past (Gibney et al. eds., 2007).

[10] The role of professional organizations will be discussed in Part IV, *infra*.

[11] *See, e.g.*, Geneva Convention Relative to the Treatment of Prisoners of War, art. 3, Aug. 12, 1949, 6 U.S.T. 3316, 75 U.N.T.S. 135 ("Third Geneva Convention").

detainees are being undermined, it is all the more important that professional ethics (in particular, medical ethics) speak clearly and that codes of ethics do not become subordinate to, or dependent upon, unilateral reinterpretations of legal doctrine. The ethics of health professionals should embrace fundamental standards of human rights and the laws of war, as recognized and interpreted by the international legal order in whose formation the United States played such a pivotal role.[12] However, if health professionals are to retain our trust, and if they are to maintain the social and cultural status engendered by their perceived humanitarian ethos, their codes of ethics should do more than simply reflect the most fundamental legal prohibitions.

Third, the focus on Guantánamo Bay conveniently distracts attention from other detention centers, such as Bagram in Afghanistan and numerous unidentified "black sites" operated by the Central Intelligence Agency (CIA) across the globe[13]—where interrogation practices and the role of health professionals have come under far less public scrutiny. There is a danger that Guantánamo Bay has or will become a staged detention center, while more egregious treatment of detainees is conducted elsewhere. Following the first newspaper reports about the existence of these black sites operated by the CIA, one experienced US interrogator observed:

> Its [sic] so nice to be secret. No trouble over human rights. So secret that most of the military or government have no idea where they are. No rights, human or otherwise have to be dealt with. Let a few inaccessible places be released through controlled media informants and then AI [Amnesty International] and all the rest will be concentrating on those places while we continue to work in the real centers.[14]

Since details of these detention centers remain undisclosed and classified, it is difficult to say much about the role of medical professionals at those sites. Although we can speak with some degree of confidence about their role at Guantánamo Bay, we should keep in mind that we are only talking about one piece of the interrogation picture.

---

[12] *See* Jonathan H. Marks, *Uphold International Law*, RALEIGH NEWS & OBSERVER, Feb. 16, 2003, at A29 (noting the irony of the United States' efforts to undermine the international legal order that the United States worked so hard to establish).

[13] The President admitted the existence of these sites in September 2006. *See* Dan Eggen & Dafna Linzer, *Secret World of Detainees Grows More Public*, WASH. POST, Sept. 7, 2006, at A18 (noting that details of the sites remain classified).

[14] Correspondence between a US Counterintelligence Liaison Officer and Jean Maria (2002–2005) (on file at the Project on Ethics and Art in Testimony, Irvine, CA) [hereinafter Arrigo Papers]. An additional copy is archived at *Intelligence Ethics Collection*, Hoover Institution Archives, Stanford University, Stanford, CA (restricted until January 1, 2010). This is, of course, just one interrogator's view of human rights. The correspondence also indicates that there have been deliberate efforts to distract and mislead the press during the war on terror. Another communication states: "[E]mbedded reporters are now being put in one vehicle and taken to staged events while the rest of the unit goes to do its job.... The use of names of the prisoners will be replaced by codes so nobody can try to trace them." Id.

2 Health Professionals and Interrogation at Guantánamo

It is possible to describe in some detail the roles that health professionals played in the design and implementation of interrogation strategies at Guantánamo Bay thanks to the tens of thousands of documents obtained by the American Civil Liberties Union (ACLU) under the Freedom of Information Act (FOIA), not to mention several other documents that have been leaked to the press. Since these roles have been described in considerable detail elsewhere,[15] I review them only briefly here.

Psychiatrists and psychologists were brought into the interrogation process not as gatekeepers or health care advocates for detainees, but as adjuncts to the interrogation mission. Although some of them clearly had no professional background or training relevant to interrogation,[16] they were considered "behavioral science consultants"[17]—assigned to teams known colloquially as "Biscuits"[18]—and their input was deemed "essential" in both the design of interrogation strategies and the interpretation of intelligence at Guantánamo Bay.[19] They advised interrogators how to ramp up interrogation stressors in order to overcome the apparent resistance of detainees to questioning.[20] The kinds of stressors used at Guantánamo Bay are now common knowledge, having been the subject of numerous newspaper reports and internal US Army (henceforth, the "Army") investigations.[21] They include sleep deprivation and manipulation, exposure to loud noise and temperature extremes, and the use of stress positions.[22] Some reports indicate that behavioral science personnel used information derived from detainees' medical records as the basis for their advice.[23] In one instance, for example, they advised interrogators to

[15] *See, e.g.*, M. Gregg Bloche & Jonathan H. Marks, *When Doctors Go To War*, 352 New Eng. J. Med. 3, 3–6 (2005); M. Gregg Bloche & Jonathan H. Marks, *Doctors and Interrogators at Guantanamo Bay*, 353 New Eng. J. Med. 6, 6–8 (2005); Steve H. Miles, Oath Betrayed: Torture, Medical Complicity and the War on Terror 43–67 (2006).

[16] *See, e.g.*, Bloche & Marks, *Doctors and Interrogators at Guantanamo Bay, supra* note 15. However, some mental health professionals were sent to Survival, Evasion, Resistance, and Escape ("SERE") school where US soldiers are trained to resist interrogation at the hands of enemy captors. *See* M. Gregg Bloche & Jonathan H. Marks, *Doing Unto Others as They Did Unto Us*, N. Y. Times, Nov. 14, 2005, at 21; *see also* Jonathan H. Marks, *Doctors of Interrogation*, 35 Hastings Ctr. Report 17, 18 (2005) (discussing whether health professionals were employed for their professional expertise or in order to add an imprimatur of decency to the process).

[17] Bloche & Marks, *Doing Unto Others as They Did Unto Us, supra* note 14.

[18] Marks, *supra* 14, at 17 (discussing whether health professionals were employed for their professional expertise or in order to add an imprimatur of decency to the process).

[19] Id.

[20] Id.

[21] Id. at 17–22.

[22] *See, e.g.*, Physicians for Human Rights, Break Them Down: Systematic Use of Psychological Torture by US Forces (2005), *available at* http://www.physiciansfor humanrights.org/library/documents/reports/break-them-down-the.pdf.

[23] Neil Lewis, *Interrogators Cite Doctors' Aid at Guantanamo Prison Camp*, N.Y. Times, June 24, 2005, *available at* http://www.nytimes.com/2005/06/24/politics/[24]gitmo.html?ex = 1277265600&en = b1960558c2ad9fa4&ei = 5088&partner = rssnyt&emc = rss.

exploit a detainee's fear of the dark.[24] Army documents also record that behavioral scientists were "on hand" to monitor interrogations, and that they were supposedly given the power to intervene if interrogations got out of hand.[25]

Although there is evidence that Biscuit personnel monitored interrogations both inside and outside the interrogation room[26]—in the latter case through one-way mirrors—there is little evidence that they intervened to prevent interrogations from going too far. On the contrary, Army documents suggest that behavioral science personnel (as well as some caregivers) stood by while detainees were abused. Mohammed Al Qahtani, the "20th hijacker,"[27] was exposed to an aggressive interrogation regime at Guantánamo Bay for up to 20 hours per day for 48 days over a 54-day period at the end of 2002 and beginning of 2003.[28] The interrogation log—obtained by *Time Magazine*—records the presence of a psychologist during parts of the interrogation.[29] However, the process still spiraled out of control, putting Al Qahtani's health in grave danger. On one occasion, Al Qahtani's pulse dropped to 35 beats per minute, and on two occasions his temperature dropped to 95°.[30] To add insult to injury, when Al Qahtani was rehydrated with three bags of intravenous fluids, interrogators refused to let him take a bathroom break, and he had no option but to wet himself.[31]

This is not the only example of medical treatment or its sequelae being deployed for strategic purposes. Force-feeding of hunger strikers at Guantánamo Bay is being conducted with the assistance of medical personnel who are caregivers, not adjuncts to the interrogation mission.[32] After some US Navy physicians refused to force-feed detainees, the Department of Defense began screening doctors assigned to Guantánamo Bay to ensure they would be willing to participate.[33] The practice of force-feeding has been defended by the Pentagon as being necessary to protect the

---

[24] Id.

[25] Marks, *Doctors of Interrogation*, *supra* note 16, at 18.

[26] Id. at 17.

[27] He was not, of course, the only Al Qaeda suspect to be branded "the 20th hijacker." *See, e.g.*, Seymour M. Hersh, *The Twentieth Man: Has the Justice Department Mishandled the Case against Zacarias Moussaoui?*, New Yorker, Sept. 30, 2002, *available at* http://www.newyorker.com/fact/content/articles/020930fa_fact.

[28] Army Reg. 15–6: Final Report, Investigation into FBI Allegations of Detainee Abuse at Guantanamo Bay, Cuba Detention Facility (*as amended* June 9, 2005), 13–21, *available at* http://www.defenselink.mil/news/Jul2005/ d20050714report.pdf.

[29] *See* Adam Zagorin & Michael Duffy, *Inside the Interrogation of Detainee 063*, Time, June 12, 2005, *available at* http://www.time.com/time/magazine/printout/

0,8816,1071284,00.html; *see also* Interrogation Log Detainee 063, Nov. 23, 2002, http://www.time.com/time/2006/log/log.pdf (presenting a partially-redacted copy of the interrogation log); *see also* Steve Miles, *Medical Ethics and the Interrogation of Detainee 063*, 7 Am. J. Bioethics 3, *available at* http://www.bioethics.net/journal /j_articles.php?aid = 1140 (discussing this interrogation from a medical ethics perspective).

[30] *See* Zagorin & Duffy, *supra* note 29.

[31] Id.

[32] Susan Okie, *Glimpses of Guantanamo-Medical Ethics and the War on Terror*, 353 New Eng. J. Med. 2529, 2530 (2006).

[33] Id.

health of detainees.[34] However, there are a number of reasons to doubt this claim. First, reports indicate that, in contrast with its use in federal prisons, force-feeding is being administered long before the health of detainees is seriously threatened by their hunger strike.[35] Second, detainees have reportedly been forced to sit in their own urine and feces while strapped into a chair for "postfeed observation."[36] Third, the Pentagon regards hunger strikes and suicide attempts as acts of "asymmetric warfare,"[37] rather than signs of desperation on the part of those being detained for an indefinite period on grounds that are often still unclear.[38] This view undermines the claim by the Assistant Secretary of Defense for Health Affairs, William Winkenwerder, Jr., M.D., that the Pentagon's "intentions are good" and that they are "seeking to preserve life."[39] How can the policy of force-feeding be *both* ethically responsible medical treatment and a response tactic in asymmetric warfare?

3 The Evolution (or Revolution) of Legal Doctrine

In order to pave the way for the use of more aggressive interrogation techniques against "high-value detainees" such as Al Qahtani, the Administration recognized that a number of legal hurdles needed to be addressed. As a result, they embarked on what I have described elsewhere as a series of exercises in legal exceptionalism, in which legal protections and prohibitions were dispensed with on the grounds that they were geographically limited (*spatial exceptionalism*), that they did not apply to a particular group (*collective exceptionalism*), or that their true meaning had been hitherto misunderstood (*interpretive exceptionalism*).[40] For present purposes, I will focus on just three examples, but there are many more.

First and foremost, the Administration wanted to make sure that interrogators deploying these techniques would not incur criminal responsibility for torture. This objective led to the August 2002 memorandum from then-Assistant Attorney General

---

[34] Luke Mitchell, *God Mode*, Harper's Magazine, July 2006, *available at* http://www.harpers.org/GodMode.html (Aug. 24, 2006).

[35] George Annas, *Hunger Strikes at Guantanamo—Medical Ethics and Human Rights in a "Legal Black Hole*," 355 New Eng. J. Med. 1377, 1379–1380 (2006).

[36] Id. at 1377; Nancy Sherman, *Holding Doctors Responsible at Guantanamo*, 16 Kennedy Inst. of Ethics J. 199, 201 (2006).

[37] BBC News, *Guantanamo Suicides "Acts of War"*, June 11, 2006, http://news.bbc.co.uk/2/hi/americas/5068606.stm.

[38] Mark Denbeaux et al., No-Hearing Hearings—CSRT: The Modern Habeas Corpus? An Analysis of the Proceedings of the Government's Combatant Status Review Tribunals at Guantanamo, Nov. 2005, http://law.shu.edu/news/final_no_hearing_hearings_report.pdf (finding Department of Defense documents indicate that "[t]he Government did not produce any witnesses in any [Combatant Status Review Tribunal] hearing and did not present any documentary evidence to the detainee prior to the hearing in 96% of the cases").

[39] Mitchell, *supra* note 34.

[40] *See* Jonathan H. Marks, *9/11 + 3/11 + 7/7 =? What Counts in Counterterrorism?*, 37 Colum. Hum. Rts. L. Rev. 559, 578–83 (2006).

Jay Bybee to then-White House Counsel Alberto Gonzalez, entitled *Re: Standards of Conduct for Interrogation under 18 U.S.C. 2340–2340A*.[41] The document narrowly defined physical torture to require pain "equivalent in intensity to the pain accompanying serious physical injury, such as organ failure, the permanent impairment of a significant bodily function, or even death."[42] For pain or suffering to rise to the level of mental torture, the memo added, "it must result in significant psychological harm of significant duration, e.g. lasting for months or even years."[43] Even if these thresholds are crossed and the interrogator *knows* they are being crossed, the memo contends that the interrogator would not be guilty of torture under US criminal law "if causing such harm is not his objective."[44] Nor would he have committed torture, according to the memo, if he "could show that he acted in good faith by taking steps such as surveying professional literature, *consulting with experts*, or reviewing evidence gained from past experience."[45] On the view set out in this memo—which was not revoked and replaced by the Department of Justice until after photographs of detainee abuse at Abu Ghraib had been published[46]—the advice of behavioral science experts would be critical, at the very least, in order to insulate interrogators from domestic criminal liability.[47]

Having tried to narrow the definition of torture, the Administration continued to emphasize that the United States does not torture.[48] However, that still left the prohibition on CID treatment or punishment as a potential impediment to more

[41] Memorandum from Jay S. Bybee, Assistant Att'y Gen., U.S. Dep't of Justice, to Alberto R. Gonzales, White House Counsel, Re: Standards of Conduct for Interrogation under 18 U.S.C. §§2340–2340A (Aug. 1, 2002), *available at* http://www.washingtonpost.com/wp-srv/nation/documents/dojinterrogation memo20020801.pdf [hereinafter Bybee Memo]. Sections 2340–2340A, which define the criminal offense of torture in the United States, were enacted in order to comply with the United States' obligations under the Convention Against Torture and Other Cruel, Inhuman or Degrading Treatment or Punishment (1984). See H.R. Rep. No. 103–482, at 229 (1994) (Conf. Rep.). The drafters of the Bybee memo drew on (and were admittedly facilitated by) understandings made by the United States when it ratified the Convention in 1994. *See* Sanford Levinson, *"Precommitment" and "Postcommitment": The Ban on Torture in the Wake of September 11*, 81 TEX. L. REV. 2013, 2036–38 (2003). The text of the ratification instrument is available at http://www.unhchr.ch/html/menu2/6/cat/treaties/convention-reserv.htm.

[42] Bybee Memo, *supra* note 41, at 1

[43] Id.

[44] Id. at 4.

[45] Id. at 8 (emphasis added).

[46] Although the document was revoked in June 2004, it was not formally replaced until December 2004, just days before the confirmation hearings of Attorney General Alberto Gonzales. *See* Memorandum from Daniel Levin, Acting Assistant Attorney General to James B. Comey, Deputy Attorney General, Re: Legal Standards Applicable under 18 U.S.C. §§2340–2340A (Dec. 30, 2004), *available at* http://www.usdoj.gov/olc/dagmemo.pdf.

[47] *See* Bybee Memo, *supra* note 41, at 8.

[48] *See, e.g.*, Statement by the President on United Nations International Day in Support of Victims of Torture, http://www.whitehouse.gov/news/releases/2003/06/20030626-3.html (June 23, 2003) (stating that the "United States is committed to the world-wide elimination of torture and we are leading this fight by example").

aggressive interrogation strategies. As a party to both the ICCPR[49] and the Torture Convention,[50] the United States has committed itself to the prohibition against CID treatment, as well as torture. The ICCPR clearly states that this is an obligation to which no exception is permitted,[51] and the Torture Convention imposes an obligation on parties to review interrogation rules to ensure that they do not result in CID treatment.[52] When the United States ratified both treaties, it made reservations defining CID to mean cruel and unusual treatment or punishment prohibited by the Fifth, Eighth, and Fourteenth Amendments to the United States Constitution.[53] The Bush Administration took the view that these reservations served not only to redefine the type of conduct that would be considered CID, but also operated to limit the geographic scope of the Unites States' international obligations so that they did not apply to aliens detained outside the United States.[54] This view created, in effect, a "legal black hole" into which Guantánamo Bay, nominally leased by the United States from Cuba, conveniently appeared to fall.[55] This was the position which Senator John McCain sought to address in the "McCain Amendment," now section 1003 of the Detainee Treatment Act of 2005.[56] Its provisions were intended to make clear that the prohibition of CID treatment applies irrespective of the nationality and geographic location of the detainee.[57] But when President Bush signed the Detainee Treatment Act into law, he issued a presidential signing statement declaring that the Administration would interpret the detainee provisions "in a manner consistent with the constitutional authority of the President to supervise the unitary executive branch and as Commander in Chief and consistent with the constitutional limitations on judicial power."[58] This firm assertion of presidential power

---

[49] ICCPR, *supra* note 3.

[50] Torture Convention, *supra* note 4.

[51] For an authoritative interpretation of the ICCPR on this point, see Human Rights Committee, General Comment No. 20 (1992), ¶ 3, *available at* http://www.unhchr.ch/tbs/doc.nsf/(Symbol)/6924291970754969c12563ed004c8ae5?Opendocument (last visited Feb. 5, 2007).

[52] Torture Convention, *supra* 2, arts. 11 and 16.

[53] For the text of the United States' ratification of the Torture Convention, *see* 36 CONG. REC. S10091 (1990), *available at* http://www.unhchr.ch/html/menu2/6/cat/treaties/convention-reserv.htm. For the text of the United States' ratification of the ICCPR, see http://www.unhchr.ch/html/menu3/b/treaty5_asp.htm (last visited Nov. 25, 2006).

[54] *See* Gonzales Nomination Transcript, *available at* http://www.humanrightsfirst.com/us_law/etn/gonzales/statements/gonz_testimony_010604.htm (last visited Mar. 30, 2006).

[55] *See* Johan Steyn, *Guantanamo Bay: The Legal Black Hole*, 53 INT'L & COMP. L.Q. 1–15 (2004).

[56] *See* Detainee Treatment Act of 2005, Pub. L. No. 109-48, §1003, 119 Stat. 2680, 2739–2744 (2005).

[57] *See* id.

[58] Statement of President George W. Bush Upon Signing of H.R. 2863, Dec. 30, 2005, *available at* http://www.whitehouse.gov/releaseas/2005/12/10551230-8.html; *see also* T.J. Halstead, Cong. Res. Serv., *Presidential Signing Statements: Constitutional and Institutional Implications*, Sept. 20, 2006, *available at* http://www.fas.org/sgp/crs/natsec/RL33667.pdf (analyzing the impact of signing statements).

naturally raised serious doubts about the practical impact of the legislation on the Administration's detention and interrogation policy.[59]

Another important doctrinal reformulation—or exercise in legal exceptionalism—concerns the Geneva Conventions. Common Article Three of the Geneva Conventions provides protections that have long been understood as the low water-mark for treatment of detainees, irrespective of their status.[60] Although so-called unlawful combatants are not entitled to the full array of protections applicable to prisoners of war, they are to be protected from cruel, humiliating, or degrading treatment *and* from outrages on personal dignity.[61] They are also to be treated humanely.[62] The formal position of the Administration, determined in February 2002, was that the Geneva Conventions did not apply to detainees who are members of Al Qaeda, because Al Qaeda is neither a state nor a party to the Conventions.[63] However, that position was unequivocally rejected by the Supreme Court of the United States in *Hamdan v. Rumsfeld* in June 2006.[64] The Department of Defense responded to this decision with a memorandum calling for a review of directives and policies to ensure compliance with Common Article Three.[65] But just a few weeks later, in September 2006, the President publicly criticized the provisions of Common Article Three for being too vague.[66] Congress addressed the President's

---

[59] It should be noted that a provision similar to the McCain Amendment also appears in the Military Commissions Act of 2006, Pub. L. No. 109-366, 120 Stat. 2600. However, the Military Commissions Act is problematic for several other reasons, some of which are discussed below. *See* notes 67–71 and accompanying text; *see also* Human Rights Watch, Q and A: Military Commissions Act of 2006, *available at* http://hrw.org/backgrounder/usa/qna1006/usqna1006web.pdf (briefly analyzing and critiquing the Military Commissions Act) [hereinafter Human Rights Watch].

[60] *See, e.g.*, International Committee for the Red Cross, *Commentary on Geneva Convention III, Article 3*, http://www.icrc.org/ihl.nsf/COM/375-590006?OpenDocument (last visited Mar. 14, 2007); Michael John Garcia, Cong. Res. Serv., *The War Crimes Act: Current Issues*, Oct. 2, 2006, *available at* http://www.fas.org/sgp/crs/intel/RL33 662.pdf; *see also* Ruth Wedgwood & R. James Woolsey, *Law and Torture*, WALL ST. J., June 28, 2004, at A10.

[61] Third Geneva Convention, *supra* note 11, art. 3.

[62] Id. A similar obligation is found in Article 10 of the ICCPR, which provides that "[a]ll persons deprived of their liberty shall be treated with humanity and with respect for the inherent dignity of the human person." ICCPR, *supra* note 3, art. 10.

[63] Office of the White House Press Secretary, Fact Sheet: Status of the Detainees at Guantanamo, Feb. 7, 2002, http://www.whitehouse.gov/news/releases/2002/02/20020207-13.html.

[64] Hamdan v. Rumsfeld, 126 S. Ct. 2749, 2794–95 (2006).

[65] Memorandum from Gordon England, Deputy Secretary of Defense to the Secretaries of the Military Departments et al., Application of Common Article 3 of the Geneva Conventions to the Treatment of Detainees in the Department of Defense (July 7, 2006), *available at* http://www.defenselink.mil/news/Aug2006/d20060814comm3.pdf.

[66] The President acknowledged that the "Supreme Court's ruling [in Hamdan] … said that we must conduct ourselves under the Common Article 3 of the Geneva Convention." He added: "And that Common Article 3 says that there will be no outrages upon human dignity. It's very vague. What does that mean, 'outrages upon human dignity?' That's a statement that is wide open to interpretation." Transcript of Sept. 15, 2006, Press Conference of the President, *available at* http://www.whitehouse.gov/news/releases/2006/09/ 20060915-2.html.

concerns later that month, passing the Military Commissions Act of 2006 (MCA).[67] The MCA purports to confer on the President the authority to "interpret the meaning and application of the Geneva Conventions."[68] It remains to be seen how the President will respond to this provision. But there is a real danger that the Executive will view it as providing *carte blanche* to define Article Three's protections narrowly. Although the MCA states that "[n]othing in this section shall be construed to affect the constitutional functions and responsibilities of ... the judicial branch of the United States,"[69] this provides little comfort given the MCA's attempts to strip the federal courts of habeas corpus jurisdiction over detainees,[70] and to prevent them from invoking the Geneva Conventions "as a source of rights" in domestic litigation.[71] If the President does narrowly redefine the scope of protections in the Geneva Conventions, it is therefore likely to be some time before a federal court will be given the opportunity to correct this. That delay will be too long, not just for detainees at Guantánamo Bay and elsewhere, but also for health professionals with whom they have contact.

Whatever the Administration's interpretation of the Geneva Conventions, health professionals would be well-advised to remember that international legal norms—as commonly understood by other nations and, in the case of the Geneva Conventions, as authoritatively interpreted by the International Committee of the Red Cross (ICRC)[72]—will be violated by more aggressive interrogation strategies long before the mental and physical health or well-being of detainees are implicated. For example, the prohibition of outrages on personal dignity in Common Article Three was clearly breached by soldiers who placed underwear on the heads of detainees or forced them to assemble naked in pyramid formation.[73] Second,

---

[67] Military Commissions Act of 2006, Pub. L. No. 109-366, 120 Stat. 2600.

[68] Id. §6(a)(3)(A).

[69] Id.

[70] Id. §7. *See also* Gerald L. Neuman, *The Military Commissions Act and the Detainee Debacle: A Response*, 48 Harv. Int'l L.J. Online 33 (2007), http://www.harvardilj.org/online/105 (arguing that Congress did not have the power to permanently abrogate the writ of habeas corpus) and Robert M. Chesney, *Judicial Review, Combatant Status Determinations, and the Possible Consequences of* Boumediene, 48 Harv. Int'l L.J. Online 62 (2007), http://www.harvardilj.org/online/110 (observing that the "slowly grinding process of developing and stabilizing our detainee laws and policies unfortunately is not yet near its conclusion").

[71] Id. at §5. In particular, this section seeks to prevent the Geneva Conventions from being invoked as a source of rights in habeas corpus or other civil proceedings against the United States, and any of its current or former officers, employees, or agents. Id.

[72] Int'l Comm. of the Red Cross, International Humanitarian Law—Treaties of Documents 1 (2005), http://www.icrc.org/ihl.nsf/CONVPRES?OpenView (ICRC's authoritative commentary on the Geneva Conventions).

[73] BG Furlow & Lt. Gen. Schmidt, Investigation into FBI Allegations of Detainee Abuse at Guantanamo Bay, Cuba Detention Facility 19 (June 9, 2005) (indicating that Guantánamo Bay detainee, Al Qahtani, "was forced to wear a woman's bra and had a thong placed on his head during interrogation"). For the infamous image of a human pyramid at Abu Ghraib, which has become emblematic of detainee abuse in the war on terror, see *New Yorker*, at http://www.newyorker.com/online/slideshows/slideshows/040510onslpo_prison_02 (last visited Feb. 10, 2007).

medical personnel may be complicit in the commission of grave breaches of the Geneva Conventions—also known as war crimes—if they advise on or monitor the use of interrogation tacticvs that qualify as torture or inhuman treatment or that "willfully cause great suffering."[74] War crimes attract universal jurisdiction.[75] So even if health professionals were not concerned about potential prosecution in the United States,[76] they would be ill-advised to ignore the possibility of being arrested and tried while visiting another country.

4 Law and Medical Ethics

The involvement of military health professionals in interrogation at Guantánamo Bay and elsewhere in the war on terror has been said to illustrate two kinds of ethical tension. Construed narrowly, the conflict is between the military and medical obligations of military health professionals (*the narrow tension*). These competing sets of obligations are often presented as a paradigm case of the so-called *dual-loyalties* problem.[77] For example, the military doctor who treats an injured soldier so that he can be returned to the battlefield confronts a tension between the best interests of his patient and the demands of the military mission. Some have argued that this kind of tension in military medicine is all too frequent and that it creates an "inherent moral impossibility."[78] They claim that "medical practice under military control [is] fundamentally dysfunctional and unethical,"[79] and, in effect, call for physicians to withdraw from military service. Others consider the tension to be challenging but not insurmountable. They tend to resolve it by giving primacy to the medical ethical obligations of a military health professional[80]

---

[74] *See* Third Geneva Convention, *supra* note 11, art. 130, *available at* http://www.unhchr.ch/html/menu3/ b/91.htm; for a discussion of the War Crimes Act in the United States, *see also* Garcia, *supra* note 58.

[75] For a more detailed discussion of universal jurisdiction and its theoretical foundations, see Jonathan H. Marks, *Mending the Web: Universal Jurisdiction, Humanitarian Intervention and the Abrogation of Immunity by the Security Council*, 42 COLUM. J. TRANSNAT'L L. 445 (2004).

[76] The Military Commissions Act also amends the War Crimes Act. Military Commissions Act of 2006, Pub. L. No. 109-366, 120 Stat. 2600. For a brief summary of the material revisions, see Human Rights Watch, *supra* note 59.

[77] *See, for example*, Leslie London et al., *Dual Loyalty Among Military Health Professionals*, 15 CAMBRIDGE Q. OF HEALTHCARE ETHICS 381 (2006).

[78] Sidel V.W., Levy B.S. *Physician-Soldier: A Moral Dilemma* in Beam T.E., Spracino L.R. (eds.), Military Medical Ethics, Vol. 1 (2003), 293–312, available at http://www.bordeninstitute.army.mil/published_volumes/ethicsVol1/ethicsVol1.html

[79] Id.

[80] *See, for example*, Dual Loyalty Working Group. *Dual Loyalty and Human Rights in Health Professional Practice. Proposed Guidelines and Institutional Mechanisms*, Washington, DC: Physicians for Human Rights (2002)

or, more controversially, to his military obligations.[81] (In the former case, a working group established under the auspices of Physicians for Human Rights has drafted a set of human rights-oriented guidelines that are intended to aid the resolution of the tension.[82])

Construed more broadly and considered at a greater level of abstraction, the tension is between the therapeutic and social purposes of medicine (*the broad tension*).[83] The military mission is just one important example of a "social purpose" that may require physicians to perform functions that are non-therapeutic and/or that may be at odds with the welfare of a patient. Medicine's social purposes abound in the civil and criminal justice system too, and in the allocation of scarce medical resources and measures adopted for the protection of public health. For example, psychiatrists are often asked to provide an assessment of a defendant's state of mind in order to help the court determine the defendant's fitness to stand trial. The assessment may not serve the interests of the defendant so, in order to perform the task at hand, the psychiatrist should endeavor to put out of his mind the consequences of the assessment for that individual. To provide a different example from the public health sphere, in some cases a physician may—when backed by force of law—administer compulsory prophylaxis (such as vaccination) or treatment against the express wishes of a patient in order to protect the health of others.[84]

In my view, the involvement of military health professionals in *lawful* interrogations—like the involvement of civilian physicians in these other lawful activities—can indeed be said to illustrate the tensions I describe. When a military health professional provides advice to interrogators on how to obtain information from an interrogatee during a rapport-building interrogation, he is performing a non-therapeutic function. He is trying to advance the military intelligence mission rather than the welfare or interests of the interrogatee. In such a case, the tensions I have described are real. As I have argued elsewhere, they cannot be convincingly explained away by contending either that physicians who perform such functions are not acting as physicians or that, because there is no doctor-patient relationship, no medical ethical obligations govern the interaction.[85] Whether health professionals are brought into

---

[81] *See, for example*, the work of the political scientist, Michael Gross, who has given primacy to the military mission by framing the tension as being between the medical ethical obligations of a physician and his duties of citizenship. Michael Gross, Doctors in the Decent Society: Medical Care, Torture and Ill-Treatment, *Bioethics*, 2004, 18(2): 181–203.

[82] Dual Loyalty Working Group. *Dual Loyalty and Human Rights in Health Professional Practice. Proposed Guidelines and Institutional Mechanisms*, Washington, DC: Physicians for Human Rights (2002)

[83] *See*, for example, Bloche and Marks, *When Doctors Go To War, supra* note 15.

[84] *See, for example*, Jacobson v. Massachusetts 25 S. Ct. 358 (1905). For a review of the recent debate on compulsory vaccination and treatment in the face of a public health emergency, *see* Jonathan H. Marks, *What Counts, supra* note 40.

[85] *See* Marks, *Doctors of Interrogation*, supra note 16, and Jonathan H. Marks, *The Bioethics of War*, Hastings Center Report, 37(2): 41–42 (2007). For arguments to the contrary, *see* Fritz Allhoff, Physician Involvement in Hostile Interrogations, 15 Cambridge Q. of Healthcare Ethics 392–402 (2006).

the interrogation process to provide advice within their field of expertise or in order to add an imprimatur of decency to the process, they are being asked to participate *because* they are professionals. The absence of a traditional doctor-patient relationship does not mean that professional ethics has nothing to say. The scope of a health professional's ethical obligations extends well beyond the confines of the paradigmatic clinical encounter.[86]

How the tensions can be resolved in the case of lawful interrogations—and have been resolved by some medical professional organizations—is a matter to which I will return shortly. However, the aggressive treatment of detainees in the war on terror that I describe in §2 violates the most fundamental norms of international law. In such a case and for the reasons I will now give, neither the narrow nor the broad tension necessarily arises—although they might, at first blush, appear to do so.

Military health professionals are, like all military personnel, required to act lawfully. Like all servicemen and women, they are only required to obey lawful orders.[87] (And should they commit war crimes, it is no defense that they were following orders if they knew the orders were unlawful or if those orders were manifestly unlawful.[88]) Strictly speaking, a military health professional who advises on or otherwise participates in an aggressive *unlawful* interrogation violates his obligations as a military professional as well as his obligations as a health professional. We recognize that a patient's express wishes need not be synonymous with or a proxy for the patient's interests. This is why a physician ought to refuse to perform a sixth or seventh cosmetic surgical procedure on an iatrophilic patient addicted to rhinoplasty. Similarly, unlawful orders are neither synonymous with nor a proxy for the military mission. So a military health professional who participates in or advises on an unlawful interrogation does not demonstrate fidelity either to medicine or the military mission. In such a case, there is no narrow tension or problem of dual loyalties. Rather, there is dual *dis*loyalty.

Similarly, the broad tension arguably does not arise in the case of an unlawful interrogation. In order to speak meaningfully about the conflict between the therapeutic and social purposes of medicine, we should probe the meaning of "social purpose" a little further. The term should not be taken to denote any instance in which a societal goal is invoked. When society has placed certain types of behavior out of bounds—either by establishing prohibitions in domestic criminal law or by entering into solemn international legal commitments—it must surely become more difficult to contend that such conduct is in pursuit of a social purpose. At the

---

[86] *See, for example*, Wynia, M. et al., Medical Professionalism in Society, New England Journal of Medicine, 341:1612–1616 (1999).

[87] Art. 92 of the Uniform Code of Military Justice. Ideally, the Code would also provide that military medical professionals can refuse to obey unethical orders too. Article 16(2) of the First Additional Protocol to the Geneva Conventions, 1125 U.N.T.S. 3 (1977) prohibits states from compelling medical personnel to perform acts contrary to medical ethics. Although the US has not ratified the protocol, it has been argued that there is now a rule of customary international law to the same effect binding all states: see Jean-Marie Henckaerts and Louise Doswald-Beck, Customary International Humanitarian Law (2005), Vol. 1, 86–88.

[88] *See, for example*, Art. 33(1) of the Rome Statute of the International Criminal Court (1998).

very least, the conduct cannot be justified as being in pursuit of such a purpose when—as in the case of torture and CID treatment—the conduct has been determined to violate absolute and fundamental norms of international human rights law and the laws of war. To some philosophers, this might appear to be an unduly legalistic or formalist interpretation of the broad tension. However, any other view would allow *génocidaires* and war criminals to defend ethnic cleansing as an exercise in social engineering.

Despite this critique of the narrow and broad tensions in the case of unlawful interrogations, I recognize that the narrow tension may be acutely perceived by military health professionals pulled into such interrogations. Furthermore, in the face of the Administration's efforts to circumvent international legal protections for detainees in the war on terror, the voice of professional ethics is especially important. Professional ethics should not be an entirely autonomous enterprise. In particular, ethical codes for physicians, psychologists, and other health professionals should incorporate basic standards that reflect fundamental protections found in international human rights law and the laws of war.[89] The Report of the American Psychological Association's Task Force on Psychological Ethics and National Security in July 2005 notably failed to do this. Proscriptions against psychologists' participation in abusive interrogation were not defined by reference to international law. They were merely tied to "applicable" US rules and regulations as "developed and refined" since 9/11.[90] When one recalls the administration's efforts to "refine" legal norms, the dangers inherent in this approach are manifest. The report also fails to recognize that since the vast majority of detainees in the war on terror are foreign nationals, the propriety of their treatment is far more likely to be judged by international standards than by domestic ones, particularly if the latter are more lax.

It is possible simply to tie ethical constraints on health professionals to international legal prohibitions—an approach taken in the United Nations Principles of Medical Ethics.[91] For example, physicians are prohibited from using their knowledge

---

[89] *See* Leslie London et al., *Dual Loyalty Among Military Health Professionals*, 15 Cambridge Q. of Healthcare Ethics 381, 385–386 (2006) (discussing the value of a human rights perspective). In the remainder of this section, I will argue that human rights should be the foundation of a health professional's ethical obligations, but not the limit of those obligations.

[90] Report of the American Psychological Association Presidential Task Force on Psychological Ethics and National Security (2005), *available at* http://www.apa.org/releases/PENSTaskForceReportFinal.pdf [hereinafter Presidential Task Force]; *see also* Tara McKelvey, *First Do Some Harm*, American Prospect, Sept. 1 2005, http://www.prospect.org/web/printfriendly-view.ww?id = 10110 (critiquing the task force, many of whose members had military or national security affiliations); Michael Benjamin, *Psychological Warfare*, Salon.com, July 26, 2006, http://www.salon.com/news/feature/2006/07/26/interrogation/index.html; Mark Benjamin, *Psychologists' Group Still Rocked by Torture Debate*, Salon.com, Aug. 4, 2006, http://www.salon.com/news/feature/2006/08/04/apa/.

[91] Principles of Medical Ethics Relevant to the Role of Health Personnel, Particularly Physicians, in the Protection of Prisoners and Detainees Against Torture and Other Cruel, Inhuman or Degrading Treatment or Punishment, G.A. Res. 37/194, Annex, U.N. Doc. A/RES/37/194 (Dec. 18, 1982), *available at* http://www.un.org/ documents/ga/res/37/a37r194.htm.

and skills to assist in an interrogation that adversely affects the health or condition of a detainee *and* is "not in accordance with the relevant international instruments."[92] These instruments would obviously include the Geneva Conventions, the ICCPR, and the Torture Convention. But giving legal norms the last word on the limits of professional conduct leaves psychiatrists and psychologists without clear guidance in the face of disagreements between lawyers and policymakers about the application of those norms. The efforts to redefine the scope and meaning of the Geneva Conventions and the prohibition of CID treatment in core human rights treaties—discussed above—provide two powerful illustrations of this point.[93]

Some codes of professional ethics impose firm constraints on health professionals, irrespective of the applicable legal norms. For example, the World Medical Association's Regulations in Times of Armed Conflict state that it is unethical for physicians to "[w]eaken the physical or mental strength of a human being without therapeutic justification" or to "[e]mploy scientific knowledge to imperil health."[94] It is difficult to understand how a physician with these prohibitions in mind would have felt able to participate in the kinds of aggressive interrogation stressors deployed at Guantánamo Bay. At the very least, the express purpose of coercive counter-resistance tactics such as prolonged isolation and sleep deprivation was to weaken the mental and physical strength of detainees.[95] In light of this, the American Medical Association (AMA) might have been expected to respond clearly and speedily to revelations of the involvement of American physicians in aggressive interrogations.

However, the AMA did not formally take a position on the role of physicians in interrogation until the summer of 2006.[96] The new ethical guidelines provide that "[p]hysicians must neither conduct nor directly participate in, or monitor an interrogation, because a role as physician-interrogator undermines the physician's role

---

[92] Id. at princ. 4.

[93] *See supra* Part III.

[94] World Medical Association, Regulations in Times of Armed Conflict ¶ 2 (2006), *available at* http://www.wma.net/e/policy/a20.htm [hereinafter Regulation in Times of Armed Conflict]. These provisions were in effect in 2002 when the aggressive interrogation strategies were introduced at Guantánamo Bay. *See* Amnesty International, Ethics Codes and Declarations Relevant to the Health Professions, ACT 75/05/00, at 18 (4th ed., 2000). Following the revelations of physician participation in interrogation in the war on terror, two more instances of unethical behavior were added to the list in May 2006. The regulations now state that it is also unethical for a physician to "[e]mploy personal health information to facilitate interrogation[,]" or to "[c]ondone, facilitate or participate in the practice of torture or any form of cruel, inhuman or degrading treatment." Regulation in Times of Armed Conflict, *supra*, at ¶2(d) and (e). The latter, in particular, should already have been obvious.

[95] *See* Bloche & Marks, *Doing Unto Others as They Did Unto Us*, *supra* note 16 (discussing the source of the aggressive interrogation strategies deployed at Guantánamo Bay).

[96] *See* Jonathan H. Marks, *The Silence of the Doctors*, The Nation, Dec. 26, 2005, *available at* www.thenation.com/docprem.mhtml?i = 20051226&5 = marks (critiquing the AMA's failure to speak out sooner).

as healer."[97] However, physicians are permitted to participate in "developing effective interrogation strategies for general training purposes," provided those strategies are humane and respectful of individuals' rights, and do not "threaten or cause physical injury or mental suffering."[98] The American Psychiatric Association adopted a similar position in May 2006, prohibiting psychiatrists from "direct participation" in interrogation, defined to include "being present in the interrogation room, asking or suggesting questions, or advising authorities on the use of specific techniques of interrogation with particular detainees."[99] The psychiatrists' association also permits its members to provide training to interrogators on "recognizing and responding to persons with mental illnesses, on the possible medical and psychological effects of particular techniques and conditions of interrogation, and on other areas within their professional expertise."[100]

Although the guidelines of both the AMA and the American Psychiatric Association therefore leave open the possibility of giving general advice and training to military and civilian personnel in either law enforcement or intelligence branches, they make clear that physicians should stay out of the interrogation room—and, for that matter, any adjoining observation room—and that they should not give advice on specific interrogation techniques for specific detainees. By contrast, the August 2006 resolution of the American Psychological Association cleared the way for continued participation of psychologists in individual interrogations at Guantánamo Bay.

That resolution admittedly improves on the organization's 2005 task force report by providing that "psychologists shall work in accordance with international

---

[97] Am. Med. Ass'n, Opinion of the Council on Ethical and Judicial Affairs: Physician Participation in Interrogation (2006), *available at* http://www.ama-assn.org/ama1/pub/upload/mm/475/cejo4i06.doc. This followed the revision to the World Medical Association's Declaration of Tokyo (Guidelines for Physicians Concerning Torture and other Cruel, Inhuman or Degrading Treatment or Punishment in Relation to Detention and Imprisonment) in May 2006 to provide that "[t]he physician shall not use nor allow to be used, as far as he or she can, medical knowledge or skills, or health information specific to individuals, to facilitate or otherwise aid any interrogation, legal or illegal, of those individuals." The revised Declaration is available at http://www. wma.net/e/policy/c18.htm.

[98] Am. Med. Ass'n, *supra* note 97. In a press release, the Chair of the AMA's Council on Ethical and Judicial Affairs, Priscilla Ray, M.D., stated that because "it is justifiable for physicians to serve in roles that serve the public interest," the "AMA policy permits physicians to develop general interrogation strategies that are not coercive, but are humane and respect the rights of individuals." *See* Press Release, AMA, New AMA Ethical Policy Opposes Direct Physician Participation in Interrogation (June 12, 2006), http://www.ama-assn.org/ama/pub/category/16446.html. Neither the policy statement nor the press release addresses the question of whether physicians would ordinarily possess the expertise to advise on what interrogation techniques might generally be effective. For a discussion of potential rationales for seeking medical advice on interrogation, see Marks, *Doctors of Interrogation*, *supra* note 16.

[99] Am. Psychiatric Ass'n, Psychiatric Participation in Interrogation of Detainees: Position Statement (2006), *available at* http://www.psych.org/edu/other_res/lib_archives/archives/200601.pdf.

[100] Id.

human rights instruments relevant to their roles."[101] However, the remainder of the document simply ties the prohibitions on psychologists' conduct to the basic legal prohibitions on torture and CID treatment. Thus, psychologists must not "knowingly engage in, tolerate, direct, support, advise, or offer training" in such treatment.[102] Nor shall they "provide knowingly any research, instruments, or knowledge that facilitates" such treatment.[103] Nor shall they "knowingly participate in any procedure in which [such treatment] is used or threatened."[104] And should they be present when torture or CID treatment occurs, they should try to stop the abuse and "failing that, exit the procedure."[105] In essence, these regulations require psychologists to obey the laws that bind us all. Beyond that, psychologists have only their consciences as a guide.

The egregious abuse of detainees at Guantánamo Bay (and elsewhere) raises real concerns about the role of psychologists in military interrogations, and emphasizes the need for firmer guidance. Dr. Gerald Koocher, President of the American Psychological Association in 2006, claims that psychologists are best placed to detect and prevent "behavioral drift" on the part of interrogators—that is, the slide into unprofessional and ultimately illegal behavior.[106] But he fails to recognize that there are powerful social and institutional pressures on health professionals associated with the intelligence mission, including military psychologists, that weigh heavily against intervening—pressures that may well have been responsible for the Biscuit psychologist's failure to intervene in the aggressive interrogation of Al Qahtani.[107]

Put simply, interrogators are not the only people subject to "behavioral drift"—it may equally affect the psychologists charged with identifying and preventing it.[108]

---

[101] *Compare* Am. Psychol. Ass'n, Resolution Against Torture and Cruel, Inhuman, and Degrading Treatment or Punishment (Aug. 9, 2006), *available at* http://www.apa.org/governance/resolutions/notortureres.html [hereinafter Resolution Against Torture], *with* PRESIDENTIAL TASK FORCE, *supra* note 90 (the former incorporating human rights standards in the manner described in the text accompanying this note, the latter stating that the Task Force "did not reach consensus on ... [t]he role of human rights standards in an ethics code").

[102] Resolution Against Torture, *supra* note 101.

[103] Id.

[104] Id.

[105] Id.

[106] Gerald P. Koocher, *Varied and Valued Roles*, MONITOR ON PSYCHOL., July–Aug. 2006, at 5, *available at* http://www.apa.org/monitor/julaug06/pc.html. The same claim was made by the Director of the American Psychological Association's Ethics Office in Stephen Behnke, *Ethics and Interrogations: Comparing and Contrasting the American Psychological, American Medical and American Psychiatric Association Positions*, MONITOR ON PSYCHOL., July–Aug. 2006, at 66, *available at* http://www.apa.org/monitor/julaug06/interrogations.html.

[107] The psychologist referred to here is discussed in the text accompanying note 29 above. See also Marks, *Doctors of Interrogation, supra* note 16.

[108] Ironically, one of the members of the APA's PRESIDENTIAL TASK FORCE has argued that its report (*see* note 90, *supra*) was itself the result of behavioral drift. Telephone interview with Jean Maria Arrigo, Ph.D., Founder, Project on Ethics and Art in Testimony, in Irvine, Cal. (Dec. 1, 2006).

Furthermore, the American Psychological Association's new guidelines create the additional problem of what I call *definitional drift*. By tying the principal constraints on psychologists' conduct to the prohibition on torture and CID treatment, the American Psychological Association's summer 2006 resolution leaves psychologists vulnerable to drifting definitions, in particular the Administration's efforts to redefine those norms. This vulnerability is particularly important in light of the Administration's emerging preference for staffing Biscuits with psychologists rather than psychiatrists[109]—a preference that predates, but has been reinforced by, the new professional guidelines for physicians in general, and psychiatrists in particular.[110]

5 Conclusion

The involvement of health professionals in interrogation is hardly new. To give just one example, congressional testimony describes the role of an American physician in a form of torture known as the "water cure" in the war in the Philippines more than a hundred years ago.[111] There too, the victims of aggressive interrogation and torture were considered undeserving of the protections of the laws of war—a precedent for current exceptionalism expressly justified on grounds that enemy "insurgents" were "not civilized."[112] However, the systematic involvement of mental health professionals in US Army interrogation practice was a significant development. Writing some months before this development occurred, M. Gregg Bloche—who trained as both a lawyer and a physician—observed that the "unreflective willingness of most Western physicians to employ clinical skills for myriad state

[109] DEP'T OF DEFENSE INSTRUCTION NO. 2310.08E, MEDICAL PROGRAM SUPPORT FOR DETAINEE OPERATIONS (2006), *available at* http://www.fas.org/irp/doddir/dod/i2310_08.pdf. "[P]hysicians are not ordinarily assigned duties as [behavioral science consultants], but may be so assigned, with the approval of [the Assistant Secretary of Defense for Health Affairs], in circumstances when qualified psychologists are unable or unavailable to meet critical mission needs." Id. at E2.2. This follows the recommendation of Maj. Gen. Martinez-Lopez in April 2005 that physicians should not be assigned to Biscuits. *See* OFFICE OF THE SURGEON GENERAL, ARMY, FINAL REPORT, ASSESSMENT OF DETAINEE MEDICAL OPERATIONS FOR OEF, GTMO, AND OIF (2005), *available at* http://www.globalsecurity.org/military/library/report/2005/detmedopsrpt_13apr2005.pdf.

[110] *See* Ken Hausman, *Military Looks to Psychologists for Advice on Interrogation*, PSYCHIATR. NEWS, July 7, 2006, at 4, *available at* http://pn.psychiatryonline.org/cgi/content/full/41/13/4 (discussing a statement made by the Assistant Secretary of Defense for Health Affairs, William Winkenwerder, Jr., to the effect that the different stances adopted by the psychologists' and psychiatrists' professional associations "contributed" to the Pentagon's preference for staffing Biscuits with psychologists).

[111] S. COMM. REC. ON THE PHILIPPINES, at 1527–1532 (1899–1921) (testimony of Charles S. Riley), *reprinted in* HENRY F. GRAFF, AMERICAN IMPERIALISM AND THE PHILIPPINE INSURRECTION (1969) 72–80 and *discussed in* Marks, *The Silence of the Doctors*, *supra* note 96, at 26.

[112] S. COMM. REC. ON THE PHILIPPINES, at 558–564 (1899–1921) (testimony of Gen. Hughes) *reprinted in* HENRY F. GRAFF, *supra* note 99, 64–72; *see also* Marks, *What Counts*, *supra* note 40, at 579.

purposes suggests that their ethical sensitivity to the problem of extraclinical consequences does not greatly exceed that of their colleagues in countries where gross human rights abuse is endemic."[113] Bearing this in mind, he emphasized the need for the training of health professionals in both ethics and international human rights norms, for institutional mechanisms to nurture professional autonomy, and for international support from (among others) professional bodies.[114]

The importance of these recommendations is highlighted not only by revelations of health professionals' complicity in detainee abuse, but also by recent statements of an experienced US interrogator in the war on terror. He notes that, in addition to the predictable pressure to support the military objectives of their colleagues, some health professionals may have financial anxieties too. In the interrogator's words:

> Most of the PAs [physician assistants] or doctors that we use have been through medical school due to military scholarships. They owe the military big bucks. If they refused to aid us then they might be brought up on charges in an internal trial and would be forced to repay the military.[115]

I do not intend to suggest that military health professionals are venal. On the contrary, the vast majority pursue careers in the military—despite the call of more lucrative private practice—for noble and altruistic reasons. However, it would be foolish to pretend either that those financial pressures do not exist or that they cannot have an impact—even subconsciously—on an individual's moral calculus. Furthermore, if social and financial pressures are not sufficient to bring on board health professionals despite their ethical qualms, interrogators may use other means to procure their cooperation and compliance with the interrogation mission.

We already know that military personnel at Guantánamo Bay were manipulated. They were told that the detainees were "the worst of the worst."[116] According to Department of Defense documents, the vast majority had been handed over to US forces by Pakistan or the Northern Alliance in exchange for large bounties—and most of them were not alleged to have committed any hostile acts against either the United States or its allies.[117] Health professionals, in particular, are not in a position to verify

---

[113] M. Gregg Bloche, *Caretakers and Collaborators*, 10 CAMBRIDGE Q. HEALTHCARE ETHICS 275, 278 (2001). In a prescient note of caution, Bloche added that, if Western physicians lack the appropriate ethical sensitivity, "their ability to avert complicity when state purposes turn troublesome or worse would not likewise differ greatly from that of their peers in more problematic settings." Id.

[114] Id. at 283.

[115] The Arrigo Papers, *supra* note 14.

[116] ERIK SAAR AND VIVECA NOVAK, INSIDE THE WIRE: A MILITARY INTELLIGENCE SOLDIER'S EYEWITNESS ACCOUNT OM F LIFE AT GUANTANAMO 193 (2005).

[117] MARK DENBEAUX ET AL., REPORT ON GUANTANAMO DETAINEES: A PROFILE OF 517 DETAINEES THROUGH ANALYSIS OF DEPARTMENT OF DEFENSE DATA 2–3 (2006), *available at* http://law.shu.edu/news/guantanamo_report_final_2_08_06.pdf. In addition, among the detainees were both children and the senescent. *See* Oliver Burkeman, *Children Held at Guantanamo*, GUARDIAN, Apr. 24, 2003, *available at* http://www.guardian.co.uk/afghanistan/story/0,1284,942347,00.html; Times Wire Reports, *Oldest Guantanamo Detainee Returns Home*, L.A. TIMES, Aug. 29, 2006, A8 (reporting that Haji Nasrat Khan, an Afghan detainee, who was "at least 71" and uses a walker, has been sent home).

the provenance of a detainee. Nor do they have the knowledge or expertise to assess the security threat posed by a particular detainee.[118] So health professionals are in a position of ignorance and uncertainty that may be exploited. The interrogator quoted above has also indicated that intelligence personnel may lie to health professionals:

> If the people are worried about doctors and psychologists aiding their own military in time of war, we can just have those who do work with us say we are not harming anyone. If they worry about our methods then we say that all plans of interrogation have approved the tactics as non 'stressful'. *As you can lie to a terrorist to get information then you can lie to any group that interferes with the job of making the people safe.*[119]

The interrogator also noted that if the use of doctors or physician assistants becomes problematic (or "too much," in his words), interrogators "would then make use of our ParaRescue or Combat Medics for medical expertise in interrogations."[120] This is important since much of the discussion to date has been about the role of psychiatrists and psychologists in interrogation. Now that the AMA and the American Psychiatric Association have issued guidelines that seek to keep doctors out of the interrogation room—and empower them both legally and practically to refuse to participate[121]—the spotlight has focused on psychologists.[122] But we would do well to remember that other types of health professionals may also be implicated.

The recent proliferation of Department of Defense manuals and directives—most notably, the new Army interrogation manual prohibiting the use of "waterboarding," hooding, and military dogs in interrogation[123]—is presumably intended to suggest that the Administration is trying to redress the errors of the past. But it is not clear how these policy documents will play out on the ground. Arguably, they may be of little relevance at the present time since detainees who have been held for years at Guantánamo Bay can no longer have actionable intelligence (even if they once did so), and there would be little point in interrogating them. However, fundamental questions remain about detainees held by the CIA, whatever their location. The CIA is contesting the ACLU's FOIA applications, so its practices are still shrouded in secrecy, and detainees in its custody will not benefit from the provisions of the new Army field manual.[124] Furthermore, in a recent radio interview, Vice President

---

[118] *See* London, *supra* note 89, at 386.

[119] The Arrigo Papers, *supra* note 14 (emphasis added).

[120] Id.

[121] International humanitarian law prohibits states from requiring medical professionals to act contrary to their codes of ethics. *See* Bloche & Marks, *Doctors and Interrogators at Guantanamo Bay*, *supra* note 16; Marks, *What Counts*, *supra* note 40 at 582.

[122] *See, e.g.*, Michael Benjamin, *Psychological Warfare*, SALON.COM, July 26, 2006, http://www.salon.com/news/feature/2006/07/26/ interrogation/index.html; Mark Benjamin, *Psychologists' Group Still Rocked by Torture Debate*, SALON.COM, Aug. 4, 2006, http://www.salon.com/news/feature/2006/08/04/apa/.

[123] *See* FM 2-22.3 (FM 34-52), HUMAN INTELLIGENCE COLLECTOR OPERATIONS ¶ 5–75 (2006), *available at* http://www.fas.org/irp/doddir/army/fm2-22-3.pdf.

[124] Although current CIA interrogation guidelines are classified, previous CIA manuals have been made public. *See, e.g.*, KUBARK COUNTERINTELLIGENCE INTERROGATION (1963), *available at* http://www.gwu.edu/~nsarchiv/NSAEBB/NSAEBB27/01-01.htm.

Cheney was asked: "Would you agree a dunk in water is a no-brainer if it can save lives?"[125] Mr. Cheney replied: "It's a no-brainer for me."[126] In the same interview, he agreed that the debate over interrogation techniques was "a little silly."[127] These comments reveal a failure at the highest levels of government to internalize the most fundamental norms of human rights law and the laws of war. In such an environment, health professionals should still be considered "at risk"—that is, in danger of becoming accomplices to the perpetration of war crimes in the counterterrorism mission. Looking forward, one of the most important questions is:

How will *they* respond?

---

[125] *See* Demetri Sevastopulo, *Cheney Endorses Simulated Drowning: Says Use of Water Boarding to Get Terrorist Intelligence is "no brainer"*, FIN. TIMES (London), Oct. 26, 2006, *available at* http://www.msnbc.msn.com/id/15433467/; *see also* Dan Eggen, *Cheney Defends "Dunk in the Water" Remark Addressing Alarm Over the Comment, Vice President Says He Was Not Referring to Waterboarding*, WASH. POST, Oct. 28, 2006, at A02, *available at* http://www.washingtonpost.com/wp-dyn/content/article/2006/10/27/AR2006102700560.html.

[126] *See* Sevastopulo, *supra* note 125.

[127] Id.

Toward a Framework for Military Health Ethics[1]

Gervase Pearce and Peter Saul[2]

As muscle work declines, large numbers of unskilled laborers are increasingly replaced by smaller numbers of highly trained workers and intelligent machines.… This process, too, is perfectly parallel in the military, where smart weapons require smart soldiers.… The idea that the Gulf War was a 'high-tech' war in which the human element in combat was eliminated is a fantasy. The fact is that the forces sent by the allies to the Gulf were the best educated and technically expert army ever sent into battle.… The new military needs soldiers who use their brains, can deal with a diversity of people and cultures, who can tolerate ambiguity, take initiative, and ask questions, even to the point of questioning authority.… The willingness to ask and think may be more prevalent in the US armed forces than in many businesses.… As in the civilian economy, fewer people with intelligent technology can accomplish more than a lot of people with the brute-force tools of the past. (Toffler and Toffler 1993, 73–77)

Even when those called professionals are something more than average people, few can be immune to the constraints surrounding the work they do. It is the institutional ethics of professionalism. If the institutions surrounding them fail in support, only the most heroic individuals can actively concern themselves with the ethical issues raised by their work. Professionalism requires attention to the ethical status of those institutions. (Friedson 2001, 12)

[1] This paper was originally prepared for a workshop hosted by the Centre for Military and Veterans' Health (CMVH) of the University of Queensland (Australia). The original title, which has been shorted for this volume, was "Towards a Framework for Military Health Ethics: An Issues Paper Examining Possible Health Related Ethical Issues Arising from Military Operations." Used with permission.

[2] The authors acknowledge the assistance of Suzanne Ross in the preparation of this paper.

F. Allhoff (ed.), *Physicians at War: The Dual-Loyalties Challenge.*

1 Introduction

This paper offers a brief examination of ethical health issues arising from military operations and outlines which, if any, of these ethical health issues apply to current Australian Defence Force (ADF) military operations. The transparency of military operations provided through real time global media reporting and the Internet, has raised public awareness of incidents that can be viewed broadly as ethical issues or dilemmas. While many of these issues are not new, it is the changing context of post cold war military operations and scale and demand of humanitarian operations that places new requirements on how the ADF best addresses these potential issues before they become critical incidents.

In identifying potential ethical issues arising from military health operations, it is recognized that military health personnel operate within a command and control organizational structure and associated culture. It is also recognized that the complexity of the issues and the environment within which military health personnel are expected to operate will raise ethical health issues not likely to be encountered to the same degree by those health practitioners operating in the average suburban practice or hospital, except when health personnel are confronted with large scale emergencies, such as those encountered with recent terrorist attacks and massacres. Some of the potential causes of these issues will arise from:

1. Role complexity (resulting in conflict within a role). This can be further distinguished as
   (a) Self conflict as a holder of a role (where there is internal conflict between expectations of knowledge or performance with what others expect of a person in that role. Perhaps best expressed by Laing (1970) "There is something that I don't know that I am supposed to know. I don't know what it is I don't know, and yet am supposed to know, and I feel I look stupid if I seem not to know it and not know what it is I don't know.")
   (b) Conflict resulting from feedback from different stakeholders (where different stakeholder have conflicting expectations "Stakeholder A praises my work, but Stakeholder B is never happy, I don't know whether what I am doing is a good enough job in meeting expectations of Stakeholder B")
2. Inter-role conflict (i.e., conflict resulting from holding more than one role)
3. Role ambiguity (i.e., uncertainty about the requirements of a role)
4. Inadequate resources, information or time for decision-making
5. Human frailties (e.g., limited energy and courage; self-interest)

This paper is divided into three major sections:

1. A brief outline of a broad framework for the context for identifying potential ethical health issues or dilemmas within the culture of a military command and control organization.
2. An overview of the role of health professionals in the military and reported ethical issues arising from this role.

3. Exploration of potential ethical issues arising from the two broad types of military operations the ADF currently sees itself in. These are:
   (a) Limited war or peacekeeping operations, where health units operate in support of the primary armed combatants. The objectives of these types of operations are set either at the national or international political level and are largely bounded by the concepts of just war and established rules of engagement determined as part of agreed international codes of operations.
   (b) Primarily humanitarian operations where the health units are the major sponsor and armed combatants act in support of the health units and in all probability major non-government organizations (NGOs) operating alongside the military health units.

Ethical issues range from strategic decisions on the size and resource support for ADF health to daily challenges such as matters of confidentiality of personal data. An ethical framework is proposed, which includes values and moral principles, to assist in identifying potential ethical issues before they reach crisis point and aid decision making within the broad range of ethical issues that are likely to be encountered. It is hoped that the ADF will consider using this to address issues currently being raised by its health practitioners.

The context of ADF's operational engagement has changed significantly over the past 20 years as they are now engaged in operations such as limited war, state endorsed peace keeping, peace making and peace building operations and operations other than war (such as humanitarian). These new operational contexts and times raises a range of operational military health issues that have and will impact on military health and operational personnel's decision making. These issues will test the ethical decision making frameworks used by personnel dealing with these issues. The scope of this paper is to identify the key military health issues that may lead to potential ethical issues and develop an ethical decision making framework that best reflects the values and principles of the ADF. In doing so, it is anticipated that this paper and its associated process will build a readiness to adapt future practice to better manage ethical health issues when they arise.

2 Interpreting Ethical Issues Within the Military

As indicated by Toffler and Toffler (1993) the changing nature of military operations requires people to be increasingly flexible and work within an environment where junior personnel are making discretionary actions or decisions. Personnel within the ADF are guided by sets of complex rules, regulations and codes of conduct that in essence depict what is acceptable behavior, which this paper will label as "ethically acceptable behavior". In short, ethically acceptable behavior is about compliance within the rules, regulations and codes of conduct. A significant dilemma arises when an individual is acting in what they perceive as an acceptable behavior, may constitute to be non-acceptable behavior to other stakeholders.

This is perhaps amplified by Toffler's comment on soldiers tolerating ambiguity, taking the initiative, and asking questions, even to the point of questioning authority. This presents the paradox of compliance while being able to question.

As noted by Freidson (2001) professional institutions such as the ADF has a major role to play in determining how ethics within the institution is viewed and lived. In order to understand the real and potential health issues that may translate into ethical health issues, it is necessary to briefly explore the notion of ethics as applied within the ADF.

Military health professionals (including doctors, nurses, psychologists, psychiatrists and dentists) join the ADF either full time or as reservists as a qualified health professional. As part of their education and training they are required to know and work within their professional code of conduct. Their training and education classically identifies potential ethical issues and provides ethical guidelines. Other ADF heath personnel (for example, medics, paramedics dental assistants and medical administrators) receive their training as a uniformed person. Health ethics training is provided as an element of their military training.

On a broader scale, a subject of ethics has recently been introduced into the Australian Defence Academy and the Australian Defence College addresses ethics. Whether or not ADF non-health officers and non-commissioned officers receive similar education and training in ethics is not clear. Current training relating to other ethical issues such as fraud, Equal Opportunity and whistle blowing appear to be in response to either legislation or significant events that have highlighted a shortcoming in practices.

Both military and health professionals have a well defined set of principles to guide their decision making when confronted by dilemmas. For example, the health profession are bound by principles of providing care, or doing no harm, or acting for the best interests of the patient (Beaty 1997; Smith 2005a). The military's principles are based on a moral obligation to be competent, loyalty to their fellow professional, and working for the good of humanity (Davenport 1987; Brunk et al. 1990). How these two sets of principles interface is not obvious. Furthermore, the ADF has a moral obligation to provide a system of not only rules, regulations and codes of conduct, but a system of training and education to guide personnel as to what is acceptable behavior.

Ethically acceptable behavior at the individual level is bundled into what is described as a person's duty. Dependent on the rank and type of duty, the rules, regulations and codes of conduct will range from the simple (the most junior rank), to the complex (senior commander).

This is similar to the work on values by major researchers in the area. Feather (1994, 32) notes that values: ae concepts or beliefs; pertain to desirable end states or desirable behaviors; transcend specific situation; guide selection or evaluation of behavior and events; and are ordered by relative importance. Feather (1994) amongst others notes that values and interpretations of good/bad and right/wrong will vary across different cultures.

Rokeach (1968, 1973, 1979) notes that values guide our actions when confronted by social or political problems. This guidance is based on our beliefs that influence or guide our evaluations of ourselves, others and the context of the problem so that we are able to rationalize our response or behavior as being acceptable in the circumstances.

3 Health Professionals in the Military Context

The ADF Defence Health Services provides health support to the Australian Defence Force. The Defence Health Services Division (DHSD) function is stated as:

> Defence Health Services provides health care and, from the health perspective, ensures the preparedness of ADF personnel for operations, as well as preparing deployable elements of Defence Health Services for deployment in support of operations. To effect this Defence Health Services Division develops strategic health policy, provides strategic level health advice and exercises technical and financial control of ADF health units. The Joint Health Support Agency coordinates the provision of high quality health support within the National Support Area. Health staff within Joint Operations Command (JOC) and the environmental commands is responsible for health aspects of deployable capability (DHSD 2007).

Anecdotal evidence suggests that the number of professional qualified full time serving health officers has declined over the past 20 years. Partly this is due to the strategic decision to rely increasingly on reserve officers to provide professional health services, as deployed medical officers (in particular as specialists); and civilian practitioners to provide services as either locums or contractors to the ADF. As well, in some humanitarian operations ADF health personnel may be joined by health professionals from NGOs or even by volunteers. The shortage of health professionals in the Australian community is also likely to have an impact on overall health workforce numbers.

It is important to note that military health practices in time of war presents unique situations not normally confronted by those in general private practice. Smith (1992, 2005a) is a leading US Navy Surgeon Captain and staff member of the Uniformed Services University of the Health Sciences who is a leading advocate of the differences arising from military medicine. His position is supported by Beam (2003a, b). It follows that health personnel working in a military environment require specific preparation to deal with the issues that arise specifically in the military context. A clear challenge confronting ADF Health Services is that a military health care system is a critical element of the ADF, but maintaining personnel levels will be increasingly challenging and in this light, the ADF will increasingly be dependent on the Australian general health care system for the provision of trained professional medical staff and gap resources and services to meet specific contingency needs. Such personnel will be even less likely than career officers and reservists to be aware of and prepared for the specific ethical issues that are posed in the military environment.

Toffler talks of smart soldiers, and Beaty (1997) talks of the need for "brilliant medics". The smart and brilliant people need to work together to understand each other's abilities and needs. As identified by commentators such as Beaty (1997),

Smith (2005b) and Klein and Kasper (2000), military health demands will continue to change, so the training and development of health personnel must also continue to change to meet these expected demands. Australia prides itself on its health practice standards. A question for the near future may be whether the ADF will be willing to use military health personnel and/or services from nations that do not have the same standards of practice.

One strong element of ADF military health practice is the working relationships and understanding developed between health and operational personnel when they work and train together. This does differ across the three services, and also differs when operating in a joint force situation. Understanding the different relationships with the different stakeholders is important in determining when and where potential ethical issues may arise.

Military health stakeholders can be broadly grouped as: patients, the general military personnel that health personnel provide a service to; the military unit commanders to whom they are accountable and responsible to within their chain of command; the wider defense force; and the societies the ADF is serving.

The stakeholders, whether acting individually or as representatives of a stakeholder group, might seek to provide guidance to act in what they see as the best interests of the different stakeholders. Despite such good intentions, the potential clashes of principles and values give rise to situations where defense health personnel will be challenged to make decisions or take actions that may fall outside of the accepted boundaries of ethical or moral behavior. Consultations conducted to date have revealed that some who legitimately see themselves speaking on behalf of particular stakeholder groups do not recognize even the potential for such conflict.

4 Exploring Ethical Health Issues

There is a wide body of literature identifying and discussing various military ethical health issues. Most of these relate to war or battlefield situations, with the majority relating to a land or army environment. The literature is largely from US, Canadian and, to a lesser degree, European commentators or authors. We suggest that health ethics issues for the ADF are similar.

Snider et al. (1999) examine the officer corps' "ethical muddle over the role of self-sacrifice in the profession's ethos" (p. 2) as part of their analysis of the professionalism, military ethic and officership within the US Army. They also suggest that this has equal relevance to other services. They note that the changing nature of operations and ambiguity of directions, regarding mission and casualties suggests that military officers are not only morally required to take risks necessary to accomplish a designated mission or task, they are morally required to take additional risks such as minimizing casualties and damage. Based on incidents ranging from World War II to Bosnia, they argue that as military officers' duty changes from war to operations other than war, the fundamental principles of duty and moral guidance appropriate for war may not be so for other kinds of operations. The diverse range of operations now confronting armed services raises clashes of incompatible moral directions or messages for behavior from the ethos or morals of the state (represented by the political leadership and community) to the institution (represented by each Service) to the individual officer. It is the operational command–health interface in different operational contexts that will determine the moral and ethically challenging issues that will jointly confront both command and health personnel.

Beam (2003a), Howe (2003), Smith (2005b) and Salisbury and English (2003) all raise a range of issues, and all at some point note the changing nature of conflicts, operations and health treatment. Suffice to note, that military health today and increasingly in the future will rely on Beaty's (1997) brilliant medic or Toffler's smart soldier. Positioning of strategic medical assets (mobile hospitals) to treat injured personnel either to return to duty or be repatriated home will be an increasing challenge. Outside the scope of this paper, is the assumption that the civilian health care system will be able to cope with repatriated military personnel in addition to its normal workload. One-off tragedies such as the 2004 tsunami, 2003 Bali bombing and 11 September 2001 attacks demonstrated that these stretched the respective counties health care resources. Any strategic or policy decision for the ADF military health system to increase its reliance on any civil health system is likely to generate increasing health ethics issues especially if the ADF finds itself in situations where the demand for use of these resources increased above its current level.

Klein and Kasper (2000) raised issues relating to health care standards that include differences in the concepts of health care, in language and legal interpretation. Smith (1995, 2005b) raised the issues of communication between hospitals and different units. This often leads to the use of non-secure or commercial radio channels and in plain language, thus limiting disclosure of information in ways that can impact on patient care and unit security; communication might not be possible because of equipment differences, such as different radio bandwidths or operating frequencies. Differences in equipment used in providing health care can create challenges. In one case, the US Army was using different (older) anesthesia techniques from those used in civil hospitals, which impacted on reserve or civil doctors being able to use the Army equipment and so effectively be able to carry out their duties.

In the main, ethical issues are more likely to arise on the ground where immediate health care is being delivered. Sidel and Levy (2003) noted five ethical dilemmas: subordinating the best interests of the patient; overriding patients' wishes; failing to provide care; blurring combatant and non-combatant roles; and preventing physicians from acting as moral agents within the military. Beam (2003a) in his chapter on the battlefield in Military Medical Ethics mentions: return to duty considerations; triage; euthanasia; and participation in interrogation of prisoners of war.

Sara Fry, a major author and researcher on ethics within nursing in humanitarian and civilian practice has identified issues arising from a conflict of values between the organization and the nursing code of ethics and between the individual nurse and the organization. Examples of the ethical issues arising from some of her research (undated) include: protecting patients' rights and human dignity; respecting/not respecting informed consent to treatment; providing care with possible risk to the nurse's health; using/not using physical or chemical restraints; staffing patterns that limit patient access to nursing care; prolonging the living/dying process with inappropriate measures; not considering the quality of a patient's life; implementing managed care policies that threaten quality of care; and working with unethical/impaired colleagues.

As a guide to the management or handling of these issues is her findings that over 30% of the nurses surveyed reported that they encountered ethical issues in their practice from one to four times per week to daily. In handling their most recently experienced ethical issue; more than 83% reported that they discussed the issue with nursing peers while over 66% discussed the issue with nursing leadership. Over 5% of the nurses reported that they did not deal with the ethical issue at all.

In her other research examining nursing ethics in humanitarian operations she noted ethical issues of: balancing the resource needs of soldiers against those of the humanitarian mission; conflicts in nurse/physician or other professional relationship; participating/not participating in euthanasia/assisted suicide; prolonging the living/dying process for the sake of training; and acting against personal and or religious views.

5 Resource Allocation

This is a strategic issue about the actual positioning and allocation of health resources including personnel during all of these operations. The results of these decisions will have direct impacts on health decisions in the field. The following are the issues of concern in relations to health resource allocation and the ethical issues arising from these are:

- Integration of health resources at an operational level, in particular when health personnel have not trained or been part of the preparations. This can lead to a lower level of teamwork and trust built up during operational readiness exercises. It also means the health personnel may not be fully informed about the health standing of the unit's personnel. In situations where the operational unit is being deployed operationally ready, this may place additional pressures between the command and health personnel leading to a range of other issues such as knowledge of whether health personal will carry a weapon for self-defense.
- Approved health and fitness standards of individuals and their capability to perform roles.
- Physical location and allocation of medical resources. Where are core health facilities located in relation to a units operating area, what level of access do injured personnel have to these facilities and what level of resource allocation is given to each of these facilities. This may potentially impact on the command-health decision of where to send personnel and the associated costs of movement.
- The experience and skill of allocated health personnel to perform a specific task do not meet or match the needs.

- When using outsourced health professionals either domestically or internationally, does the command have the same level of communication with these personnel and do these personnel have the same understanding of military levels of fitness.
- In cases where generally qualified health professionals act in specialist roles for which they are not fully qualified, the command may not be aware of this which may impact on decisions, or if the command is aware of this, they will be making decision on limited information.
- Use of paramedic trained personnel in place of doctors and nurses and the level of ethical awareness given to these personnel.

6 Interoperability

The primary issues relating to interoperability relate to the differences in values and the potential problems relating to pre-deployment training and rotation training. An aspect of this will relate to operations with personnel from non-English speaking countries and those from poorer resourced nations who will have different standards of health care and pay structures for their personnel. At the other extreme include operations with the US, whose health resources and budgets exceed that of the ADF.

In addition to cross-cultural issues, potential issues include:

- Mission creep—the changing nature of the objectives and needed resources change without notification to all units in particular health units. Command and health personnel may have different objectives resulting from mission creep.
- Conflicts in professional relationship arising from different standards of care.
- Differing attitudes to participating/not participating in euthanasia/assisted suicide.
- Prolonging the living/dying process to provide training or experience.
- Proceeding with levels of intervention beyond that normally used to either gain experience or train personnel.
- Coalition differences especially dealing with the end of life decisions and issues of litigation.
- Engagement in other practices and behaviors, often related to economic outcomes, that are deemed unethical within Australian practices and behaviors, but are deemed acceptable practices and behaviors by another states personnel.

7 Triage

This is an operational level issue and one that will potentially arise daily, but can be managed with appropriate policy and leadership. The nursing and medical codes of conduct present clear guidance on triage, based on degree of injury. However, in environments such as Iraq, Rwanda and Afghanistan the triage policy differentiates by patient ethnicity not degree of injury.

Differences in triage may arise from command directives and/or control of scarce medical resources available to on the ground health personnel. Further compounding this issue is the real time delays in communication and information flows between the on the ground health personnel and the command. This may relate to earlier issues such as the location of primary health care facilities and the availability of transportation of patients.

Potential issues include:

- Priority in treatment of injured personnel based on whether they are military (ADF, coalition and enemy), civilian attached to military forces (e.g., diplomatic, interpreters, media) or other civilians
- Level of treatment or care provided in each case (i.e., use of resources especially in cases where physical resources such as drugs for pain are scarce)
- Level of treatment to be given where hygiene or sterile conditions cannot be guaranteed and the level of infectious disease (e.g., HIV/AIDS is known to be high)
- Providing different levels of care to different patients, which may involve life/death decisions, e.g., providing extended care for a near death person which limits the care provided to other patients whose condition may deteriorate or take longer to recover as a result

8 Confidentiality

Patient confidentiality is a well recognized tenet of our health system. Confidentiality within the Australian health and defense system is covered by a number of Acts and policies such as the Privacy Act, Mental Health Act and Defence instructions. The involvement of different parties with differences in power and in how that power is used, and differences in which legislation the groups are aware of and give priority to can generate ethical conflicts. This may become particularly difficult where the attached health person is of a significantly lower rank than the commander but is legally or ethically required to implement legislated obligations that might not apply to the commander, or might not be given priority by the commander.

Potential issues include:

- Disclosure of the results of drug testing or other indications of substance or alcohol abuse.
- Access to personnel health records or documentation, especially where the health person is either a non-commissioned officer or other rank.
- Dispute between the health professional and command in terms of treatment or care.
- Accurate and complete recoding of events of incidents that may be critical for future use, either for a medical claim or legal proceedings.
- Challenges associated when the actual command is ill or not medically or psychologically fit to continue. While not common, the cited case was that of HMAS Voyager.

9 Other

This is a broad category of potential issues that do not readily fit under the other headings.

Potential issues include:

- Lack of ethical awareness and training of health personnel who are not members of professional bodies, e.g., paramedics, other ranks and non-commissioned officers.
- Lack of preparation of health personnel in dealing with death and life/death situations, especially injuries sustained from violent situations. This may limit personnel effectiveness to operate in these circumstances, in particular if this detracts from health personnel's decision making or advice giving to the command.
- Lack of understanding or knowledge of ADF requirements by contracted health providers may require more of the command's attention in managing health related issues. Military health personnel have completed formal military training and are aware of ADF procedures and standards.
- Determining the level of engagement of the local community at body identification in the cases of badly decomposed bodies from mass graves. Decisions relating to at what stage of body decomposition do health personnel stop seeking or allowing possible family members actual identification of a corpse.
- Need for re-burial of or hygiene with bodies from mass graves, which is in conflict with local religious or cultural practices.
- Command–health processes with the identification of post deployment stress or psychological distress arising from operations. The posting of personnel on return from deployment and a culture of not reporting possible post deployment stress conditions may heighten this. Failure to address this may impact on the operational fitness of affected personnel.
- Fitness to deploy decisions, especially in light of current overseas ADF activities and personnel numbers.
- Greater awareness by the average military person of their rights and possible claims against the ADF, especially as a veteran which may allow some less principled personnel to take advantage of such a system. In these cases the health–command relationship needs to make decisions on a person where the actual information may be biased or the person concerned is playing the health-command system against each other.
- Decisions relating to conducting autopsy in the field under the less than ideal conditions (e.g., on site such as a crash site or bomb site or in third world facilities)
- Decisions and problems associated with retaining body parts for further analysis for say an investigation or evidence.

10 Humanitarian Operations (Medical Led) Potential Ethical Issues

Humanitarian operations are a diverse range of operations from the catastrophic regional tsunami, to individual localized events such as cyclones to provision of aid in response to either a UN or regional request. It can also cover the transfer of operations from peacekeeping to nation building such as those currently underway in the Solomon Islands.

A significant element of these operations, is that the armed forces are there to support and protect not just ADF health personnel, but other aid agencies or NGOs who will respond to these types of disasters.

It is clear that the major ethical challenges will arise from the different values of NGOs and the ADF. This will require new thinking in terms of interoperability between the ADF and major health related NGOs

Potential issues include:

- Operating alongside NGOs in particular when assisting with aid has raised issues of confusing the roles of military personnel with NGO personnel which has placed strains on relationships and sharing of information. It can also have greater impact if ADF personnel rely on NGO health support, as NGOs charter is to support those in need, not those providing the support.
- Differences in the level of care provided as part of humanitarian aid and that required for military operational levels of care.
- Determining the level of engagement of the local community at body identification in the cases of badly decomposed bodies. Decisions relating to at what stage of body decomposition do health personnel stop seeking or allowing possible family members actual identification of a corpse and associated training to prepare health personnel for such a task.
- Command–health processes with the identification of post deployment stress or psychological distress arising from humanitarian operations. The posting of personnel on return from deployment and a culture of not reporting possible post deployment stress conditions may heighten this. Failure to address this may impact on the operational fitness of affected personnel.

11 Towards a Framework of Military Health Ethics

Examination of the literature on military health ethics highlights that there are three fundamental systems with associated principles and values:

- The individual's system, including the individual's principles and values and the beliefs they bring with them to the ADF or any given situation
- The professional system, including the principles, values and beliefs endorsed by each professional body or entity represented through the education and

training o individual professionals (e.g., medical, nursing, psychologist, dentist, seaman, logistician, cavalry, infantryman, aviator, etc.)
- The ADF system, with its own principles, values and beliefs (which can vary with the particular service involved and even between units with a service)

To a lesser extent other systems involved include: the broader Australian community and the values espoused as being Australian; the values of dominant multinational force partners; and the values of the community where operations are taking place.

The ethical issues noted above primarily arise from a clash of principles or values; or conflicts between two of the fundamental systems noted above. In rare cases this may arise from a clash of all three systems. Therefore, any framework needs to identify these primary systems and highlight to all parties where these systems will come into potential conflict.

It is hypothesized that currently that the principles and values of command and military health professionals have been developed separately and do not combine to create a set of shared health values and ethics across the organization.

References

Beam, Thomas. 2003a. Medical Ethics on the Battlefield: The Crucible of Military Medical Ethics, In *Military Medical Ethics*, vol. 2, ed. Thomas Beam, 367–402. Washington, DC: Borden Institute.

Beam, Thomas, ed. 2003b. *Military Medical Ethics*, vols. 1 and 2. Washington, DC: Borden Institute.

Beaty, Scott. 1997. The Revolution in Military Medical Affairs. *Parameters* 27.4 (Winter 1997/1998): 60–72.

Brunk, Gregory, Donald Secrest, and Howard Tamashiro. 1990. Military Views of Morality and War: An Empirical Study of the Attitudes of Retired American Officers. *International Studies Quarterly* 34.1: 83–109.

Cook, Martin L. 2002. The Proper Role of Professional Military Advice in Contemporary Uses of Force. *Parameters* 32.4: 21–33.

Davenport, Manuel M. (1987). "*Professional or Hired GUNNS* Loyalties are the Difference," In M. Walkin et al. (eds.), *Military Ethics*. Washington, DC: National Defense University.

Defence Health Services Division (DHSD). 2007. *About Defence Health Services Division*. 8 February. http://www.defence.gov.au/DPE/dhs/about/about_dhsd.htm. Cited 1 June 2007.

Feather, Norman T. 1994. Values and National Identification: Australian Evidence. *Australian Journal of Psychology* 46.1: 35–40.

Freidson, Eliot. 2001. *Professionalism: The Third Logic*. Chicago, IL: University of Chicago Press.

Fry, Sara T. and Johnstone Megan-Jane. 2002. *Ethics in Nursing Practice: A Guide to Ethical Decision Making*, 2nd ed. Oxford: Blackwell.

Fry, Sara T., Henry R. Luce, and Joan M. Riley. Undated. *Ethical Issues in Clinical Practice: A Multi-State Study of Practicing Registered Nurses*. http://jmrileyrn.tripod.com/nen/research.html#anchor195458. Cited 1April 2006.

Gross, Michael L. 2004. Bioethics and Armed Conflict: Mapping thee Moral Dimensions of Medicine and War. *Hastings Center Report* 34.6: 22–30.

Howe, Edmund. 2003. Dilemmas in Military Medical Ethics Since 9/11. *Kennedy Institute of Ethics Journal* 13.2: 175–188.

Klein, Leo and Martin Kasper. 2000. The Medical Mission in NATO Operations. *NATO's Nations and Partners for Peace* 1: 102–104.
Laing, Ronald David. 1970. *Knots*. New York: Pantheon Books.
Miles, Steven H. 2004. Abu Ghraid: Its Legacy for Military Medicine. *Lancet* 364: 725–729.
Rokeach, Milton. 1968. *Beliefs, Attitudes, and Values: A Theory of Organization and Change*. San Francisco, CA: Jossey-Bass.
Rokeach, Milton. 1973. *The Nature of Human Values*. New York: Free Press.
Rokeach, Milton, ed. 1979. *Understanding Human Values: Individual and Societal*. New York: Free Press.
Salisbury, David and Allan English. 2003. Prognosis 2020: A Military Medical Strategy for the Canadian Forces. *Canadian Military Journal* (Summer): 45–54.
Sekerka, Leslie E. 2005. Battling Moral Mediocrity in the Military: An Integrated Proactive Approach to Ethics Management. *Ethics and Integrity of Governance: A Transatlantic Dialogue*. http://soc.kuleuven.be/io/ethics/program/workshops/workshop3.htm. Cited 1 April 2006.
Sidel, Victor W. and Barry Levy. 2003. Physician-Soldier: A Moral Dilemma? In *Military Medical Ethics*, vol. 1, ed. Thomas Beam, 294–312. Washington, DC: Borden Institute.
Smith, Arthur M. 1992. Military Medicine: Not the Same as Practicing Medicine in the Military. *Armed Forces and Society* 18.4: 576–591.
Smith, Arthur M. 1995. Joint Medical Support: Are We Asleep at the Switch? *Joint Force Quarterly* (Summer): 1012–1109.
Smith Arthur M. 2005a. Competing Imperatives for Military Medicine at War: An Examination of the Potential for Moral Disengagement. *Navy Medicine* 96.1: 21–25.
Smith, Arthur M. 2005b. Has the Red Cross-Adorned Hospital Ship Become Obsolete? *Naval War College Review* 58.3: 121–131.
Snider, Don M., John A. Nagl, and Tony Pfaff. 1999. *Army Professionalism, the Military Ethic, and Officership in the 21st Century*. Strategic Studies Institute, US Army War College. http://www.strategicstudiesinstitute.army.mil/pubs/display.cfm?PubID = 282. Cited 1 April 2006.
Toffler, Alvin and Heidi A. Toffler. 1993. *War and Anti-war*. Boston, MA: Little Brown.
UN Peacekeeping. Undated. http://www.un.org/Depts/dpko/dpko/index.asp. Cited 1 April 2006.

Part II
Physicians and Torture

Physician Involvement in Hostile Interrogations[1,2]

Fritz Allhoff

1 Introduction

Military conflicts inevitably lead to the detention and interrogation of adversaries (or perceived adversaries), and American military action in Afghanistan and Iraq has resulted in the protracted and scrutinized detention and interrogation of varied personnel. Detention and interrogation, in turn, inevitably lead to moral and legal questions, and these questions have been especially poignant during and following the aforementioned campaigns. Controversially, the Bush administration did not afford Geneva Convention protections to "enemy combatants"; these protections would have increased the standard of care (e.g., legally, medically, etc.) afforded to detainees and would have limited the interrogation options available to military personnel. Also controversially, reports have alleged that military interrogators have practiced "stress and duress" tactics which include: "sleep management" (i.e., sleep deprivation), "dietary manipulation" (i.e., food withholding), "environmental manipulation" (e.g., exposure to extreme temperatures, presence of dogs, etc.),

[1] This paper was originally published as Fritz Allhoff, "Physician Involvement in Hostile Interrogations," *Cambridge Quarterly of Healthcare Ethics* 15.4 (2006): 392–402. Reprinted with permission.

[2] I would like to thank the following people for their helpful discussions and feedback on the ideas in this paper: Jean Maria Arrigo, William Casebeer, Michael Davis, Jan Goldman, Michael Gross, David Guinn, Kenneth Kipnis, Justin List, Jonathan Marks, Albert Pierce, Michael Pritchard, Len Rubenstein, Allen Weiner, Matthew Wynia, John Yoo, Daniel Zupan, and two anonymous reviewers from the *Cambridge Quarterly of Healthcare Ethics*. Their correspondences should obviously not be taken to imply that any of them agrees with my conclusions. This paper was presented at The Australian National University and at the 2005 meeting of the Australasian Association of Philosophy; I would like to thank those present for their comments, especially Dirk Baltzly, Jeanette Kennett, and Thomas Pogge. Finally, much of this paper was written during a fellowship in the Institute for Ethics of the American Medical Association, and I thank the AMA for supporting my research. Obviously the views expressed in this paper should not be taken to reflect those of the American Medical Association (and, in most cases, are directly contrary to those views).

F. Allhoff (ed.), *Physicians at War: The Dual-Loyalties Challenge*.

forced maintenance of uncomfortable positions for extended periods of time, isolation (sometimes for longer than 30 days), hooding, etc.[3]

Whether these tactics are tantamount to torture is debatable. They are certainly unpleasant but, in my view, fall short of archetypical instances of torture. While the invocation of 'torture' might seem merely semantic, it has substantial rhetorical force which has been often been carelessly and uncritically employed. For this reason, I propose to label interrogations which incorporate these tactics as hostile (which they clearly are) as opposed to torturous (which they arguably are not).[4] To be sure, many of the arguments that I will advance in this paper are as applicable to torture as to hostile interrogations. However, I want to try to preserve the distinction so as to reflect current allegations.

Before turning to a moral evaluation of physician involvement in hostile interrogations, it might be useful to briefly consider the morality of the interrogations themselves. If the interrogations are immoral, then physician contributions to their efficacy are presumably immoral *a fortiori*.[5] So, if someone wanted to defend the morality of physician involvement in these interrogations, he/she would have to carry two burdens: first to show that the interrogations themselves are morally permissible and then to show that *even if* they are morally permissible, it is morally permissible for *physicians* to participate in them. For the scope of this paper, I will confine my argumentation to this second project. Methodologically, however, I take this first project to be as important as the second, though I have already

[3] See, for example, Dana Priest and Barton Gellman, "US Decries Abuse but Defends Interrogations: 'Stress and Duress' Tactics Used on Terrorism Suspects Held in Secret Overseas Facilities," *Washington Post* (December 26, 2002): A1, 14, 15; Neil A. Lewis, "Iraqi Prisoner Abuse Reported after Abu Ghraib Disclosures," *New York Times* (December 12, 2004b): A12; Neil A. Lewis, "Fresh Details Emerge on Harsh Methods at Guantanamo," *New York Times* (January 1, 2005): A3, 11; Major General George R. Fay, *AR 15–16 Investigation of the Abu Ghraib Detention Facility and 205th Military Intelligence Brigade (The Fay Report)*, http://news.findlaw.com/hdocs/docs/dod/fay82504rpt.pdf, cited April 13, 2005; Steven H. Miles, "Abu Ghraib: Its Legacy for Military Medicine," *The Lancet* 364 (2004): 725–728; and M. Gregg Bloche and Jonathan H. Marks, "When Doctors Go to War," *New England Journal of Medicine* 352.1 (2005): 3–6; Joe Stephens, "Army Doctors Implicated in Abuse: Medical Workers Helped Tailor Interrogations of Detainees, Article Says," *Washington Post* (January 6, 2005): A8.

[4] Other authors have chosen other modifiers for such interrogations. For example, Jonathan Marks prefers "aggressive interrogations" and Matthew Wynia has used "harsh interrogations." I think that "hostile interrogations" is superior to these locutions for various reasons. First, some of the tactics employed are withholdings or deprivations which, by definition, are not aggressive since they are omissions rather than commissions. I think that 'harsh' is less problematic, though it carries a range of definitions which range from "unpleasant" to "severe or cruel." While the former is clearly appropriate, the latter is debatable (i.e., it begs important questions), so this usage is not without its perils. 'Hostile' can mean "characteristic of an enemy," "demonstrative of ill will," or "unfavorable to health or well-being"; any of these definitions would, I think, be appropriate.

[5] This does not, of course, *necessarily* follow: sometimes we might be morally required to participate in immoral practices in order to minimize overall harm or wrongness. However, given the structure of this debate and the positions put forth by its commentators, I will assume that if hostile interrogations are impermissible then physician involvement is, *a fortiori*, impermissible.

undertaken it in greater detail elsewhere.[6] Therefore, in this paper, I propose to consider whether there are any *special* reasons for physicians to not participate in hostile interrogations, *even if* such interrogations are morally justifiable.

2 Physician Involvement in Hostile Interrogations

It should be recognized that there are a host of moral issues that confront physicians in times of war, though I will herein focus only on the issue of their involvement in hostile interrogation.[7] First, we might consider what allegations have actually been made against physicians: the International Committee of the Red Cross (ICRC) has reported that the medical staff at Guantanamo Bay has shared patient records with military personnel who planned interrogations, and the ICRC has called these actions "a flagrant violation of medical ethics."[8] In response, the Pentagon has claimed that its detention operations are "safe, humane, and professional" and that "the allegation that detainee medical files were used to harm detainees is false."[9] Gregg Bloche and Jonathan Marks further allege that documents and interviews have shown not only that medical personnel shared confidential documents with potential interrogators, but that "physicians assisted in the design of interrogation strategies, including sleep deprivation and other coercive methods tailored to detainees' medical conditions. Medical personnel also coached interrogators on questioning technique."[10] Whether these allegations turn out to be true is, of course, an empirical matter and not one in which I am able to make any contribution. However, their truth is irrelevant to the *moral* debate which investigates whether such acts (actual or counterfactual) are morally permissible.

I propose to proceed in two stages. First, I want to consider moral arguments against physician involvement in hostile interrogations and to show why these arguments are problematic. Second, I wish to advance positive arguments against the thesis that medically-trained interrogators are physicians. Just for precision, let us designate

[6] See Fritz Allhoff, "Terrorism and Torture," *International Journal of Applied Philosophy* 17.1 (Fall 2003): 105–118. Reprinted in *Understanding Terrorism: Philosophical Issues*, ed. Timothy Shanahan (Open Court Press, 2005), 243–259. See also Fritz Allhoff, "A Defense of Torture: Separation of Cases, Ticking Time-Bombs, and Moral Justification," *International Journal of Applied Philosophy* 19:2 (2006): 243–264.

[7] For a discussion of some of these other issues, see Michael Gross, "Bioethics and Armed Conflict: Mapping the Moral Dimensions of Medicine and War," *Hastings Center Report* 34.6 (2004): 22–30; a reply to Gross by Leonard S. Rubenstein, "Medicine and War," *Hastings Center Report* 34.6 (2004); and Edmund G. Howe, "Dilemmas in Military Medical Ethics Since 9/11," *Kennedy Institute of Ethics Journal* 13.2 (2003): 175–188.

[8] Neil A. Lewis, "Red Cross Finds Detainee Abuse in Guantanamo," *New York Times* (November 30, 2004a): A1. Quoted in Bloche and Marks (2005), 3.

[9] Lewis (November 30, 2004a), A1. Quoted in Bloche and Marks (2005), 3.

[10] Bloche and Marks (2005), p. 3.

the controversial activities as the following: physicians' sharing of medical records (especially with would-be interrogators), physicians' development of interrogation strategies (especially strategies that make special use of medical knowledge and/or medical susceptibilities of detainees), and physicians' direct participation in hostile interrogations (whether in an oversight or advisory role or else physical participation in the interrogations). What arguments could be offered against these practices?

The most obvious argument would be that these practices run contrary to the moral nature of medicine and the moral obligations of physicians. Since the advent of medical ethics, harkening back to Hippocrates, medicine has been argued to be an inherently moral enterprise. Correspondingly, physicians have been ascribed various moral responsibilities; the most notable of these have been beneficence, non-malfeasance, confidentiality, honor, and loyalty.[11] Certainly we think that physicians should help patients (beneficence) and that they should not harm them (non-malfeasance). Confidentiality is also an important moral good insofar as it is necessary for optimal medical care: if patients cannot trust that their physicians will maintain confidences, patients will be less likely to disclose relevant medical information and physicians will not be able to provide as effective treatment. Physicians have always been among society's more esteemed members, and they (arguably) therefore have a greater obligation to serve as role models and to carry themselves honorably. Finally, we expect physicians to be loyal to their patients and to serve the interests of those patients, uncompromised by extraneous influences or conflicts of interest. Physicians who turn over medical records to potential interrogators would arguably violate all five of the aforementioned moral ideals, thus such an act would be morally problematic. Physicians who devise hostile interrogation strategies would at least be violating the principle of non-malfeasance, and active participation in these interrogations would be similarly morally problematic.

First, I would like to explore the extent to which endorsement these of core medical values actually precludes physician participation in torture, though these results will be readily transferable to the less controversial hostile interrogations. The American Medical Association's *Code of Medical Ethics* is quite unequivocal on this question:

> Physicians must oppose and must not participate in torture for any reason. Participation in torture includes, but is not limited to, providing or withholding any services, substances, or knowledge to facilitate the practice of torture. *Physicians must not be present when torture is used or threatened.* Physicians may treat prisoners or detainees if doing so is in their best interest, but physicians should not treat individuals to verify their health so that torture can begin or continue.[12]

---

[11] See, for example, "The Hippocratic Oath," *Ancient Medicine: Selected Papers of Ludwig Edelstein*, eds. Owsei Temkin and C. Lilian Temkin (Baltimore, MD: Johns Hopkins University Press, 1967), 6; American Medical Association, *Code of Medical Ethics: Current Opinions with Annotations* (2004–2005 ed.), (Chicago, IL: AMA, 2004), xiv, 295–296 (10.01); Albert Jonsen, *A Short History of Medical Ethics* (Oxford: Oxford University Press, 2000).

[12] American Medical Association, "2.067: Torture" (2004), pp. 24–25 (emphasis added). This statement continues that "Physicians should … strive to change situations in which torture is

Certainly these statements inveigh against participation in the three controversial practices that I have mentioned. However, I find the injunction against physician presence during torture to be peculiar and problematic. If torture is morally permissible (or even if it is merely occurrent), then I would maintain that the traditional values of medical ethics *mandate* physician presence during the interrogations. This contention has been vehemently criticized,[13] but it seems to me to directly follow from the principle of beneficence: insofar as this principle motivates concern for the welfare of the detainee, then physician oversight is morally obligatory to ensure the safety of the interrogatee. Obviously the well-being of the interrogatee is jeopardized during torture (and, less extremely, in hostile interrogations), and there is a chance that, absent physician intervention, he/she might die, suffer irreversible damage, etc. For example, imagine that, during an interrogation, an interrogatee were to go into cardiac arrest and that, pursuant to AMA opinions, no physician were present. The interrogatee might easily suffer a *preventable* death, and I think that this would be entirely unacceptable.[14]

The rub, of course, is the principle of non-malfeasance: physicians must not revive interrogatees just so that the interrogatees can be tortured even more, ultimately being made the worse off for the physician intervention. A couple comments are appropriate here. First, it seems unlikely to me that more torture would be worse than death (though, in some cases, this might be the case). Therefore, resuscitating someone merely so he/she can face more torture does not necessarily violate the principle of non-malfeasance *if*, absent resuscitation, he/she would have been even worse off (e.g., dead). And, again, the principle of beneficence would seem to require these interventions.

I take it that the argument made against this claim would effectively be epistemic: physicians would not know whether resuscitation would lead to further hostile interrogations and therefore whether interrogatees would be made worse off from physician intervention. However, this is not a *moral* argument and would be impotent against the claim that physicians *should* resuscitate (and, *a fortiori*, be *present* during the interrogation) *if* resuscitation were in the best interest of the interrogatee. But even contra the epistemic worry, I have the intuition that, in most cases, interrogatees would be better off *even if* their resuscitation led to more torture (or, less controversially, to more hostile interrogating) simply because their lives would usually be ones worth living so long as the interrogations would eventually cease and they could resume a quasi-normal (if detained) life. Regardless, I certainly

---

practiced or the potential for torture is great." I object to this claim on the grounds that the American Medical Association has neither the authority nor license to make political (or non-medical moral) statements; its magisterium is medicine (including medical ethics) and its remarks should be therein confined.

[13] Kenneth Kipnis and Matthew Wynia, personal communication (2005).

[14] Of course the death would also have been preventable if the torture were not to occur, but this is irrelevant to the current question which is whether, *given* the occurrence of torture, physicians are obligated to prevent preventable deaths.

think that the principle of beneficence *requires* at least minimal physician participation in hostile interrogations, at least in those cases where physician intervention would be in the medical interest of the interrogatee.

3 Are Medically-Trained Interrogators *Physicians*?

In the previous section, we investigated how traditional medical values would constrain physician involvement in hostile interrogations, though I argued that these values actually *mandate* at least minimal participation. However, we have so far been *assuming* that traditional medical duties or responsibilities apply to medically-trained interrogators, and this is an assumption against which I will now argue. Ultimately, my conclusion will be that medically-trained interrogators are *not* physicians, and therefore are exempt from whatever medical duties or responsibilities might otherwise be incumbent upon them. To motivate this discussion, let us consider actual remarks made by David Tornberg, Deputy Assistant Secretary of Defense for Health Affairs: Tornberg argues that medically-trained interrogators who helped to plan interrogations are not acting *qua* physicians (i.e., have not entered into a patient-physician relationship) and are therefore not bound by confidentiality, beneficence, non-malfeasance, etc.[15] Tornberg further contends that a medical degree is not a "sacramental vow", but rather a certification of technical merit. Some military physicians and Pentagon officials have claimed that their medically-trained personnel act as *combatants*, not physicians, when they put their medical knowledge to use for military ends.[16]

As a possible defense of this position (which they ultimately reject), Bloche and Marks propose to consider civilian parallels wherein the "Hippocratic ideal of undivided loyalty to patients fails to capture the breadth of the profession's social role."[17] The general problem, that of dual loyalties of the physician, warrants far more discussion than I can afford it in this paper, but the simple point is that there are at least some cases in contemporary society where physicians have duties or responsibilities beyond those merely to their patients; examples include forensic psychiatry, occupational health, public health, etc.[18] We certainly could look at the hostile interrogation debate as one of dual loyalties. The idea here would be to say that medically-trained interrogators have duties or responsibilities to the interrogatees as well as to something else (e.g., the military chain of command, national security, etc.) and that the latter duties trump the former.I think that this approach would be profitable, and I certainly think that these extra-medical invocations

---

[15] Bloche and Marks (2005), 3.

[16] Bloche and Marks (2005), 4.

[17] Bloche and Marks (2005), 4–5.

[18] For more discussion of these issues, see Physicians for Human Rights, *Dual Loyalties & Human Rights* (Boston, MA: 2002, Physicians for Human Rights). See also Gross (2004).

could successfully countervail medical duties or responsibilities.[19] However, I wish to defend the more extreme claim that there are *no* medical duties or responsibilities that the medically-trained interrogator has to the interrogatee, or at least no "special" duties or responsibilities that present themselves *merely* in virtue of the interrogator's medical knowledge and that could not be accommodated by general moral approaches (e.g., consequentialist or deontological). In other words, I do not even see the tension here being one of a *physician* having dual loyalties (i.e., to the interrogatee and elsewhere) because I do not think that the medically-trained interrogator is a physician at all (or acts *qua* physician during the interrogation).

Whether the medically-trained interrogator has special duties or responsibilities to the interrogatee depends on two central questions. First, has the interrogator entered into a patient-physician relationship with the interrogatee? Second, even if he/she has not, would there be other arguments (i.e., ones not based on invocation of non-existent patient-physician relationship) which would inveigh against the use of medical knowledge in a way that could bring harm to the interrogatee? One quick way to get around the issue of the patient-physician relationship is to note that physicians have the prerogative to refuse to enter this relationship. According to the American Medical Association's *Code of Medical Ethics*: "Physicians are free to choose whom they will serve. The physician should, however, respond to the best of his or her ability in cases of emergency where first aid treatment is essential."[20] The first statement here is quite unequivocal, though the latter qualification is somewhat confusing. I read it as a non-binding suggestion because, otherwise, it would contradict the first statement (which then should have been written as "physicians are free to choose whom they will serve so long as ..."). (The invocation of 'essential' is also confusing: essential for what?) Elsewhere, the *Code of Medical Ethics* says: "[I]t may be ethically permissible for physicians to decline a potential patient when ... [a] specific treatment sought by an individual is incompatible with the physician's personal, religious, or moral beliefs."[21] While the language is not entirely congruent with the issue we are trying to consider, I read this statement as affording physicians the license to decline patients on moral grounds since the physician might think that *any* treatment would be inappropriate for the interrogatee. The physician might think this because he/she could ascribe to a moral view which would license the hostile interrogations.

While I think that the *Code of Medical Ethics* supports a physician's prerogative not to enter into a specific patient-physician relationship, this prerogative could also be defended by simple moral philosophy. Since this relationship is a deontic one

[19] It should be acknowledged that some people find this claim controversial. For example, some philosophers ascribe to some form of Michael Walzer's spheres of justice doctrine which holds that, for example, only *medical* considerations are relevant to medical decisions. On this model, other considerations, such as national security, could not countervail medical considerations since the former are impotent against the latter.

[20] American Medical Association, "8.11: Neglect of Patient" (2004), 226.

[21] American Medical Association, "10.05: Potential Patients" (2004), 305.

(i.e., one defined by duties or responsibilities), its formation would presumably be grounded in deontological ethics. Taking Kant as the standard torchbearer of this enterprise, we could observe that it would be a violation of the physician's autonomous will to *force* him/her enter into a relationship if he/she does not want to; such a forcing would be morally impermissible. So, whether we invoke the *Code of Medical Ethics* or Kant, I think that compelling arguments can be made for the physician's right to decide whether to enter into a particular patient-physician relationship (the patient would obviously also have to consent in order to establish the relationship). Therefore, we have at least one argument supporting the claim that medical interrogators do not have medical duties to interrogatees: so long as the physicians do not wish to assume the relationship, the duties will not apply. If we limit our considerations to medically-trained interrogators who *willingly* assume their hostile roles (as opposed to merely assume them once commanded to), we might reasonably infer that these interrogators do not wish to assume a patient-physician relationship with the interrogatee and therefore are exonerated from the associative moral duties.[22]

These previous paragraphs have tried to establish that physicians can simply *choose* not to enter into a patient-physician relationship and that, absent this constitution, they are exempted from the associative moral duties. However, I do not take these comments to be overwhelmingly convincing, though I do think that they merit consideration. For one thing, the citations from the AMA *Code of Ethics* are not even *arguments* at all, they are merely *statements* (and, furthermore, statements that might not be interpreted in the way that I have suggested). Since the *Code of Ethics* only issues statements, we have no reasons (as might be offered by premises and a purported inferential structure) to accept them aside from the fact that the American Medical Association endorses them. This is, to my mind, the devastating weakness of the *Code of Ethics* for philosophical purposes since philosophy requires argumentation and not simply stipulation by fiat. And any deontological argument which prioritizes individual autonomy (viz., the autonomy not to enter into a patient-physician relationship) will be impotent against anyone who does not ascribe to such a moral theory. So, while I think that these ideas should be taken seriously, I cannot yet claim to have decisively settled the issue.

Therefore, I propose to directly argue against the view that medical knowledge confers moral duties, including the moral duty to establish a patient-physician relationship and absorb the associative moral burdens. Or, to explicitly reference

---

[22] Of course, it is an empirical question how these interrogators actually view their relationship with the interrogatees. Certainly there will be some interrogators that do view interogatees as patients and, in these cases, there might be plausible arguments as to why a patient-physician relationship would be therein constituted. But this is irrelevant for present purposes as we are assuming that the interrogator does not have this attitude. The moral project needs merely to show that hostile interrogations by medically-trained interrogators are morally permissible given some plausible affective state of the interrogator (whether actual or counterfactual). My assumption here seems weak enough to at least be afforded this plausibility.

the current administration's position, I want to defend the notion that a medical degree is *merely* a certification of technical merit and not a "sacramental vow."[23] My conclusion, already mentioned, is that medically-trained interrogators have *no* medical duties or responsibilities to interrogatees, and I take this to be a stronger claim than the one which would hold that such duties exist but are countervailed by other duties (e.g., toward the public good). I will offer three arguments in favor of this position: the logical argument, the metaphysical argument, and the argument from analogy (with other professions).

First, consider the logical argument. People who claim that medically-trained interrogators are violating medical duties often say something like: the medically-trained interrogator has medical knowledge, *therefore* he/she has certain moral duties. (Sometimes this is expressed as: medically-trained interrogators have certain moral duties *in virtue of* their medical knowledge—this equivalent expression just inverts the premise and conclusion.) At the risk of being tedious, this argument has one premise (viz., that the medically-trained interrogator has medical knowledge) and one conclusion (viz., that he/she has certain moral duties). As currently formulated, the argument is at least formally invalid (i.e., we might represent the argument as P, therefore Q, which is formally invalid). Furthermore, many philosophers endorse a fact-value divide such that we cannot validly move from descriptive premises to a normative conclusion; this principle is not above debate, but something always looks fishy about attempts to circumvent it.[24] Accepting this principle, the argument is again going to be invalid since the premise is descriptive and the conclusion is normative.

The most obvious way to try to repair the argument's doubly alleged invalidity would be to say that it is enthymatic: if we can restore the suppressed premise, then we can get the argument to come out valid. What is the suppressed premise? One likely candidate is: if the medically-trained interrogator has medical knowledge, then he/she has certain moral duties. A coupling of this premise with the original premise will yield the conclusion by simple application of *modus ponens*, thus making the revised argument valid. But is it sound? I think that the validity can only be restored if we insert a dubious premise, which leads to my second argument: the metaphysical argument.

So consider this new premise: "if the medically-trained interrogator has medical knowledge, then he/she has certain moral duties." For the argument to be sound, this premise would have to be true. But is it? I do not think so, because I find this premise

[23] Bloche and Marks (2005), 4. This is a position that is hastily dismissed by Bloche and Marks who argue that such a position is "self-contradictory" because a "military physician's contributions to interrogation—to its effectiveness, lawfulness, and social acceptance in a rights-respecting society—arise from his or her psychological insight, clinical knowledge, and perceived humanistic commitment." Bloche and Marks (2005), 5.

[24] The principle is generally credited to David Hume, see his *A Treatise of Human Nature* 2nd ed., ed. Paul H. Nidditch (Oxford: Oxford University Press, 1978), III.I.i. A contemporary discussion is in W.D. Hudson's *The Is/Ought Question: A Collection of Papers on the Central Problems in Moral Philosophy* (London: Macmillan, 1969).

(and ones like it) to have dubious metaphysical commitments. More formally, such a premise holds that since A knows P, A is morally required to ϕ.[25] Or, in other words, the knowledge of P is *sufficient* to obligate an agent to ϕ. But this just seems obviously wrong. It cannot be the case that *mere* knowledge of some (non-moral) proposition (or set of propositions) can obligate someone to do something. Rather, *normative principles* are the sorts of things that create moral obligation. For example, if I am obligated to ϕ, the *reason* has to be that ϕ maximizes happiness, that its negation cannot be willed to be universal law, etc.; obligation can follow from these sorts of normative claims. But how could obligation possibly follow from propositional knowledge alone? Certainly such knowledge could be *necessary* for moral obligation: insofar as we endorse the "ought implies can" principle, we cannot be obligated to that which we are unable. And, insofar as knowledge could be a necessary precondition for ability (e.g., I *cannot* save the drowning child unless I *know* where he/she is), we would not have moral obligation absent knowledge of the appropriate propositions. But the necessity of knowledge for moral obligation is irrelevant here. Rather, the proponent of medical knowledge's ability to create moral duties must defend the *sufficiency* of knowledge for moral obligation, and this is metaphysically problematic since knowledge alone cannot *create* moral obligation. Medical knowledge alone is not sufficient to create moral obligations absent some *moral principle* that would yield those obligations. And remember that, at least for the sake of argument, we are supposing that some moral principle could license the hostile interrogations themselves if not physician participation in them. While I take this argument to be devastating against the opposing view, let us also consider a third argument: the argument from analogy.

The argument from analogy proceeds by looking at how moral obligations can be said to work in other professions; maybe we can learn something about medicine (i.e., the controversial one) by looking at less controversial professions. For example, take engineering ethics, though similar examples could be illustrated by appealing to other professions. The analogous question would be: do engineers have moral obligations *merely* in virtue of their technical knowledge? For example, do chemical engineers, *qua* chemical engineers, have duties not to construct chemical weapons? I would argue no: it would only be impermissible to construct these weapons if such constructions were morally impermissible as dictated by some plausible normative principle. In my view, there is nothing *intrinsic* about their technical knowledge that would morally prohibit them from doing something. Rather, the moral wrongness of any application of their technical knowledge must reside in some incriminating moral principle. If this is true and if this engineering case is analogous to the medical case, then it would be implausible to suggest that medically-trained interrogators have moral duties or responsibilities in virtue of their medical knowledge.

---

[25] Though this formalization might appear as though all duties require positive acts, this need not be the case as ϕ could be an omission instead of a commission.

Is the case analogous? Or, in other words, is there anything that makes medicine *special* as a profession? First off, I tend to be against things being special (i.e., exceptions to general principles) on the grounds that I prefer homogenous conceptions of value. Someone might try to say that medicine is special on the grounds that it aims, most fundamentally, at healing, and that healing is an inherently moral project. Engineering, she might continue, is not inherently moral since it merely aims at, let us say, building things. So, even if the critic were to share my intuition in the engineering case, she might argue that it is irrelevant in the medical case. I disagree that medicine *necessarily* (i.e., conceptually) aims at healing: I take the field of medicine (as any other field) to be merely constituted by an accumulation of facts, and facts do not *do* anything, much less heal people. Rather, medical knowledge (as with all knowledge) can be applied to *any* ends, whether healing or harming. If those with medical training *should* heal, it is because pleasure is better than pain, because people consent to healing and not harming, and so on, not because there is any *intrinsic* feature of medical knowledge such that it should be applied to healing. So, contra the critic, I would argue that the analogy stands.

One objection to my three arguments might be that they are against the wrong thesis: I have been considering whether medical *knowledge* alone gives rise to medical duties, and we might instead think that this is the wrong question to be asking. To wit, another question might be whether it is a physician's *role* (as opposed to merely his knowledge) that gives rise to the medical duties. While the structure of my answer to this question is already in place, some further remarks are warranted. The idea of role-differentiated morality is fairly intuitive: many of us think that duties or responsibilities are sometimes dictated by the roles that we occupy. For example, we might think that parents have a stronger duty to provide for their own children than do complete strangers, and that law enforcement is more justified in using lethal force than the general public would be. While these ideas could be discussed in more length, I take them to be so intuitively plausible that I will not pursue their justification.

The application of these concepts to our current investigation is straightforward, and the question now becomes: is there something about the role of the medical interrogator that could ground medical duties or responsibilities? Presumably, this challenge assumes that this question is logically distinct from the one I have been asking, which is whether medical knowledge alone grounds medical duties or responsibilities. However, even accepting the thesis of role-differentiated morality (which I do), I do not think that the interrogator's role is relevant to our inquiry.

What is the role of the interrogator? Certainly it is not that of a physician: the interrogator's primary task is to facilitate the acquisition of information, not to heal. So, as a matter of empirical fact, I assert that the role the interrogator actually plays is not that of physician, but rather that of *interrogator* (hence the job title). The relevant objection to this assertion is that we are not concerned with empirical fact, but rather with the normative realm. And of course I agree. So now we must ask whether the interrogator *should* assume the role of physician, and therefore the associative moral duties. And, again, I think that the answer is no.

Remember that we are assuming, at least for the sake of argument, that hostile interrogations are morally justified. Therefore, absent any other considerations, the interrogator's role is justified *a fortiori* (as a necessary element of those interrogations). What about other considerations? We might propose that the medically-trained interrogator is *obligated* to assume some special role which would ground medical duties or responsibilities, but I argued against this claim in §2. It seems to me that we can exhaust logical space by postulating a third option: that the medically-trained interrogator is somehow thrust into the role of healer, even if he/she would rather not assume this role, and therefore bound by the duties and responsibilities thereof. But why would this be true? If it were true, it would have to be in virtue of his medical training since that is the only feature that could serve as a differentia between him and anyone else. Whether the duties and responsibilities derive directly from the interrogator's medical training or are else mediated through some role is irrelevant since either position would be committed to the *sufficiency* of medical training for these duties and responsibilities.[26] And this, of course, is the claim against which I have argued.

Finally, let me offer a few remarks on the notion of professionalism and oaths, as these notions have been invoked in criticisms against my position.[27] As I hope to have made clear, I view the medically-trained interrogator as acting outside of the profession of medicine and thus exempt from whatever standards might therein apply. If professional societies do/should play some role in safeguarding the profession, then they might well take issue with admitting medically-trained interrogators into their ranks. For example, we might imagine that these people return from their military assignments and want to practice medicine: should they be licensed by local boards? Maybe we think that their ability to heal has been compromised or else that we simply do not *want* such people as part of the profession. I do not really have views on these issues, other than to say that they are irrelevant to my current inquiry (albeit interesting in their own right). Relatedly, we might wonder whether medically-trained interrogators are violating some oath (e.g., Hippocratic) they might have at one time taken. Here I have two comments. First, we could easily imagine medically-trained interrogators who never took such an oath and therefore, *ex hypothesi*, would not be breaking one. If the only argument against medically-trained interrogators is merely a contingent avowal of some oath, then this does not strike me as a particularly powerful objection. For example, we could just identify prospective medically-trained interrogators earlier and make sure they never uttered the words. Then what would be the objection? But the second comment might be more substantial: I interpret oaths as governing behavior within a profession, and I think that medically-trained interrogators lie outside of professional medicine. To be sure, there are some duties that would "follow" medically-trained interrogators as they leave the profession (e.g., the duty to maintain confidences established

[26] This is just a consequence of propositional logic: If P is sufficient for Q and if Q is sufficient for R, then P is sufficient for R.

[27] These criticisms have been made especially by Dirk Baltzly, Jeannette Kennett, and Thomas Pogge.

while part of the profession). However, I think that those duties can only attach to particular relationships forged while in the profession and cannot provide blanket edicts that universally apply after departure from the profession. So, whether the medically-trained interrogator never enters the profession of medicine or else leaves to go interrogate, I think that arguments predicated upon professionalism and oaths are impotent in rendering moral indictments against him/her.

4 Conclusion

In this paper, I have pursued two main goals. First, I argued that traditional medical values mandate, as opposed to forbid, at least minimal physician participation in hostile interrogations. Second, I argued that traditional medical duties or responsibilities do not apply to medically-trained interrogators. In support of this conclusion, I argued that medically-trained interrogators could simply choose not to enter into a patient-physician relationship. Recognizing that this argument might not be convincing, I then proposed three further arguments against the claim that medical knowledge creates special duties: the logical argument, the metaphysical argument, and the argument from analogy. Finally, I argued that invocations of role-differentiated morality, professionalism, and oaths could not circumvent the central argumentation of this paper.

References

Allhoff, Fritz. 2003. Terrorism and Torture. *International Journal of Applied Philosophy* 17.1: 105–118.

American Medical Association. 2004. *Code of Medical Ethics: Current Opinions with Annotations*, 2004–2005 ed.Chicago, IL: AMA.

Arrigo, Jean Maria. 2004. A Utilitarian Argument Against Torture. *Science and Engineering Ethics* 10.3: 1–30.

Bloche, M. Gregg and Jonathan H. Marks. 2005. When Doctors Go to War. *New England Journal of Medicine* 352.1: 3–6.

Dershowitz, A. 2001. Is There a Torturous Road to Justice? *Los Angeles Times* 8 November 2002: B19.

Dworkin, R. 1977. *Taking Rights Seriously*. Cambridge, MA: Harvard University Press.

Fay, Maj. Gen. George R. 2005. *AR 15–6 Investigation of the Abu Ghraib Detention Facility and 205th Military Intelligence Brigade (The Fay Report)*. http://news.findlaw.com/hdocs/docs/dod/fay82504rpt.pdf. Cited 13 April 2005.

Gewirth, A. 1981. Are There Any Absolute Rights? *Philosophical Quarterly* 31: 1–16.

Gross, Michael L. 2004. Bioethics and Armed Conflict: Mapping the Moral Dimensions of Medicine and War. *Hastings Center Report* 34.6: 22–30.

Howe, Edmund G. 2003. Dilemmas in Military Medical Ethics Since 9/11. *Kennedy Institute of Ethics Journal* 13.2: 175–188.

Hudson, W.D. 1969. *The Is-Ought Question: A Collection of Papers on the Central Problems in Moral Philosophy*. London: Macmillan.

Hume, David. 1978. *A Treatise of Human Nature*, 2nd ed., ed. Peter Nidditch. Oxford: Oxford University Press.

Jonsen, Albert. 2000. *A Short History of Medical Ethics*. Oxford: Oxford University Press.

Levin, Michael. 1982. The Case for Torture. *Newsweek* 13 (7 June 1982).

Lewis, Neil A. 2004a. Red Cross Finds Detainee Abuse in Guantanamo. *New York Times* A1 (30 November 2004).

Lewis, Neil A. 2004b. Iraqi Prisoner Abuse Reported After Abu Ghraib Disclosures. *New York Times* A12 (12 December 2004).

Lewis, Neil A. 2005. Fresh Details Emerge on Harsh Methods at Guantanamo. *New York Times* A3, 11 (1 January 2005).

Miles, Steven H. 2004. Abu Ghraib: Its Legacy for Military Medicine. *The Lancet* 364: 725–728.

Nozick, Robert. 1974. *Anarchy, State, Utopia*. New York: Basic Books.

Physicians for Human Rights. 2002. *Dual Loyalties & Human Rights*. Boston, MA: Physicians for Human Rights.

Priest, Dana and Barton Gellman. 2002. U.S Decries Abuse but Defends Interrogations: 'Stress and Duress' Tactics Used on Terrorism Suspects Held in Secret Overseas Facilities. *Washington Post* A1, 14, 15 (26 December 2002).

Rawls, John. 1999. *A Theory of Justice*, rev. ed. Cambridge, MA: The Belknap Press of Harvard University Press.

Rubenstein, Leonard. 2004. Medicine and War. *Hastings Center Report* 34.6: 3.

Indecent Medicine Revisited: Considering Physician Involvement in Torture[1]

Richard Matthews

1 Introduction[2]

Although physician involvement in torture has been systematically documented and condemned by Amnesty International, Human Rights Watch, Physicians for Human Rights, and other human rights organizations, less attention has been paid to the arguments that favor the participation of physicians in torture. Perhaps this is because of a widespread sense that torture is so completely antithetical to medical ethics as to require no discussion. Doctors who torture or otherwise contribute in deliberately harming individuals would then be so beyond the pale as not even to require reasoned criticism. However, the literature is not uniformly opposed to physician participation. Gary Jones (1980) explicitly argues for doctor participation in torture when states of emergency exist and no other effective means are available to resolve the crisis. Because effectiveness in crisis resolution is crucial and because effective torture requires medical involvement, clinical and research resources are needed to increase the likelihood of success. More recently, Michael Gross (2004) argues that physicians have a civic duty to aid their security forces in the interrogation of certain suspects.

Gross's position is as follows: first, in what he calls "decent societies", physicians may be governed by religious norms and commitments to collective well-being rather than individual rights. Prioritization of the common good legitimately weakens the prohibition against torture and consequently creates a moral obligation for physicians to participate in torture if the relevant emergency circumstances arise. For Gross, absolute prohibitions against torture only work by presupposing liberal norms about the absolute worth and dignity of the individual. Whereas

[1] §§1–7, with only minor editorial changes, were originally published as Richard S. Matthews, "Indecent Medicine: In Defense of the Absolute Prohibition against Physician Participation in Torture," *American Journal of Bioethics* 6.3 (2006): W34–W44. Reprinted with permission. §§8–10 have been added to this essay and are primarily a reply to Fritz Allhoff (2005b) and (2006); the latter is reprinted in this volume).

[2] I would like to thank Fritz Allhoff and Emma Woodley for their generous and careful criticisms of this revised version. The paper has benefited enormously from their aid.

F. Allhoff (ed.), *Physicians at War: The Dual-Loyalties Challenge*.

decent societies respect human rights generally, Gross asserts that they are entitled to use torture when the interest of the common good so requires because in decent societies the public good occasionally must override individual rights. As members of decent societies, the relevant doctors have moral obligations to aid in preservation of the common good. Hence, standard medical principles of beneficence, maleficence and autonomy do not apply where the relevant public need exists. Rather, doctors are required to consider not only the good of their patient, but also the question of benefits and harms to the wider community.

It should be clear that these positions run contrary to 60 years of progress in medical ethics and international law relating to the definition of and sanctions for torture, as well as to sustained ethical reflection on the subject beginning at least with Beccaria's (1764) attack on torture in the eighteenth century. The Declaration of Tokyo (1975), the United Nations Declaration on the Protection of All Persons From Being Subjected to Torture and Other Cruel, Inhuman or Degrading Treatment or Punishment (1975), the United Nations Principles of Medical Ethics (1982), as well as the Convention against Torture and Other Cruel, Inhuman or Degrading Treatment or Punishment (1984) absolutely prohibit the use of torture by state officials in interrogations, for the sake of punishment or revenge, or for any other purpose. The Declaration of Tokyo, the Principles of Medical Ethics and many other national and international medical associations specifically prohibit physician participation in torture, whether as state agents, or in any other capacity. These prohibitions are non-derogable even in times of national crisis.

It is clear that a successful argument would weaken the struggle to end torture, for if it were sound, absolute prohibitions against torture would be invalid. Consequently, the absolutist position might be unethical. A utilitarian might argue, for example, that weakening the prohibition against torture might enhance general well-being by permitting greater flexibility of response to internal or external threat.

I present four counterarguments. The first is directed against Gross. He is wrong to conclude that physicians in decent societies are obliged to participate in torture. Gross incorrectly analyses the nature of "decent societies", a term he borrows from the book *The Law of Peoples* (Rawls 1999), because he fails to recognize that decent peoples are obligated to obey international norms such as those established by the United Nations, the World Medical Association, and other international bodies. Moreover he fails to recognize that there are moral limitations, defined by an ideal or established international human rights regime and international humanitarian law, which no decent society could violate under any circumstances. According to Rawls, the absolute prohibition against torture is such a limit.

Gross's position does not stand or fall with the decent society argument. As with Jones, the ultimate foundation is utilitarian. But their versions of utilitarianism raise additional substantial problems. First, it is not clear how and to what extent doctors in decent societies are to participate in torture. Arguably there are no limits to the ways in which they might be expected to aid in interrogations. Although he alludes to current Israeli use of "moderate physical pressure" in interrogations and to the constraints that would emerge in having to defend the use of torture in a decent society, Gross provides no clear restrictions on physician involvement

(Gross 2004, 189). The same problem arises for Jones; both positions are far too permissive. If any of the possible physician contributions to torture are justifiable on consequential grounds, then all of them are. Furthermore, not only is the utilitarian argument too permissive, but it requires unacceptable changes both in the principles and virtues of medical ethics.

Another problem concerns the necessity defense as a justification for torture. All utilitarian arguments for torture tacitly or explicitly turn on necessity. I show that necessity is a red herring and that on careful consideration utilitarian thinkers should forbid torture. Finally, there is the problem of institutional and cultural degradation. Effective use of torture presupposes advanced medical, technical, and scientific research. It requires training facilities, prisons, interrogation centers along with trained torturers and any necessary bureaucratic and institutional supports. These can only be put in place well in advance of any hypothetical "emergency situation". They suggest a normalization of torture that degrades the medical, legal and human rights culture of any society that employs it.

2 A Decent Society Cannot Permit Torture

As mentioned, Gross takes his account of the decent society from John Rawls' (1999) *The Law of Peoples*. Owing an explicit debt to Immanuel Kant's *Perpetual Peace* (1795), this work "hopes to say how a World Society of liberal and decent Peoples might be possible" (Rawls 1999, 6). Avowedly utopian, the discussion of constitutional liberal and decent societies examines the behavior of societies under relatively ideal conditions, and does not endorse any existing or past society. Its purpose as a realistic utopia is the extension of the limits of practical political philosophy (Rawls 1999, 35) and its aim is the elimination of oppression and injustice, both internal to a given State, and in wars between States. Rawls argues that in the event of the establishment of just or "decent" societies, the conditions for the great evils of human history would vanish. Rawls's book is thus about abolishing social ills, not defending them.

A decent society is one which treats its citizens and minorities reasonably well, even if it does not function according to the liberal norms that Rawls believes to be constitutive of the best kind of society. The following properties of the decent society are particularly relevant to the subject of torture:

- It offers other peoples, including ethnic minorities within its own borders, fair terms of political and social cooperation.
- It respects its international treaties and obligations.
- It respects specified restrictions in the conduct of its wars, in particular those covered by just war considerations (Rawls 1999, 37).

Just and decent societies are committed to international human rights and do not violate them. For Rawls, a society cannot be decent if it chooses to flout international human rights, whatever its reasons for doing so. It is only in virtue of its acceptance of its international obligations that the society is decent. So such a society cannot define its human rights entirely on its own terms and certainly cannot employ tactics such as torture that are absolutely forbidden at international law.

A Rawlsian decent society acknowledges a right of dissent on the part of its citizens, and is obliged to give reasoned and public responses to the dissenters. Therefore, if a given group disagrees with state-sanctioned torture, then the decent society must take into account this dissent and provide a public argument in favor of the deployment of torture. In the event that the disagreement persists then since it tolerates dissent the decent society does not compel them to participate.

Take, for example, the *Islamic Code of Medical Ethics* (1981). It commits Islamic doctors to benevolence and non-malfeasance on religious and non-liberal grounds even in time of war. It requires the physician to protect the life of enemy detainees and to treat their injuries. It specifically emphasizes that medical personnel and professions are not to allow the use of clinical, technical, or scientific resources for the purposes of infliction of any kind of harm. No military or political reasons can countermand this. In consequence physicians and medical personnel are absolutely forbidden from participating in torture in any way. Rawls insists that in the event that a decent society were to reject the Islamic Code of Ethics or some similar non-liberal variant, it would be obliged to give arguments in public as to why this was so, and to permit dissent even once its arguments were aired. Failure to do this entails the conclusion that the society is some form of non-benevolent paternalism (i.e. an authoritarian society) (Rawls 1999, 72). It would therefore not be decent. Because dissent is permitted in the decent society, there could be no legal obligation for physicians to participate in torture.[3]

Gross pays little attention to the role played by human rights in Rawls' account of the decent society and assumes they are coextensive with liberal rights. He fails to recognize that liberal rights are defined within constitutional liberal democracies, but that human rights are more general. Obviously the decent society is not bound by liberal conceptions of the equality of the individual, for this would make it liberal rather than decent. However, it is bound by human rights. According to Rawls, the Law of Peoples and human rights restrict the reasons that any state may legitimately use in going to war to that of self-defense, and they restrict the means by which war may be conducted. Just as significantly, they restrict the internal autonomy of a state with respect to its own people or to ethnic, political or other minorities within that state (Rawls 1999, 79). The fulfillment of human rights is a necessary condition of the decency of the society's political institutions and legal order (Rawls 1999, 81).

So, consider Gross's claim that physicians of decent societies might be morally obligated to participate in torture. He seems to think that torture is absolutely prohibited only by constitutional liberal democracies, whereas for Rawls and in

[3] Gross wavers on the issue of dissent. On the one hand he supports some kind of conscientious objection. Yet he also holds that there are moral obligations to torture of the sake of the common good of the society. It is not clear that these are compatible.

international law the prohibition against torture is a non-derogable human right. Recall that Gross's argument is based on the idea that a decent society has a human rights regime, but is concerned with general social well-being rather than with the rights of individuals, and so may make decisions that harm the individual in the interests of the social well-being of the whole. In particular, a decent society is entitled, if not obligated, to violate the interests of specific individuals when this is believed to be necessary for the sake of the well-being and survival of the state. Because the decent society, in Gross's view, is entitled to act in this way, and because doctors who are citizens of decent societies have moral obligations to meet the norms of these societies, they also share the obligation to participate in torture where such a need exists.

This position is incompatible with Rawls. It pays no attention to the importance of the international obligations of decent societies. Nor is the torture of suspects consistent with Rawls' requirement that the decent society offer fair terms of political and social cooperation to ethnic minorities because torture suspects cannot be the beneficiaries of any fair legal proceedings. I have already indicated that decent societies do not violate their international treaty obligations and that they respect international human rights. Furthermore, a Rawlsian decent society accepts the usual just war constraints in prosecuting its wars, and thus cannot use unjust means such as torture. Finally, international human rights place restrictions on the internal autonomy of states. Should a State violate any of these constraints, it is simply indecent. Torture constitutes, both in contemporary international law, and in any Rawlsian human rights regime, a grossly unacceptable class of practice. Indeed, as Gross recognizes, in contemporary international law, torture is non-derogable; it cannot be justifiably employed for any reason at all, including on grounds of necessity (CAT articles 1 and 2). It is also forbidden in Rawls' utopian community of *Peoples*. A decent society will prohibit torture as contrary to human rights norms and international humanitarian law. It will not use any form of torture to repress its internal minorities, nor can it employ torture on external enemies.

Now, because the decent society cannot justifiably use torture internally on its own citizens or ethnic minorities or externally on members of other peoples, there is no further argument to make to suggest that physician citizens of decent societies are obligated to contribute to torture. If torture is a human rights violation and if human rights violations are completely prohibited by the Law of Peoples, then no state or individual can justifiably employ or participate in torture. The antecedents are both true for Rawls. Consequently, no state or state-employed physician can participate in torture.

Gross' position is not that decent societies would use torture arbitrarily (Gross 2004, 200), and not even that torture would necessarily be legal within a decent society. It is rather that under conditions of necessity it may be the only moral thing to do, and therefore that interrogators and physicians will be morally obligated to use torture to meet such emergencies and then will have to defend their actions before the court of public opinion.

To claim that doctors in decent societies are morally obligated to participate in torture in emergency circumstances is false. If the society is decent in Rawls's sense, then torture will never be permitted. The fact that physicians act with a view to common well-being does not override their obligations under international human rights and medical ethical norms. If torture is permitted, then the society that uses it is either an outlaw society and must be opposed by both liberal and decent societies, or it is burdened and requires assistance (Rawls 1999, 90). Torture is an unconditionally forbidden international human rights violation both in the real world and in any reasonable Law of Peoples. Because Rawlsian decent societies are defined in terms of their adherence to the international human rights regime of a reasonable Law of Peoples, they forbid torture unconditionally. And because decent societies always prohibit torture no matter by whom and regardless of the circumstances, then clearly the physicians of decent societies are likewise forbidden.

3 Limits on Physician Behavior Are Unclear or Non-existent

What the previous argument shows is that Gross cannot appeal to Rawls's concept of the decent society either for a defense of torture or for the claim that doctors are obliged to torture under some circumstances. But it does not show that Gross is wrong altogether. Both he and Jones employ a utilitarian argument in favor of physician involvement in torture. Doctors are obligated to assist their security services in the torture interrogation of suspected terrorists in the event that an emergency threatens and no other means of combating the emergency are available. Here it is just a matter of a balancing of the harm done in torturing the suspect against the good consequences arising from successful interrogation.

Before proceeding we should have some idea of the kinds of things that physicians have done in torturing individuals or abetting their torture. According to Human Rights Watch, physicians and other medical personnel may contribute to torture in at least the following ways:

- Directly participating or assisting in abuse, such as in the case of dentists applying dental torture, or doctors injecting abusive drugs
- Attending torture sessions in order to intervene when the victim's life is in danger
- Developing abusive methods to produce the results desired by the interrogators, such as psychiatric techniques
- Providing indirect assistance and legitimacy to abuse, by monitoring the health of victims undergoing torture or ill-treatment, or examining and/or treating victims before and after torture sessions, without attempting to stop the abuse
- Failing or omitting to correctly diagnose sequelae of torture, thereby frustrating attempts at documenting evidence of abuses (Human Rights Watch 1994)

The British Medical Association adds that doctors have also designed torture devices, shared important clinical information with torturers to help identify physical and psychological weaknesses, delayed or refused to treat victims of torture, or refused to investigate or register victim complaints (British Medical Association

1992, 33–34). This list is not exhaustive and may be limited only by the imagination of the torturer(s) and efficiency considerations.[4]

Although Gross argues that physicians in decent societies are, under some circumstances, obligated to participate in torture, he is never clear what this entails. Which, if any, of the above torture practices does he rule out? Which are required? Late in his essay Gross claims that:

> If, when faced with a "ticking bomb", torture can save more lives than would otherwise be the case if it were not used in an interrogation and, if it meets the condition of necessity outlined earlier, then the physician must do his part during an interrogation (Gross 2004, 199).

Torture can only be employed in interrogations, and therefore can only be used to acquire information vital to resolving an emergency. Physicians have to be present to help ensure the torture works. Modern torture, which involves the infliction of severe physical and mental suffering on its victims, requires medical assistance if it is to be effective. Successful interrogations require the victims to remain alive and coherent long enough to reveal good information. If interrogators inadvertently kill their victim prior to acquiring the information, then they cannot achieve their goals. The same is true if the victim is so psychologically destroyed as to be no longer capable of communication. In either event the purpose(s) of interrogation cannot be achieved.[5] To ensure that neither case occurs, medical personnel have to be available.

So what is the physician's "part"? Unfortunately, Gross is unclear. He fails to define torture in any sophisticated way and only discusses one of the many possible roles that medical personnel might play in torture. This is worrying as his reliance on the necessity defense may mean that physicians are obligated to contribute to torture in all the possible variations. The question as to what is required and what prohibited is therefore crucial.

Of the practices named by Human Rights Watch and the British Medical Association, Gross explicitly names only the following: in Israeli interrogations physicians determine the fitness of a suspect for interrogation. Gross also seems to approve of "moderate physical pressure,"[6] but whether this entails the conclusion

---

[4] For a wealth of information on involvement and practice of medical personnel in torture, see the essays in *The Journal of Medical Ethics* 1991; 17: Supplement.

[5] As Gross analyzes the use of torture in interrogations, I restrict myself to the analysis of "interrogational" torture. I leave aside other torture functions, such as its use in the purposive spread of terror or as the punishment of convicted criminals. But one should resist thinking that torture ever serves only one single function. Regardless of the intention of the torturer, the use of torture in interrogation will inevitably spread terror to the community to which the victim(s) belong and will also inevitably be seen as an illicit punitive measure. To borrow terms from the philosophy of technology, torture is multivalent and multifunctional.

[6] "Moderate physical pressure" has been much maligned and for good reason. There is the problem of the subjectivity of pain, which means that suffering inflicted on one person may be experienced more severely than the same torture inflicted on another. Furthermore Mordechai Kremnitzer notes that "inherent in every physical, even if 'moderate', blow is the potential of injury and even death. All depends on the strength of the hitter, the thickness of the victim's skull and the ever-present possibility of missing the mark." See Kremnitzer 1989, 22

that physicians should mete out the "pressure" is not addressed. Still worse, nothing in his argument clearly forbids more extreme measures (other than perhaps his worryingly vague remarks that decent societies will not permit 'abuses' because torturers and physicians will be required to give an account of their actions to their peers (Gross 2004, 199).[7] Because torture is defensible under conditions of necessity, any of the listed actions might be required provided the emergency is severe enough, and provided that the means offer a reasonable possibility of achieving the desired ends. That is, there are no clear limits set on what may be done, or how severely.[8] For instance, one might think, given that proper public evaluation of their behavior presupposes knowledge of the facts surrounding the torture, that falsification of medical records would be ruled out by the requirement that physicians and torturers defend their actions in front of their peers. But the harmful consequences of public disclosure of torture might be sufficient to outweigh the social benefits to be gained by public evaluation. Disclosure might, for example, inflame a population to further violence against the state and thereby create additional and even greater threats. Simultaneously it may introduce civic discontent among the non-target population from the mere fact that the torture is practiced. If the torture was judged to be necessary, and if disclosure of the torture in court or elsewhere might provoke an intensification of violence and civic unrest, then consequential considerations might support document falsification. If any form of participation in torture is permitted under conditions of necessity, then it is difficult to deny that all forms are allowed.

Jones is no better. He claims that torture is morally obligatory in interrogations conducted to resolve ticking bomb situations, but the only restriction is that "the minimal amount of pain necessary to obtain the information should be inflicted" (Jones 1980, 11). He neglects to discuss the notion of minimal pain and so does not consider that this can vary enormously depending upon the resistance capacities of the interrogation suspect and the extremity of the situation. If the stakes are high enough, anything might be allowed. He explicitly supports biomedical research into torture. Hence medical personnel ought to design torture technologies and otherwise assist in the development of efficient interrogation techniques.

This is not a slippery slope objection. I am not maintaining that if we start with permitting physicians to examine the suitability of prisoners for torture, then physicians will end up performing more egregious acts. That is a doubtful empirical claim whose truth will vary on a case-by-case basis. Rather, I am making a logical point concerning the activities which are entailed by consequentialist arguments for

---

[7] It is not clear that this requirement is plausible, given that interrogations are carried out under conditions of secrecy and under the provisions of some form of Official Secrets Act. I find it hard to imagine that one's peers would ever have access to the information necessary for them to ask the right questions.

[8] In his recent book, *Bioethics and Armed Conflict* (Gross 2006) Gross appeals to the just war principles of military necessity and proportionality to address this question of limits. I do not believe that these can provide a satisfactory solution to the problem, but cannot provide the argument here.

physician participation in torture. Lack of careful consideration of the limits on physician participation fails to rule out any form of involvement in torture at all. If the situation is appropriately exigent and the cost-benefit equations turn out in the relevant way, then any of these practices can be required.

4 Allowing Torture Requires Wide-Ranging and Unacceptable Changes in Medical Ethics Norms

Standard accounts of medical ethics and medical ethical codes list beneficence, non-malfeasance, autonomy, and justice as fundamental principles. These require physicians to: act in the best interests of the patient; do no harm to the patient unless some greater therapeutic benefit can be thereby achieved; respect the desires and interests of the patient even if these are contrary to the beliefs and interests of the physician; and treat patients in a fair manner regardless of their economic, political, ethnic, sexual, or other status.

Physicians who in any way participate in torture violate all of these principles in obvious ways. Torture cannot be benevolent, for by definition it is carried out contrary to the interests and well-being of the patient. It is an infliction of a serious harm to satisfy a perceived state interest. Torture is essentially malevolent. It has the function of deliberately inflicting substantial harms upon the victim. As such, any physician involved in torture is maleficent. Torture is also a violation of the autonomy of the individual. The sole point of inflicting torture on interrogation suspects is to compel them to do something they would not otherwise do. No suspect is consensually tortured. Finally, torture suspects are typically singled out in virtue of some form of group membership, whether as an alleged member of some terrorist group, part of the wrong ethnic community, or some other similar reason. As such, the choice to inflict harm must violate fairness constraints.

If (at least some) physicians are obliged to torture, they are simultaneously required to violate all of the most basic principles of medical ethics. They are thus either immoral, or medical ethical principles must be revised to account for such obligations. This is to redefine the role of the physician. The physician is no longer understood essentially as a healer; rather therapeutic roles will be required to coexist uneasily with incompatible and maleficent ends. The physician is forced to occupy two roles—those of healer and security agent. As a result physicians have to employ their medical expertise for non-medical purposes. This in turn places doctors in the contradictory normative position of being enjoined both to do no harm and to inflict harm. It also requires the physician both to be benevolent and maleficent.

As a result, resolution of the inconsistency becomes a difficult problem. It is a commonplace of logic that, from inconsistent premises any conclusion whatsoever follows. This means that inconsistent premises cannot be action-guiding and cannot help an individual to decide appropriate actions. To place physicians simultaneously in the role of healer and violator is to put them in just such a contradictory situation. Should they then ask whether medical or security norms ought to prevail, there is no rational answer to be given unless one can find a suitable higher norm that would place such competing obligations in a hierarchy. Gross's decent society argument was one such unsuccessful attempt. The final two sections of the paper show that Gross's and Jones's utilitarian arguments also fail either to resolve this hierarchy dilemma or to provide any argument in favor of physician participation in torture interrogation of suspects.

5 Utilitarians Hotly Dispute the Use of Torture, and a Careful Utilitarian Analysis Prohibits Torture Even in the Case of the Ticking Bomb

Because decent societies prohibit the use of torture, Gross cannot invoke decent society membership as a ground for requiring doctors to participate in torture. So we should consider a further and more fundamental sub-argument, which is in fact the most common justification for torture: the necessity defense. The core argument is that torture is defensible provided that it is used to prevent imminent and grievous harm to others, that there are no other alternatives available, and on condition that it does not cause harm disproportionate to the harm that is to be avoided. (Gross 2004, 190)

There are many models used to describe ticking bomb situations. Gross uses an empirical example from Israel, but given the contentious nature of such historical cases, we can move to hypothetical cases to express the same point. Henry Shue has a good example:

> Suppose a fanatic, perfectly willing to die rather than collaborate in the thwarting of his own scheme, has set a hidden nuclear device to explode in the heart of Paris. There is no time to evacuate the innocent people or even the moveable art treasures—the only hope of preventing tragedy is to torture the perpetrator, find the device, and deactivate it (Shue 1978, 141).

Given the example, many would be inclined to agree that in cases like this, straightforward utilitarian considerations will demand that we torture the fanatic. By hypothesis, the events are so immediate that only the quick and effective torturing of the individual will suffice to get the requisite information and disarm the bomb. How then can we justifiably refrain from torturing the fanatic? We are only going to harm one (or perhaps a few) individuals. A simple cost benefit calculation weighing the harms incurred by all those killed, wounded and economically disadvantaged by the bomb in contrast to the harm suffered by the torture victim(s) will show, as Gross and Jones maintain (but not Shue),[9] that torture is the morally requisite

[9] Shue's position is that he does not know how to deny the appropriateness of torture in the ticking-bomb situation. He thinks on practical grounds that such situations never arise and therefore ultimately the ticking-bomb situation is moot.

course of action. Far more people are advantaged through having their lives and interests preserved then are harmed by the torturing of the individual. The stipulation that there are no other available alternatives is crucial, for a good utilitarian will always take the alternative that provides for the least suffering, and so would condemn the use of torture in the event that other possibilities for disarming the bomb were available. Because torture is, *ex hypothesi*, the only means available for resolving the crisis, are we (and physicians) not obligated to torture the suspects to acquire the desired information?

Gross and Jones are not alone in responding affirmatively. Fritz Allhoff claims that torture is permissible to save lives provided that "the use of torture aims at acquisition of information; the captive is reasonably thought to have the relevant information; the information corresponds to a significant and imminent threat; and the information could likely lead to the prevention of torture" (Allhoff 2005a, 255).

However Twining notes that it is perfectly possible for utilitarians to support an absolute prohibition against torture, even while granting that the ticking bomb case might call for torture when considered in the abstract. This is because utilitarians may consider the consequences of giving such seemingly unlimited powers to state agents to be still worse than even the worst ticking bomb scenarios; it encourages absolute and authoritarian governments, destroys civil liberties, and will inevitably be employed not just in the ticking bomb situation, but in less extreme situations. Consequently, it renders the society less just and decent than it would otherwise be (Twining and Twining 1973, 348). David Lowry considers the historical case of the British struggle against the IRA in Northern Ireland and notes some specific problems the situation raised that should concern utilitarians who wish to justify the use of interrogational torture. Among other things, the British military and security services inadvertently tortured individuals unconnected with the bombings and radicalized the Catholic population of Northern Ireland, bringing more bombers into the ranks of the IRA and actually increasing its strength, not to mention contributing strongly to much higher levels of violence to the point of being a partial cause of a virtual state of civil war (Lowry 1973, 562). In practice the use of torture is highly imperfect and carries with it consequences that the abstract ticking bomb scenario fails to consider.

The problem that Lowry notes, and Gross disregards, is that the simplified ticking bomb scenario ignores difficulties such as which harmful consequences to recognize. The arguments for torture focus on the immediate tactical aim of preventing the explosion of some bomb, and do not take into account long term and unintended consequences that often easily outweigh any informational gains arising from the use of torture. The ticking bomb case focuses solely on what one might call the primary consequences (defusing the bomb) and the claimed most successful means (here, torture) and ignores the side effects, such as further increased violence in the target population and consequent additional attempts to create additional bombs. In Lowry's view, utilitarians have to take the "side effects" of a practice to be just as important as its primary effects (Lowry 1973, 578). Therefore, if we successfully stop a nuclear bomb at one instant, but in doing so create the conditions for further attempts with similar weapons at some later point in time, then at best we are no further ahead, and at worst we have taken steps backward and increased the risks to our society.

The point here is that the utilitarian argument only entails the use of torture in the ticking bomb case if we refuse to consider all the effects of our actions. If we restrict ourselves to the unacceptably artificial case in which there is only one action and one effect, then the argument in favor of the use of torture may follow. But utilitarian calculations are always more complex than such a superficial thought experiment allows. Once we consider further impacts, a good utilitarian case can be made that torture should not be employed even to remove ticking bombs.

6 Effective Use of Torture Presupposes Its Normalization in the Community and Thus Involves No Appeal to an Imminent Emergency

The final problem involves more extended reflection on the issue of the destruction of ethical and cultural norms which must occur if torture is to be effectively employed. Here, the problem is that the effective use of torture requires advance preparation. Such advance preparation in turn presupposes some level of systemic deployment of the use of torture, not its *ad hoc* use only in the unpredictable extreme situation.

To begin with, consider again the invocation of necessity in support of the use of torture. This need not be classically utilitarian, but might be more broadly consequentialist. For example, it might instead invoke some kind of right of a state or people to use any means necessary to preserve itself in emergency situations and might eschew utilitarian or deontological justification altogether. Such means will include a requirement that torturers and physicians break the laws of their own states under conditions of necessity. This is clearly the case Gross contemplates, for he recognizes that torture is illegal in Israel, and therefore that the use of torture cannot conform to Israeli law. However, he maintains that torture is excusable or defensible in the event of the ticking bomb conditions outlined previously and therefore that the prohibition against torture is derogable (Gross 2004, 190, 200).

This is a difficult and paradoxical position in which to place an interrogator or physician. Torture is illegal and thus prohibited by the society and the defense of necessity can be used to mitigate punishment but not to exculpate the torturer(s) (Gross 2004, 190). And yet on grounds of membership in the society the torturer and physician supposedly have a moral obligation to break those laws in time of need. An intuitive example might help to make the point. We have an obligation not to speed, because driving at high speeds threatens the health and safety of other people. But if a person in our car suddenly has a heart attack and is in dire need of medical help, speeding may be the only way to keep them alive. In this event, breaking the law might be morally required. Having broken that law, we may well have to explain our reasons to a court. But the court will surely find our actions justifiable under the circumstances (provided that we do not kill, injure, or place other individuals at great risk) because, if the law was not broken, then great harm that could otherwise have been prevented would have likely resulted. If this is true for saving the heart attack victim, why is it not also true for torturing to save the lives of others? For Gross, the same argument is at the heart of his case for torture and for physician involvement in the torture. The torture will be defensible in the event that the court accepts the action was necessary to disarm the bomb.

Leaving aside the general utilitarian considerations already discussed above, one should consider the importance of imminence in the necessity defense. The actions may only be excused if the danger is imminent and if no other alternatives are available. If the heart attack victim is not at risk of immediate death, then speeding would not be justifiable. The problem is that immanence carries with it the notion of unpredictability. We do not know when such situations will arise, and when they do we find that we have no alternative but to break the law in order to minimize harm. If we are in a situation of immanent danger, then we have no alternatives.

But torture is not like this. Indeed Gross and Jones may not notice this, but their arguments presuppose its normalization. They insist that in the event of a ticking bomb, interrogators and physicians have an obligation to torture (provided there are no reasonable alternative strategies). But in order to effectively meet the threat, a host of advance political, medical, economic, and institutional conditions need to be in place. William Casebeer recognizes the problem:

> Most consequentialist justifications for the permissibility of torture neglect to consider the institutional and character-based harm that we do to ourselves when we actually attempt to build a system for torture interrogation that the utilitarian would find praiseworthy. Perversely, consequentialist justifications for torture interrogation require well-trained torturers who know where and when to apply pain, but establishing the institutions required in order to sustain such well-honed practice is fraught with perils that the utilitarian would condemn, all things considered (Casebeer 2005, 262).

The problem is that of cultural degradation. As I understand Casebeer, if a state is to torture effectively, it cannot do so in an *ad hoc* and unplanned manner. It must train for it and put in place a set of laws, policies, and institutions that will best allow interrogators to take advantage of torture. Badly trained or wholly untrained torturers will kill suspects inadvertently, get bad information, and in other ways undermine the purposes of torturing the victim. An untrained torturer is much more likely to exacerbate any ticking bomb situation than is any trained torturer.

In practice, the effective exploitation of torture in the event of an emergency presupposes its institutionalization. Jean Maria Arrigo identifies the following special institutional requirements: trained medical personnel, biomedical and psychological research into torture techniques, and the establishment of a torture interrogation unit along with accompanying training facilities. He also notes that if the torture program is to be effective it has to be coordinated with the police, judiciary, the military, and other relevant government departments (Arrigo 2004, 546).

Gross does not address the cultural impact of allowing torture at all. However, and unlike Casebeer and Arrigo (both of whom oppose interrogational torture in practice), Jones is enthusiastic about such institutional changes. He clearly recommends that research resources be put to the task of developing more efficient means of torture and consequently implicitly advocates substantive changes in medical research ethics in addition to clinical practice (Jones 1980, 12). Successful scientific development of torture techniques would require animal experimentation, clinical trials, and the other apparatus of rigorous scientific research. Such research could not meet the existing norms of ethics governing medical research. Among other things, to test the effectiveness of torture researchers would have to ignore the consent of the research subjects. Otherwise they would not be torturing their subjects at all.

The requirement that torture be effective presumes that a wide range of institutions and policies are in place in the absence of any imminent threat. If a state is going to deal effectively with emergencies, it is better off on utilitarian grounds if it prepares in advance for all of the possibilities than not. But if the effective fight against ticking bomb situations requires a state to prepare now for as yet unanticipated future threats, then experience, research, and training will have to proceed regardless of whether a ticking bomb situation ever occurs. For if the emergency is not imminent then, strictly speaking, there is no guarantee that one will in fact develop.

If the preparations have to be in place in advance of the imminent threat, then the ticking bomb is no longer ticking or, worse, the way in which a state defines threats extends beyond the imminent situation to include potential bombs as well. But in either event preparations for torture would have to be normalized, as is arguably the case in every single state in which torture is practiced. If it is not normalized, if medical personnel are not trained to support it, and if considerable work is not done to determine which methods are more and which are less successful, then the likelihood that torture will fail is greatly increased. So an additional failing of the ticking bomb scenario is that it tacitly presupposes the institutionalization and more general acceptance of torture than necessity considerations permit.

The necessity defense can only be invoked in the exceptional situation, not as the rule. Yet torture can only be used effectively if considerable institutional support is put in place to support it, which means that torture has to involve more than merely the exceptional situation. It will necessitate the creation of a norm or more probably a family of norms governing the behavior of the relevant individuals. In the context of a society in which torture is illegal and immoral yet excusable, this creates an impossible situation. It demands the institutional regularity of all the supports of torture, and thus demands considerable state involvement in establishing the conditions under which it might be excusably used, while at the same time maintaining its illegality. These additional considerations suggest that the utilitarian dispute in the previous section in fact has to be resolved against the ticking bomb scenario even in the most extreme cases, for unless one is a crude utilitarian, the establishment of torture-supporting institutions and their impact upon national and international ethical norms constitutes a genuine further set of harms. To maximize the possible effectiveness of torture, authoritarian institutions have to be put in place with consequent threats to and diminishment of civil liberties. As the institutional considerations suggest, this has to be done in the absence of an imminent threat and thus poses significant institutional risks to civil liberties and professional ethics whether in medicine, the police, judiciary or elsewhere.

7 Conclusion

If the previous reflections are correct, then none of the arguments in favor of torture that I have considered are valid. Gross's unusual argument that doctors have a civic duty to participate in torture when required by the good of the decent society fails because Rawlsian decent societies by definition prohibit torture as a violation both of human rights and of a reasonable Law of Peoples. Both Gross and Jones are far too permissive. They fail to rule out physician involvement in any form of torture (provided that exigency conditions are satisfied). The utilitarian arguments in favor of torture fail because utilitarianism is at least as compatible with the rejection of torture, and once carefully formulated in terms of both immediate and long term consequences requires us to recognize the substantial social and political harms arising from the use of torture even in ticking bomb situations. Finally, the necessity defense is problematic because it can only be invoked for isolated acts carried out under conditions of immanent necessity. Yet the effective use of torture presupposes an organized institutional framework with a practiced expertise in the use of torture. Indeed, in the cases explicitly mentioned by Gross and Jones, the physician functions as an indispensable institutional support to an interrogator in a prison or interrogation wing, a scenario which is not compatible with cases in which a sudden event overwhelms a state, supposedly leaving it with no alternative but to torture to preserve its interests and protect its citizens.

Accordingly none of these arguments support the use of torture by anyone, let alone mandate the participation of physicians. The absoluteness of the prohibition against torture remains untouched. Specific existing norms absolutely prohibiting physician involvement in torture even under conditions of emergency remain sound.

8 Empiricism and the Torture Debate

Since writing this original paper, I have continued to think about my views on these topics and, in particular, wanted to offer a response to Allhoff (2005b, 2006) and other recent literature. In the next three sections, I will further develop my position.

It has become apparent to me that opponents and torture defenders differ on methodology. The division concerns the moral significance of the history and practice of torture. Torture defenders never offer any detailed analysis of its sequelae and neglect to explore its institutional nature and its historical impacts. In my view they treat torture in a vacuum—a perspective that I believe to be inadequate for applied ethics. There are no exceptions to this. The most one finds is a reference to a favorable newspaper article or the statement of a government official.

Since many arguments for torture claim to be consequentialist, it is disturbing to see no empirical attention to its nature and consequences. Given that torture defenders construct cost-benefit analyses which claim to show that the benefits outweigh the costs, this absence of empiricism is damaging. There is a great deal of evidence available. The medical, psychological, and psychosocial sequelae are well-documented. A significant historical literature details its complex cultural, political, and social impacts. This literature demonstrates that the violence torture inflicts extends across whole communities and has nothing to do with the hypothetical lone "terrorist" imagined in pro-torture arguments. Torturing a single individual always assaults many—the individual, their families into at least the second generation, their friends and colleagues, as well as the communities from which they come. Reference to this literature is wholly absent from pro-torture arguments (see, for examples, Gorman 2001; Kagee 2004; Kordon 1997; Saporta and Van der Kolk 1992; Somnier et al. 1992; Vesti and Kastrup 1992). Furthermore, the testimony of torture survivors and former torturers is wholly unanalyzed (see, for examples, Amery 1995; Bunster 1993; Lomax 1995; Timmerman 1981, 2006). On the rare case when such accounts are even mentioned, they get dismissed as irrelevant appeals to emotion (for example, see Dershowitz 2004, 265).

The basic error is the belief that the question of the permissibility of torture is logically independent of its empirical history and possibilities. The dependence of pro-torture arguments on ticking bomb hypotheses is one example. Construction of a logical possibility demonstrates nothing about historical possibility. To discuss that, the history matters. Another example is Allhoff's (2005b, 257) assertion that the occurrence of ticking bomb scenarios is logically independent of the question as to torture's permissibility under such circumstances. Elsewhere he asserts the irrelevance of the truth or falsehood of the allegations about US torture to questions about the permissibility of torture. He believes that their empirical character makes them irrelevant (Allhoff 2006, 393). Stephen Kershnar's (2005, 223) willingness to claim that the events at Abu Ghraib have given interrogational torture a "bad name" is another example. There is no good name for torture to have, but to see this, attention to the empirical details is critical.

This *a priorism* leads to unsupported and false assertions. For example, Allhoff claims, with neither empirical nor historical support, that it is controversial whether American torture techniques should be described as tortures. The reason for this seems to be only intuition and the public statements of certain US government officials. The risk of an inappropriate appeal to authority is strong here. Similar problems arise with Jean Bethke Elshtain (2004, 85), Seumas Miller (2005, 179), Gross (2006, 227), and others who deny that "psychological" methods and stress positions are torture or claim that they are less severe than "physical" methods. There is a considerable historical, medical, and survivor literature available on the impacts of psychological torture methods. This literature uniformly rejects such unsupported intuitive judgments (see Lorentzen 1998; Conroy 2000; Malinowski 2006; McCoy 2006; Ratner and Ray 2004; Lunde and Ortmann 1992; Hinshelwood 1996; Lomax 1995; and Pokempner 2006 as a subset of the available evidence). Given this evidence, and absent a detailed empirical and conceptual argument to the contrary, the phrase "hostile interrogation" is just a euphemism for torture (cf., Allhoff 2006).

Careful empirical analysis of this same literature also undermines the category of interrogational torture. It demonstrates that torture is a multifunctional coercion strategy with inevitable gendered, terroristic, and intersubjective elements. Interrogation is a possible contingent purpose, but it is parasitic on these prior elements. The "pure" case of interrogational torture is an empirical impossibility—it would be the class of tortures that do not terrorize. Yet medical, sociological and historical reflection shows that while torture need not yield information, it can only terrorize populations. The category of interrogational torture only exists because of a lack of attention to the empirical details. If interrogational torture is an unacceptable category, then torture defenders either have to abandon defenses of torture, or they have to construct arguments for practices that are far more violent and messy. Either way, they should work with the empirical details.

As an applied ethical debate, the moral analysis of torture should proceed on analogy with other issues in environmental or biomedical ethics. That is, the science and the empirical facts matter. Ethical writing on germ-line engineering that pays no attention to the genetics would be inadequate. Even if valid, such arguments are unsound. The same point holds for torture, yet for some reason torture defenders pay no attention to any of the empirical issues. This worries me, because it raises the possibility that torture defenders do not understand torture. Again, attention to the institutional, historical, structural and medical complexities of torture is needed to avoid this criticism.

9 Can Torture Be Beneficent and Non-maleficent?

Allhoff (2006) argues that both non-malfeasance and beneficence require physicians to assist medically in torture sessions. Still, more disturbingly, he insists that they must assist not merely in the event that torture is permissible, but also when it is "occurrent." So, even if torture is an unjustifiable wrong, physicians have an obligation to assist in it. For, if they do not, then there is a greater risk of increased suffering, injury, and death than there would otherwise be. Preventable deaths and injuries will occur during torture sessions if physicians refuse to participate (Allhoff 2006, 294). Consequently, to refuse to assist in torture interrogations is wrong because it permits greater evil to occur than would otherwise happen. This puts physicians, nurses and psychiatrists in the strange position of having a greater obligation to participate in torture than even the torture interrogators—the latter at least have the option to refuse to torture where it is impermissible. Medical personnel are not so fortunate.

It is a mistake to think that the torturing physician, nurse, or psychiatrist acts with the interests of the torture victim in mind. Victims are never put in torture chambers for their own good; they are there so that some set of state interests might be achieved. Physicians are present to facilitate torture and aid in securing state interests. Furthermore, should perceived state security needs require the torture team to inflict suffering up to and including death, the torture physician will be obligated to help. The suffering the torture team inflicts is not motivated by the well-being of the victim, but by effectively securing some goal. Physician participation simply helps to make this more successful.

Allhoff's failure to pay attention to the multiplicity of roles that physicians play in torture matters here as well, since they are all consistent with perceived state security needs, but can only be harmful to the victim. In the torture setting, even resuscitation is compatible with malfeasance, as it is done to ensure the success of the interrogations. Suppose a psychiatrist develops a plan to play upon specific sexual phobias of an individual and then counsels a combination of sodomy with routine photographing of the torture as a potentially effective torture technique—this introduces an evil that would not otherwise exist. Consequently, there is no lesser evil decision concerning the health of the victim and the actions are simply malfeasant. The same goes for every role that medical personnel play. If the physician resuscitates a victim in order to face further suffering, then avoidable evils are introduced, and it is additionally likely that the victim will still die. This is fundamentally malevolent. Are physicians obligated to participate in every way? Allhoff, unfortunately, gives no answer.

The victim's interests have no significance in the torture session. In cases of torture, victim health and state interest are in logical conflict. Serving the one violates the other. Should physicians serve the former, then they harm state interests. If they prioritize the latter, they violate the victim. There is no middle road here. That in some cases physician intervention during torture may save the life or reduce injury is a contingent accident. For, to the extent that the victim's interests are primary, the physician, nurse or psychiatrist will attempt to prevent harm being done to the torture victim at all; to the extent that state interest is believed to trump the well-being of the torture victim, considerations of the victim's well-being will be irrelevant. This is not to say that physicians may not monitor health and try to keep torture victims alive, but this has to do with state rather than victim interest. In the emergency situation as torture defenders conceive it, state interest trumps that of the individual *a priori*.

Given that torture is intrinsically malevolent and given the automatic priority of state over victim interest in torture, there is no non-malfeasant state torture. Physician participation is similarly malfeasant and contravenes any plausible medical ethics.

10 Substituting Medically-Trained Interrogators for Doctors

Allhoff (2006) is aware that the previous arguments are not strong and develops an unusual argument to avoid the biomedical dilemmas. If doctors have a legal and professional obligation not to participate in torture, then states should refrain from using doctors and nurses for torture. Rather, they should make medical training an essential component of torture training (Allhoff 2006, 395). Should states choose this route, then the subject of torture is no longer a concern for doctors, nurses and psychiatrists at all. They become matters for military, intelligence and perhaps police ethics. Under these circumstances, there would be no medical professional code violations and no oath-breaking at all.

I believe this further exacerbates the violence. Physiological and psychological torture research has been going on for at least 60 years. Allhoff's suggestion guarantees that it will continue and intensify. This history is exceptionally violent and, given that it specifically studies the breaking of human beings, cannot be ethically performed—especially not under the ill-defined state-of-emergency conditions which supposedly justify torture. Removal of all of the elements of torture programs from the biomedical sphere simply creates a cadre of research personnel to support the torturers. Institutionalization problems are bad enough for the regular biomedical ethical community. The creation of a clinical and research community devoted to torture increases the harms, since the clinical and research norms of biomedical ethics could not apply to what must be an extensive program of research. The development and continuing refinement of the body of knowledge necessary to support torture will require a more or less constant flow of victims as well. To appreciate all of this, John Conroy (2000), Jennifer Harbury (2005), Alfred McCoy (2006) and Steven Niles (2006) are essential reading.

Allhoff (2006, 397–398) supposes that the propositional knowledge acquired by physicians, nurses and psychiatrists is a technical skill and thereby value-neutral. This is a further example of the *a priori* thinking which we have to abandon in applied ethics. Allhoff here invites us to treat technical, medical, and scientific knowledge in an historical and moral vacuum. This is exactly what we should never do. This is, however, an element from one side of an important epistemological debate. To evaluate this claim would require an excursion into the realism/anti-realism debate as well as some of the important claims from continental philosophy. The concept of value-neutrality of knowledge, particularly of medical expertise, is deeply controversial.

References

Allhoff, Fritz. 2005a. Terrorism and Torture. In *Philosophy 9/11: Thinking about the War on Terrorism*, ed. Timothy Shanahan. Peru, IL: Open Court Publishing.

Allhoff, Fritz. 2005b. A Defense of Torture: Separation of Cases, Ticking Time Bombs, and Moral Justification. *International Journal of Applied Philosophy* 19.2: 243–264.

Allhoff, Fritz. 2006. Physician Involvement in Hostile Interrogation. *Cambridge Quarterly of Healthcare Ethics* 15.2: 392–402.

Amery, Jean. 1995. Torture. In *Art from the Ashes: A Holocaust Anthology*, ed. Lawrence L. Langer, 121–137. New York: Oxford University Press.

Arrigo, Jean-Maria. 2004. A Utilitarian Argument Against Torture, Interrogation, and Terrorists. *Science and Engineering Ethics* 10.2: 543–572.

British Medical Association. 1992. *Medicine Betrayed: The Participation of Doctors in Human Rights Abuses*. London: Zed Books.

Bunster, Ximena. 1993. Surviving Beyond Fear: Women and Torture in South America. In *Surviving Beyond Fear: Women, Children and Human Rights in Latin America*, ed. Marjorie Agosin, 98–125. New York: White Pine.

Casebeer, William. 2005. Torture Interrogation of Terrorists: A Theory of Exceptions (With Notes, Cautions, and Warnings). In *Philosophy 9/11: Thinking about the War on Terrorism*, ed. Timothy Shanahan, 261–272. Peru, IL: Open Court Publishing.

Cesare, Beccaria, *On Crimes and Punishments* (Indianapolis, IN: Hackett, 1986 [1764]).

Conroy, John. 2000. *Unspeakable Acts, Ordinary People: The Dynamics of Torture*. New York: Alfred A. Knopf.

Dershowitz, Alan. 2004. Tortured Reasoning. In *Torture: A Collection*, ed. Sanford Levinson, 257–280. Oxford: Oxford University Press.

Elshtain, Jean Bethke. 2004. Reflections on the Problem of Dirty Hands. In *Torture: A Collection*, ed. Sanford Levinson, 77–92. Oxford: Oxford University Press.

Gorman, William. 2001. Refugee Survivors of Torture: Trauma and Treatment. *Professional Psychology, Research and Practice* 32.5: 443–451.

Gross, Michael. 2004. Doctors in the Decent Society: Torture, Ill-treatment, and Civic Duty. *Bioethics* 18.2: 181–203.

Gross, Michael. 2006. *Bioethics and Armed Conflict: Moral Dilemmas of Medicine and War*. Cambridge, MA: MIT.

Harbury, Jennifer. 2005. *Truth, Torture and the American Way: The History and Consequences of US Involvement in Torture*. Boston, MA: Beacon.

Hinshelwood, Gill. 1996. Women, Children, and the Family. In *Amnesty International, A Glimpse of Hell: Reports on Torture Worldwide*, ed. Duncan Forrest, 187–196. New York: New York University Press.

Human Rights Watch. 1994. *Torture and Ill-Treatment: Israel's Interrogation of Palestinians from the Occupied Territories*. New York: Human Rights Watch.

Jones, Gary. 1980. On the Permissibility of Torture. *Journal of Medical Ethics* 6 (March 1980): 11–13.

Kagee, Ashraf. 2004. Present Concerns of Survivors of Human Rights Violations in South Africa. *Social Science and Medicine* 59.3: 625–635.

Kant, Immanuel, *Perpetual Peace*, M. Campbell Smith, trans. (London: Swan Sonnenschein & Co, 1903 [1795]).

Kershner, Steven. 2005. For Interrogational Torture. *International Journal of Applied Philosophy* 19.2: 223–241.

Kordon, Diana. 1997. Impunity's Psychological Effects: Its Ethical Consequences. *Journal of Medical Ethics* 17 Suppl.: 29–32.

Kremnitzer, Mordechai. 1989. The Landau Commission Report — Was the Security Service Subordinated to the Law, or the Law to the 'Needs' of the Security Service? *Israel Law Review* 23.2–23.3: 216–279.

Lomax, Eric. 1995. *Railway Man*. London: Jonathon Cape.

Lorentzen, Lois-Ann. 1998. Women's Prison Resistance: Testimonials from El Salvador. In *The Women and War Reader*, eds. Lois-Ann Lorentzen and Jennifer Turpin, 192–203. New York: New York University Press.

Lunde, Inge and Jorgen Ortmann. 1992. Sexual Torture and the Treatment of Its Consequences. In *Torture and Its Consequences: Contemporary Treatment Approaches*, ed. Metin Basoglu, 310–331. Cambridge: Cambridge University Press.

Lowry, David. 1973. Ill-treatment, Brutality, and Torture: Some Thoughts on the Treatment of Irish Political Prisoners. *DePaul Law Review* 22: 216–279.

Malinowski, Tom. 2006. Banned State Department Practices. In *Torture: Does It Make Us Safer? Is It Ever OK? A Human Rights Perspective*, eds. Kenneth Roth, Minky Worden, and Amy Bernstein, 139–144. New York/London: The New Press.

McCoy, Alfred. 2006. *A Question of Torture: CIA Interrogation, from the Cold War to the War on Terror*. New York: Metropolitan Books.

Miller, Seumas. 2005. Is Torture Ever Morally Justifiable. *International Journal of Philosophy* 19.2: 179–192.

Niles, Steven. 2006. *Oath Betrayed: Torture, Medical Complicity, and the War on Terror*. New York: Random House.

Pokempner, Dinah. 2006. Command Responsibility for Torture. In *Torture: Does It Make Us Safer? Is It Ever OK? A Human Rights Perspective*. eds. Kenneth Roth, Minky Worden, and Amy Bernstein, 159–172. New York/London: The New Press.

Ratner, Michael and Ellen Ray. 2004. *Guantanamo: What the World Should Know*. Vermont: Chelsea Green Publishing.

Rawls, John. 1999. *The Law of Peoples*. Cambridge, MA: Harvard University Press.

Saporta, Jose Jr. and Bessel A. Van der Kolk. 1992. Psychobiological Consequences of Severe Trauma. In *Torture and Its Consequences: Current Treatment Approaches*, ed. Metin Basoglu, 310–331. Cambridge: Cambridge University Press.

Shue, Henry. 1978. Torture. *Philosophy and Public Affairs* 7.2: 124–143.

Somnier, Finn, Peter Vesti, Marianne Kastrup, and Inge Kemp-Genefke. 1992. Psycho-Social Consequences of Torture: Current Knowledge and Evidence. In *Torture and Its Consequences: Current Treatment Approaches*, ed. Metin Basoglu, 56–68. Cambridge: Cambridge University Press.

Timmerman, Hector. 2006. Torture: A Family Affair. In *Torture: Does It Make Us Safer? Is It Ever OK? A Human Rights Perspective*, eds. Kenneth Roth, Minky Worden, and Amy Bernstein. New York/London: The New Press.

Timmerman, Jacopo. 1981. *Prisoner Without a Name: Cell Without a Number*. New York: Alfred A. Knopf.

Twining, W.E. and P.E. Twining. 1973. Bentham on Torture. *Northern Ireland Legal Quarterly* 24: 307–356.

Vesti, Peter and Marianne Kastrup. 1992. Psychotherapy for Torture Survivors. In *Torture and Its Consequences: Current Treatment Approaches*, ed. Metin Basoglu, 348–362. Cambridge: Cambridge University Press.

Convention Against Torture and Other Cruel, Inhuman, or Degrading Treatment or Punishment (entered into force 26 June 1984). http://www.unhchr.ch/html/menu3/b/h_cat39.htm. Cited 4 June 2007.

Declaration on the Protection of All Persons from Being Subjected to Torture and Other Cruel, Inhuman or Degrading Treatment or Punishment. (Adopted by General Assembly Resolution 3452(xxx) of 9 December 1975. http://www.unhchr.ch/html/menu3/b/h_comp38.htm. Cited 4 June 2007.

Principles of Medical Ethics Relevant to the Role of Health Personnel, Particularly Physicians, in the Protection of Prisoners and Detainees Against Torture and Other Cruel, Inhuman, or Degrading Treatment or Punishment. (Adopted by General Assembly Resolution 37/194 of 18 December, 1982.) http://www.unhchr/ch/html/menu3/b/h_comp40.htm. Cited 4 June 2007.

The World Medical Association Declaration of Tokyo: Guidelines for Physicians Concerning Torture and Other Cruel, Inhuman, or Degrading Treatment or Punishment in Detention and Imprisonment. (Adopted by the 29th World Medical Assembly, Tokyo, Japan, October 1975. http://www.wma.net/e/policy/c18.htm.) Cited 4 June 2007.

Torture and the Regulation of the Health Care Professions*

John Lunstroth

1 Introduction

The press is filled with reports of torture committed by members of the US government. All too frequently these reports contain disturbing references to "health care" personnel such as medical doctors, psychologists, social workers and others. Although the reports of global US-sponsored torture are often presented as though it is something new in response to security concerns after 9/11, in fact the US has had explicit policies condoning torture and torture facilities since the early cold-war period, and medical personnel have always been involved.[1]

Stories about doctors involved with torture routinely contain statements that doctors are bound by a "code of ethics" that prohibits them from participating in torture. The question is, though, of what use is the code of ethics if doctors are a necessary part of torture and torture is practiced by 150 countries?[2] Are there situations in which doctors are required, but the medical code of ethics is not allowed? Are there two kinds of doctors, those that can assist in torture, and those that cannot? Are there laws regarding torture that exempt doctors?

The idea of doctors involved with torture is morally troubling because national security norms allow for acts towards life that are abhorrent to the values of Hippocratic medicine. National security concerns itself with protection of the sovereign state in the international arena. It is partially constrained by constitutional rule

*The citations for this essay have been rendered according to law journal conventions—as opposed to those exercised in the rest of the Volume—per the preferences of the author and his primary audience.

[1] *See generally*, Steven Miles, OATH BETRAYED: TORTURE, MEDICAL COMPLICITY, AND THE WAR ON TERROR (2006); Physicians for Human Rights et al., *Dual Loyalty & Human Rights In Health Professional Practice: Proposed Guidelines & Institutional Mechanisms* (2002), at http://www.physiciansforhumanrights.org/library/documents/reports/report-2002-duelloyalty.pdf, accessed December 16, 2006; British Medical Association, THE MEDICAL PROFESSION AND HUMAN RIGHTS: HANDBOOK FOR A CHANGING AGENDA 43–162 (2001). Naomi Klein, *'Never Before!' Our Amnesiac Torture Debate*, The Nation, December 8, 2005, accessed online December 12, 2006 at *http://www.thenation.com/doc/20051226/klein*.

[2] Amnesty International, *Stop Torture* (2001), at http://web.amnesty.org/library/index/engACT760012001?open&of=eng-326, accessed June 20, 2007.

F. Allhoff (ed.), *Physicians at War: The Dual-Loyalties Challenge*.

of law (in the US), but since the sovereign is an international actor, the norms that directly constrain it are gathered under the rubric of public international law. Generally speaking, international law has two relevant bodies of norms regarding life those regarding war (law of war, or international humanitarian law) and those regarding human rights. The law of war, at both the theoretical and practical levels (*ius ad bellum* and *ius in bello*, respectively) recognizes and accepts the possibility of physical and mental injury of all severities, including death. Such injury is deemed acceptable for soldiers and civilians, although civilian injuries are to be minimized. It accepts that wars and other sanctions can result in severe health pressures on civilian populations from loss of civil and public health infrastructure, disruption of food production and distribution, and so on. Thus, national security norms devalue human life both at the individual and population level in the interest of protecting the sovereign. Interrogations that devolve into, or are planned as, torture or cruel, inhuman and degrading treatment or punishment are undertaken both for external security (e.g., Guantanamo detainees) and for internal security (law enforcement).

The troubling aspect of medical personnel involved with torture involves more than a conflict of the normative regimes of different social institutions (national security and medicine). It is troublesome because it points to a profound problem in the social role, self-identification, and regulation of the profession of medicine. Medical education is intended to convey a minimum set of scientific competencies in graduates of medical schools. It is well understood to be seriously lacking in what is referred to as "the humanities." This is significant because "medical ethics" is, if anything, associated with, or an aspect of, the humanities. Medical ethics, the norms that are potentially in direct conflict with national security, are not essential to the values of education in scientific medicine. Therefore, there is at best only an accidental relationship between medical ethics and medical education. Doctors who have Hippocratic ethics, have them in spite of medical education, not as a result of it. Compounding the problem is the regulatory structure of medicine. Licensure in the US is state-based, but the medically trained personnel required for national security ends work in an international environment far removed from state- and patient-based practice. The social conception of doctors in the state-based, early 20th century, paradigm is as a unified profession, and such problems construed as dual-loyalty problems. Doctors are put in situations where they are said to have loyalty to their patient and to their employer at the same time. But if the loyalty to patients is based on medical ethics, then it is clear only a subset of doctors could ever have dual-loyalty problems as an ethical matter. Since ethical norms against torture do not apply to some medically trained persons, it is important to know if any legal norms apply. Because the interrogations that are at issue take place in the normative regime of national security, legal norms (including human rights norms) prohibiting torture are strong, but the enforcement mechanism is weak. In light of the foregoing, the idea of medical ethics categorically prohibits the involvement of medical doctors in torture can clearly be seen to be a social construction with little substantive force.

I examine the questions raised by the weakness of medical ethics in the face of strong national security norms. In the first section of the paper I consider national security norms regarding torture. What was once a clear US legal norm against torture has been considerably weakened in the wake of 9/11. Many moral arguments have been asserted in its favor justifying the Bush Administration's *de facto* use of torture as a national security policy. Since medical personnel are required for interrogations that include torture and cruel, inhuman and degrading treatment or punishment, the ethical and legal position of the medical personnel has been also made more unclear. In the second section of the paper I examine both the legal and ethical norms applicable to medically trained persons, especially medical doctors. Medical ethicists and legal commentators both are loath to assign to medical personnel any more than an ethical duty not to support torture. The lack of clear norms in both national security and the medical institutions regarding interrogations that require medical inputs, and the lack of clear norms guiding medical personnel acting in national security settings, has brought into stark relief the insufficiency of the existing norms regulating medical personnel in these situations.

I conclude by proposing two independent regulatory approaches to the problem of health care providers[3] (HCPs) and torture. I begin with the observation that HCPs are regulated by the states, that state-based regulation does not by design look beyond state borders, and that it fails on two fronts. First, it does not distinguish between the two types of employment facing its graduates, work primarily for patients, or primarily for an institution. Beyond the general training, those whose primary loyalty will be to patients should be on one track, those whose primary loyalty will be to institutions should be on another track, and the licensing scheme should recognize that. Second, the legally mandated adherence of the licensee to a code of ethics is weakened to virtual non-existence at the state border. The state should criminalize torture for every HCP that trains or ever has privileges in the state. Each of these failures or inefficiencies can be remedied by statute in such a way that the state functions to implement the otherwise weak code of ethics.

2 The National Security Norm

Interrogation is national security tool. Torture and cruel, inhuman and degrading treatment or punishment (hereinafter "torture") describe certain kinds of interrogation.[4] Torture is prohibited in international and domestic law. International laws criminalizing

[3] I use the terms "health care providers," "health care personnel," "medically trained personnel," and similar terms interchangeably to refer to persons with medical training and a license to "see patients" as independent professionals. *See* Section 3, infra.

[4] Torture includes being beaten and tortured to death, the rape of men, women and children of both sexes, and other techniques such as water-boarding, electric shocks to genitalia, and use of extreme temperatures (Abu Ghraib); and severe beatings, threats by vicious dogs, and the violent insertion of naso-gastric tubes into hunger-strikers (Guantanamo). Torture is distinguished from cruel, inhuman and degrading treatment or punishment. *See, e.g.*, Ireland v. The United Kingdom—

it include the Geneva Conventions, the International Covenant on Civil and Political Rights (ICCPR), the Rome Statute (establishing the International Criminal Court), and the Convention Against Torture and Cruel, Inhuman and Degrading Treatment or Punishment (CAT). In international law the status of the law against torture is absolute. It is a peremptory norm, a norm *ius cogens*, meaning that, although derogation from other norms is allowed under certain circumstances, it is in the class of special norms from which no derogation is allowed. There are no exceptions to the prohibition against torture.[5]

Torture and cruel, inhuman and degrading treatment or punishment (CID) is criminalized in the US for civilians, the military and military contractors in several statutes.[6] In addition to a purely domestic prohibition, the War Crimes Act of 1996 incorporates provisions of the Geneva Conventions, including common Article 3, which prohibits "violence to life and person, in particular murder of all kinds, mutilation, cruel treatment and torture; ... outrages upon personal dignity, in particular humiliating and degrading treatment."

Aiding and abetting torture is also a crime, punishable as though the person aiding and abetting was a principle.[7] The law of aiding and abetting is lengthy and detailed, but it is clear HCPs that participate at any stage of the torture, whether present or not, can be found liable under these rules. For example, the Court held, in Kvocka et al. (Trial Chamber), November 2, 2001, para. 262:

> The aider or abettor of persecution, as a 'special intent' crime, must not only have knowledge of the crime he is assisting or facilitating. He must also be aware that the crimes

---

5310/71 [1978] ECHR 1, §167 (8 January 1978). *But see*, Anthony Cullen, *Defining Torture in International Law: A Critique of the Concept of Employed by the European Court of Human Rights*, 34 Cal. W. Int'l L.J. 29 (2003) (there exists on the one hand violence which is to be condemned both on moral grounds and also in most cases under the domestic law of the Contracting States [and] it appears on the other hand that it was the intention that the Convention, with its distinction between "torture" and "inhuman or degrading treatment", should by the first of these terms attach a special stigma to deliberate inhuman treatment causing very serious and cruel suffering). *See also*, General Assembly of the United Nations, Resolution 3452 (XXX), Article 1, 9 December 1975 ("Torture constitutes an aggravated and deliberate form of cruel, inhuman or degrading treatment or punishment").

[5] The Geneva Conventions and Protocols, at http://www.icrc.org/Web/Eng/siteeng0.nsf/html/genevaconventions, accessed 12/17/2006; International Covenant on Civil and Political Rights, G.A. res. 2200A (XXI), 21 U.N. GAOR Supp. (No. 16) at 52, U.N. Doc. A/6316 (1966), 999 U.N.T.S. 171, entered into force Mar. 23, 1976; Covenant Against Torture and Other Cruel, Inhuman or Degrading Treatment or Punishment, G.A. res. 39/46, annex, 39 U.N. GAOR Supp. (No. 51) at 197, U.N. Doc. A/39/51 (1984), *entered into force* June 26, 1987 (Signed by the US April 18, 1988, ratified October 21, 1994); ROME STATUTE OF THE INTERNATIONAL CRIMINAL COURT, U.N. Doc. 2187 U.N.T.S. 90, entered into force July 1, 2002.

[6] Uniform Code of Military Justice (UCMJ, Arts. 77–134); The War Crimes Act of 1996 (18 USC. §2441); the federal anti-torture statute (18 USC. §2340A); Torture Victims Protection Act of 1991, 28 USC.A. §1350 (2004); Military Extraterritorial Jurisdiction Act of 2000 (Public Law 106–778).

[7] Crimes and Criminal Procedure, Title 18 USC.A. §2 (Principals). *See also*, Human Rights Watch, *Case Law of the International Criminal Tribunal for the Former Yugoslavia*, Art 7(1), at http://hrw.org/reports/2004/ij/icty/index.htm, accessed 12.16.2006.

being assisted or supported are committed with a discriminatory intent. The aider or abettor of persecution does not need to share the discriminatory intent, but must be aware of the broader discriminatory context and know that his acts of assistance or encouragement have a significant effect on the commission of the crimes. Each and every act of discrimination need not be known or intended by the aider or abettor. The aider or abettor of persecution will thus be held responsible for discriminatory acts committed by others that were a reasonably foreseeable consequence of their assistance or encouragement.

The destruction of 9/11 shook the foundations of the foregoing laws in the US, as the executive branch of the federal government took a very aggressive stance and declared "war on terrorism." Although there are many narratives as to what subsequently happened, and the details are still coming to the surface, it is safe to say the Administration sought to evade the absolute prohibition on torture. The scandals of Guantanamo, Bagram, Abu Ghraib, the CIA "black prisons," and other incidents followed, as well as many lawsuits.[8]

In response to the scandals, the republican Congress passed the McCain Amendment, legislation that purports to limit torture and CID. Unfortunately, it came with problems. Some commentators see it as acknowledgement torture is now official US policy. Simultaneously the Graham-Levin Amendment was passed permitting the use of information received during torture and making it harder for torture victims to access the US courts to sue US torturers. Later, in the summer of 2006, the Supreme Court of the US ruled that common Article Three of the Geneva Conventions was the law of the US, unless Congress passed a law limiting it. The republican Congress responded to the Supreme Court by passing, in October 2006, the Military Commissions Act. In this legislation Congress gave indemnity to all US personnel who may have been in violation of the War Crimes Act (prohibiting torture and other violations of the Geneva Conventions), took the right of habeas corpus from all non-citizens with no contacts with US territory, and amended the War Crimes Act to make finding a violation based on torture more difficult.[9] Under the new laws, taken in conjunction with the Presidential signing statements and proposed amendments to the Armed Forces Manual sections dealing with torture, it appears torture and CID (albeit by different names) have become the official policy of the US.[10]

The forceful attempts by the Administration to change the law of torture in the US has resulted in an extraordinary moral analysis of torture. Academics and pundits of all stripes weighed in to justify and oppose the behavior and desires of

[8] Center for Constitutional Rights, *War Crimes Complaint Against Rumsfeld, et al.*, at http://www.ccr-ny.org/v2/GermanCase2006/germancase.asp, accessed December 18, 2006. The complaint includes allegations of war crimes against the lawyers (professionals) who provided the legal justification for derogating from the absolute prohibitions against torture and CID.

[9] *See*, Kathleen Duignan, *The Military Commissions Act of 2006: 'Play it Again, [Uncle] Sam.'* The Jurist (December 12, 2006), at http://jurist.law.pitt.edu/forumy/2006/12/military-commissions-act-of-2006-play.php, accessed 12/19/06.

[10] *See, e.g.*, David Cole, *Sanctioning Lawlessness*, The Nation (October 23, 2006), at http://www.thenation.com/doc/20061023/cole, accessed 12/23/2006 ("abusive interrogations").

their government, and ambiguate the issue.[11] Most arguments focus on the "ticking bomb" scenario. A thorough analysis of the various "ticking bomb" justifications is beyond the scope of this paper.[12] Legally the ticking-bomb scenario is moot. It is illegal to perform torture or CID. It is important to recall it *is* illegal because of the murkiness in moral analysis caused by the Bush Administration. HCPs, and other sensible people, may be led to think torture and CID have somehow become acceptable because the administration argues forcefully "we" ought to be able to torture in the war on terror because the enemy is ferocious, exceedingly dangerous, and does not fight by the rules of the Geneva Conventions. There are no ticking bomb exceptions to the absolute prohibition on torture, except as perhaps found in US law now, but those laws contravene international law and probably will not withstand constitutional scrutiny in the long run. The position against the ticking bomb scenario was recently enunciated by the Israeli Supreme Court. It held:

> 64. In one case we decided the question whether the state is permitted to order its interrogators to employ special methods of interrogation which involve the use of force against terrorists, in a "ticking bomb" situation. We answered that question in the negative. In my judgment, I described the difficult security situation in which Israel finds itself, and added:

---

[11] An analysis of the effect on expert morality of the "sovereign sentence" would be extremely interesting, especially in light of ancient link between the form of government (as law) and the idea of justice. *See, e.g.*, Peter Fenves, *The Sovereign Sentence: Kant and the Deportation of Justice*, in LAW, JUSTICE, AND POWER: BETWEEN REASON AND WILL 97–114 (Sinkwan Cheng, ed. 2004). For example, Aristotle argued that law is a reflection of justice (but not in all cases). *See* John Lunstroth, *Linking Virtue and Justice: Aristotle on the Melian Dialogue*, 12 International Legal Theory 99 (2007). Therefore, if the government changes the law, the popular perception of what is just will also change, i.e., morality will have been legislated. For an anti-torture analysis, with reference to liberal arguments pro and con, *see* David Luban, *Liberalism, Torture, and the Ticking Bomb*, Virginia Law Review 1425 (2005). *But see*, Mirko Bagaric and Julie Clarke, *Not Enough Official Torture in the World? The Circumstances in Which Torture is Morally Justifiable*, 39 USF.L. Rev. 581 (2005) (arguing the ticking-bomb scenario provides moral justification for legalizing torture).

[12] Is torture and CID morally justified? Torture involves three sacrifices. The obvious sacrifice is the individual who will be tortured. Less obvious are the other two sacrifices. The torturer's moral status is sacrificed, and the rule of law is sacrificed. Utilitarianism is about "happiness," but happiness as that term might be used by Aristotle, not Billy Graham. It refers to the ability of the polity to flourish. I argue that the sacrifice of the rule of law is too great to make in terms of the "happiness" of society. Rather, if torture is thought at the actual time and place of the scenario to be the only way to get the information, the legal burden is better to fall on the torturers. Torture and CID should be illegal, and the exception made on a case by case basis by a jury of peers. *See, e.g.*, Paola Gaeta, *May Necessity Be Available as a Defence for Torture in the Interrogation of Suspected Terrorists?* 2 J. Int. Criminal Justice 785 (2004). As the recent admonition of the chief warrant officer who stuffed a general in a sleeping bag and suffocated him to death, after he had been "softened up" by 2 days of beatings with a rubber hose, testifies, the moral insufficiency of the American people is not to be underestimated. Human Rights First, *Command's Responsibility: Detainee Deaths in US Custody in Iraq and Afghanistan*, at http://www.humanrightsfirst.org/us_law/etn/dic/mowhoush.asp, accessed 12/18/06. The rule of law is [said to be] synonymous with civilization and it underlies the rights cosmopolitan liberals value most—equality and liberty—and it cannot be sacrificed without profound penalty. *See also id.*, David Luban, *Liberalism, Torture, and the Ticking Bomb*; Mirko Bagaric and Julie Clarke, *Not Enough Official Torture in the World?*

> "We are aware that this judgment of ours does not make confronting that reality any easier. That is the fate of democracy, in whose eyes not all means are permitted, and to whom not all the methods used by her enemies are open. At times democracy fights with one hand tied behind her back. Despite that, democracy has the upper hand, since preserving the rule of law and recognition of individual liberties constitute an important component of her security stance. At the end of the day, they strengthen her and her spirit, and allow her to overcome her difficulties (HCJ 5100/94 *The Public Committee against Torture in Israel v. The State of Israel*, 53(4) PD 817, 845).[13]

HCPs are called on to facilitate, participate in and cover up torture and CID in many ways. They can be involved in planning torture,[14] both generically and for specific prisoners; in carrying out torture, e.g., by administering drugs, monitoring health status, or withholding care; and in the follow-up, e.g., by administering health care to injured prisoners, by saying nothing and by falsifying medical records and death reports.[15] Given the highly ambiguous status of the laws against torture in the US, and the DOD policy of screening HCPs that are assigned to places where torture is carried out to exclude those who oppose torture,[16] all HCPs that work for the military, whether in uniform or not, are on notice that they may be asked to aid and abet torture or CID. This is important because it goes to the requirement that in order to aid and abet there must be some assent to the illegal behavior. In other words, it negates defenses to charges of aiding and abetting torture or CID in which lack of *mens rea*, of intention to participate, is alleged. There is nothing that gives HCPs exemption from the statutes that prohibit torture or CID, or that prohibit aiding and abetting torture and CID.

---

[13] HCJ 769/02 The Public Committee against Torture in Israel v. The Government of Israel—Summary of Judgment 42 (December 14, 2006), at http://elyon1.court.gov.il/eng/verdict/search_eng/verdict_by_case_rslt.asp?case_nbr_html=HCJ 769%2F02, accessed December 18, 2006.

[14] For the development by the Central Intelligence Agency of the *Kubark Counterintelligence Interrogation* (CIA manual), *see* Alfred McCoy, A Question of Terror: CIA Interrogation, from the Cold War to the War on Terror 1–59 (2006). *See also*, Drake Bennet, *The war in the mind*, The Boston Globe (November 27, 2005), at http://www.boston.com/news/globe/ideas/articles/2005/11/27/the_war_in_the_mind, accessed November 28, 2005; Shankar Vedantam, *Medical Experts Debate Role in Facilitating Interrogations*, Washington Post A19 (November 14, 2005).

[15] *See, e.g.*, Miles, Oath Betrayed, *supra* note 1, at 41–140; British Medical Association, The Medical Profession, *supra* note 1, at 56–129; Physicians for Human Rights, *Dual-Loyalty, supra* note 1, at 26–50. *See also, e.g.*, Linda M. Keller, *Is Truth Serum Torture*, 20 Am. U. Int'l L. Rev. 521 (2005); David Weissbrodt, Ferhat Pekin and Amelia Wilson, *Piercing the Confidentiality Veil: Physician Testimony in International Criminal Trials Against Perpetrators of Torture*, 15 Minn. J. Intl L. 43 (2006). For an example of how physicians can help bring perpetrators to justice, *see* Katherine J. Eder, *The Importance of Medical Testimony in Removal Hearings fro Torture Victims*, 7 DePaul J. Health Care L. 281 (2004).

[16] George Annas, *Hunger Strikers at Guantanamo—Medical Ethics and Human Rights in a "Legal Black Hole,"* 355:13 N. Eng. J. Med. 1377, 1380 (2006).

In summary, torture is highly illegal, in spite of the attempted derogation by the US.[17] HCPs who work for the US government are on notice they may be asked or ordered to aid and abet torture; i.e., are and will be at risk to become criminals.

3 Legal Norms in Medicine

In the US the health care professions are regulated by the states. The theory justifying regulation of the professions is primarily derived from the duty of the state to protect citizens from potentially dangerous agencies using its police and *parens patriae* powers.[18] The US Department of Labor lists 42 categories of healthcare and medical technology occupations, including M.Ds. and D.Os.[19] All are regulated on a state by state basis through a "practice act" that regulates the profession. Regulation is usually accomplished through licensing, but certification and registration are also used. Most practice acts can be characterized as "statutory self-regulation." That is, the profession is delegated the power of the state to regulate itself through a board that promulgates and enforces rules, issues licenses, and "protects" the profession's turf in the legislature. Only persons with valid state licenses can practice legally, and then only in the states in which they are licensed.[20]

Each practice act has a "scope-of-practice" (SOP) section that describes what health care acts the licensee may legally undertake after being licensed. Some SOPs include the authority to make independent decisions affecting the welfare of the client. That is, some SOPs recognize that the licensee has been trained to "see patients" without supervision for defined services. It is this group of HCPs I refer to in this paper.

Licensure is granted upon demonstration of a minimal set of competencies. The minimal set of competencies is generally related to the scope of practice of the license, and generally speaking overlap between licenses is kept to a minimum, with one major exception. The license granted M.Ds. has frequently been interpreted to cover all health care disciplines, except as carved out by statute.

In most cases, as a condition of being granted a license by a profession that is statutorily self-regulated, the HCP also agrees to be bound by the profession's code

---

[17] *But see*, Marti Koskeniemmi, *Hierarchy in International Law*, EJIL web site, 4 ("In times of social or political tension the development of … legal discourse is disturbed and grey zones … appear. The stable structures of 'lawful/unlawful' that organize so much of social control are blurred and possibly reversed: property becomes theft, theft property"); Foucault, Discipline and Punish, infra note 22 (describing the condition of the state in which torture is legal in a way that remarkably mirrors press reports of the Bush Administration's attitudes to the acts committed on detainees in the "global war on terror").

[18] Lawrence Gostin, Public Health Law: Power, Duty, Restraint 47–59 (2000).

[19] US Department of Labor, Bureau of Labor Statistics, Occupational Employment and Wages, November 2004, at http://www.bls.gov/oes/current/oes290000.htm (accessed 11/23/06).

[20] John Lunstroth, *Voluntary Self-Regulation of Complementary and Alternative Medicine Practitioners*, 70:1 Albany L. Rev. 101 (2006).

of conduct. In this way a code of conduct that is voluntary becomes mandatory. The condition of the privilege of the license is that a breach of the code of conduct can result in forfeiture of the privilege, and other civil and criminal penalties. The profession can seek promulgation of, and regulate, civil and criminal penalties as a delegee of state police powers. These mandatory codes of conduct, codes of conduct that have legal effect, more or less stop at the state's border. They are parochial geographically, and have no more than incidental effect in the federal and international domains.[21]

HCPS can be distinguished by their type of employment. Among other things, they can make a living treating individuals for health or enhancement, they can be involved in larger social structures in the health care system distributing resources, they can be engaged in human subjects research, they can work as independent contractors using their expertise for any purpose, or they can be involved in international organizations such as the military. These types of employment can be aligned on a scale. At one end is the HCP treating individuals for health issues with more or less full legal and professional authority to use their professional judgment, and at the other is the employment situation in which professional authority is heavily circumscribed by virtue of employment (not the SOP) and in which the professional has legal, ethical and institutional loyalty to their employer.

There is no one point on the spectrum in which these two poles become separate. Most HCPs who see patients have to limit their practice according to health care

---

[21] The Medical Board of California rejected a complaint against a military doctor licensed in California, the chief medical officer at Guantanamo, Captain John Edmondson, on grounds the Army's surgeon general had not found misconduct, and therefore it had no jurisdiction. Janice Hopkins Tanne, *Lawyers will appeal ruling that cleared Guantanamo doctor of ethics violations*, 331 British Med. J. 180 (2005) (Edmondson is licensed in California and Georgia, and as of December 20, 2006, no complaints have been registered in his profiles on the web sites of the respective medical boards.). *But see*, David Nicholl et al., *Forcefeeding and restraint of Guantanamo Bay hunger strikers*, 367:9513 The Lancet 811 (2006) (letter signed by 262 doctors claiming Guantanamo medical personnel were in violation of medical ethics as expressed in World Medical Association's Declaration of Tokyo). David Nicholl, lead author of the letter to The Lancet and chairman of the British Medical Association's ethics committee, was a complainant in the California case. *See also*, Andre Sofair and Peter G. Lurie, *Military Medicine and Human Rights*, 364 The Lancet 1851 (2004) (placing value on license revocation for HCPs "found guilty"). But Stephen Xenakis, a former brigadier general in charge of the Southeast Regional Army Medical Command, and subsequently a member of Physicians for Human Rights USA, doubts the efficacy of complaints against individual doctors. He thinks the "best answer is for the professional associations to … put pressure on the Department of Defense to change … policy." *Quoted in*, Owen Dyer, *Force Feeding at Guantanamo breaches ethics, doctors say*, 332 British Med. J. 569 (March 11, 2006). *See also*, Michael Wilks, *Guantanamo: a call for action: Doctors and their professional bodies can do more than they think*, 332 British Med. J. 560 (March 11, 2006). After some dithering for the Bush Administration, the AMA came out against force feeding of detainees and physician participation in torture and CID. Dyer, *Force Feeding at Guantanamo, id.*; American Medical Association, *Letter to the Editor of the Nation: AMA Unconditionally Condemns Physician Participation in Torture* (December 20, 2005), at http://www.ama-assn.org/ama/pub/category/15937.html, accessed December 20, 2006.

coverages, may work for MCOs, or are otherwise somewhat circumscribed in their professional judgment. On the other hand, HCPs who work designing resource distribution policy for an insurance company, as researchers, or in the military may see patients as independent practitioners. In these latter situations the loyalty to the employer or enterprise is such that if that HCP were to see a patient in the context of their job (not independently) there would be serious legal, ethical and employment issues related to their divided loyalty.[22]

The regulatory scheme described above was developed in the late 19th century. Then physicians treated cases of human disease in their patients on a one-on-one basis. There were no conflicts of loyalty. The practical realities of medical training and practice have long outgrown their regulatory framework.

The ability of the profession to regulate itself has important and interrelated limitations. First, the authority of the medical board only extends to current licensees. If an M.D. loses her license for any reason, and then practices medicine, the state board has no authority over that person. Rather, she will have committed a violation of a civil or criminal law, and investigation and enforcement will be by local law enforcement. Second, the authority only extends to the state borders. In general, if an M.D. licensed in one state travels to another state and practices medicine, that M.D. is violating the law of the second state, but not the first. The regulation of medicine stops at state borders.

The Department of Defense, Health Affairs Policy 05-006, Medical Program Principles and Procedures for the Protection and Treatment of Detainees in the Custody of the Armed Forces of the United States (June 3, 2005) (the "Policy"), provides an example of how a federal employer subjects state-licensed doctors to superseding rules that can contradict the state-based professional regulations. All Armed Forces health care personnel with detainee contact are to receive training in the principles and policies described in the Policy.[23]

The Policy covers "health care personnel of the Armed Forces" including physicians, nurses, contractor personnel, and, significantly, "[h]ealth care personnel engaged in non-treatment activities, such as forensic psychology or psychiatry, behavioral science consultation, forensic pathology, or similar disciplines."

It distinguishes between HCPs that have a "professional provider-patient treatment relationship with detainees," and those that do not. Those that do "shall not undertake detainee-related activities for purposes other than health care purposes." Those that *do not* have a "professional provider-patient treatment relationship," i.e., HCP "engaged in non-treatment activities, such as forensic psychology[,] … shall not also engage in any professional provider-patient treatment relationship with detainees."

The Policy provides principles that are only applicable to those HCPs charged with the provider-patient relationship, and principles applicable to all HCPs. HCPs

[22] *See, e.g.*, International Dual Loyalty Working Group, Dual Loyalty & Human Rights In Health Professional Practice; Proposed Guidelines & Institutional Mechanisms (2002). http://www.phrusa.org/healthrights/dl.html.

[23] *See* Department of Defense, Health Affairs Policy 05-019, *Training for Health Care Providers in Detainee Operations* (October 13, 2005).

who have a treatment relationship "have a duty to protect [the detainee's] physical and mental health and provide appropriate treatment for disease." Furthermore, it contravenes DoD policy for such HCPs "to be involved in any professional provider-patient treatment relationship with detainees the purpose of which is not solely to evaluate, protect or improve their physical and mental health."

For all HCPs, it is a contravention of DoD policy:

- To apply their knowledge and skills in order to assist in the interrogation of detainees in a manner that is not in accordance with applicable law
- To certify, or to participate in the certification of, the fitness of detainees for any form of treatment or punishment that is not in accordance with applicable law, or to participate in any way in the infliction of any such treatment or punishment

Given that the law of the US is at best ambiguous, and at worst directly authorizes torture and CID (albeit by different names), then this policy well illustrates that HCPs can be called on to aid and abet torture and CID. That is most clear for those HCPs that do not have a "provider-patient relationship." They are not limited to simply providing health care services. But those that do have such relationships can use their knowledge and skills "in accordance with the law." If the amended Armed Forces Manual, taken in conjunction with the McCain Amendment, indeed authorizes torture and CID, then this policy clearly allows HCPs to provide services before, after and during the torture or CID. Against this is the backdrop of the military command structure. If a uniformed officer refuses orders, he or she can be court-martialed. In other words, DoD policy may require HCPs to violate international criminal law prohibiting torture and CID.

The state-based regulatory scheme described above is no longer responsive to societal needs. That section of the social contract no longer reflects the relationship between medically trained persons and society.[24] It is now clear each health care

[24] *See, e.g.*, Chalmers Clark, *infra* note 28, at 5 (arguing the "medical profession is a socially endowed moral autonomy," deriving its power from the trust of the public (the social contract), and that such trust diminishes to the extent the profession does not prioritize patient benefit). A discussion of the contemporary social contract between the medical profession and the polity would be valuable, especially in light of the recognition of an emerging international norm of democratic governance (or, the right to democratic governance). This norm, or its cognates, such as the proposed "principle of democratic inclusion," posit the just society as one in which the polity has the right to engage in the setting of its ethical, social and legal norms, domestically and internationally. In other words, the interested polity is no longer just the polity of the US, but includes the international community broadly construed. *See, e.g.*, Susan Marks, THE RIDDLE OF ALL CONSTITUTIONS: INTERNATIONAL LAW, DEMOCRACY, AND THE CRITIQUE OF IDEOLOGY (2000). The DC Circuit recently held that the fundamental right to bodily integrity includes the right for an individual to determine which medicine he or she takes, regardless of its efficacy; threatening the structure established by the Drug Amendments of 1962 on which the research enterprise is largely based, and threatening FDA jurisdiction over the *efficacy* (not safety) of drugs. Abigail Alliance for Better Access to Developmental Drugs v. von Eschenbach, 445 F.3d 470, 484–486 (D.C.Cir.2006); rehearing denied at 469 F.3rd 129. When one considers the foregoing developments in light of the fact only some 10% of doctors work in the fee-for-service model on which "medical ethics" is based, and the fact that in no other countries do doctors have the

profession can regulate itself, that the state legislatures and boards of health are competent to regulate the ordinary practice of medicine, and that in significant cases the existing state-limited regulatory model is insufficient.

4 Ethical Norms

The basis of moral outrage when doctors support torture or CID is the idea that status as a doctor is conditioned on adherence to the principles of medical ethics "first do no harm" (*primum non nocere*) and primary loyalty to the patient. References to "medical ethics" are made as though their mere existence establishes a sacred duty that can never be breached by a doctor, as though it has the status of positive law.[25] The statements are often made in such a way as to place the moral culpability on the institution or other that forced the doctor to engage or be complicit in torture.

---

same social authority they do in the US, it is reasonable to conclude that the social meaning of medicine as a profession has moved so far from its roots as to completely undercut the shared assumptions (the meeting of the minds) on which the original social contract with the profession was based. There is no longer any substantial consideration for the social grant of authority to the medical profession (broadly construed). The deal must be renegotiated. General arguments that society should *strengthen* medical authority underestimate economic and institutional pressures on graduates of medical schools and lack sufficient nuance to achieve their ends. *See, e.g.*, Michael Gottlieb, *Executions and Torture: The Consequences of Overriding Professional Ethics*, 6 Yale J. Health Pol'y & Ethics 351 (2006); note 28, *infra*. On another level, the ideology of the medical profession is ripe for more transformative critique. *See* Susan Marks, The Critique of Ideology, id., at 121–151 (drawing on Marx's idea of critique, as opposed to criticism, as developed by Horkheimer, Habermas and Foucault). *See, e.g.*, Michel Foucault, The Birth of the Clinic: An Archeology of Medical Perception (Sheridan Smith, tr. 1994) (a critique of medicine, including the medical profession); Harry Marks, The Progress of Experiment: Science and Therapeutic Reform in the US, 1900–1990 (1997) (a critique of medical epistemology). *See also*, Michel Foucault, Discipline and Punish: The Birth of the Prison 3–69 (Alan Sheridan, tr. 1977) (a critique of torture).

[25] *See, e.g.*, Steven Miles, Oath Betrayed, *supra* note 1, at *xii* (Miles refers to his entire book as a "work of medical ethics"); Michael Wilks, *A Stain on Medical Ethics*, 366 The Lancet 429 (2005). George Annas and Michael Grodin, in an unsuccessful approach to the subject that combines Parsonian idealism about doctors, a belief in the mythic power of medical ethics, and the [contradictory] explicit recognition the label "doctor" does not convey moral purity, argue that doctors should play a leading role in the [proposed] international penal oversight of medical research. Their ultimate aim of a medical oversight body is sound, though. *See* George Annas and Michael Grodin, *Medical Ethics and Human Rights: Legacies of Nuremberg*, 3 Hofstra L. & Pol'y Symp. 111, 119 (1999) ("The medical profession is perhaps the best candidate to take a leading role here because it has an apolitical history. It has consistently argued for at least some neutrality in wartime to aid the sick and wounded. It has a basic humanitarian purpose for its existence. Physician acts intended to destroy human health and life are a unique betrayal of both societal trust and the profession itself. It is also much easier for governments to adopt inherently evil and destructive policies if they are aided by the patina of legitimacy that physician participation provides.') *See also*, Steven Miles, The Hippocratic Oath and the Ethics of Medicine 166–168 (2004).

In fact, HCPs who engage or are complicit in torture or CID may very well have violated legal norms but this is rarely mentioned. The statements referencing "medical ethics" elide the hard problem of whether applicable legal norms reach the doctor. For example, Human Rights Watch, in an article on the legality of torture, provides one of many examples of the socially constructed position of medically trained persons involved in torture:

> The administration of any of the drugs identified as having the potential for causing a person to talk is an involved medical procedure requiring delivery of the drug intravenously over a period that can range from two to twelve hours. The international Principles of Medical Ethics Relevant to the Role of Health Personnel provide that the participation of doctors or other medical practitioners in the administration of such drugs for interrogation purposes would violate medical ethics.[26]

This statement is written by an expert on international law and it speaks as though "medical ethics" has the authority of a *ius cogens* legal norm, i.e., the most powerful international legal norm. This position on ethics is presented as self-evident, but it also refers back to an international code of medical ethics, as though that code is sufficient pedigree to establish the ethical norm as positive law. It is as though the doctor is merely a passive agent, and to use one in this fashion would cause the doctor to be in violation of "medical ethics." The suggestion is that the doctor would never willingly be involved in torture, and if one was present or utilized during torture, the doctor is without culpability because doctors *a priori* do not engage in torture. This message has a powerful legal subtext. If a doctor cannot engage in torture, he can never be found criminally liable because criminal liability requires a "criminal mind." Legal norms concerning torture do not apply to doctors, only ethical norms.[27] This is social construction at its finest. The reference to "medical ethics" serves to shift responsibility from the HCP to the persons or institutions undertaking the torture.

There is yet another subtext in the quote. It implies that doctors would not intentionally violate the code of ethics in the sense that doctors, because of their training and the Oath, are morally superior and would never engage is such unethical and unprofessional behavior. This is the moral correlate to the legal subtext. That this assertion is dubious is testified to by the *professionalism* crisis. Over the past 15 years, a tremendous number of articles have been written about the need to include humanization in medical education. The danger that medical students will leave residency devoid of interpersonal skills (virtue, character) is well-recognized. A few 6-week classes in the course of an intense 4–9 years educational in *science* is insufficient to develop character.

---

[26] Human Rights Watch, *The Legal Prohibition Against Torture*, at http://www.humanrightswatch.org/press/2001/11/TortureQandA.htm, accessed 1/23/06.

[27] For a somewhat hobbled discussion of how to morally characterize the positive norm *ius cogens* against torture, *see, e.g.*, Jeremy Waldron, *Torture and Positive Law: Jurisprudence for the White House*, 105 Columbia L. Rev 1681 (2005).

Provisions of an ethics code must resonate with the individual professional to be effective. Medical school and oaths cannot create character. The problem is compounded many-fold by the power relations found in the military. In those positions there are clear chains of command, and the HCP is another cog in a wheel that must obey orders and conform to institutional culture. In the powerful, intensely illegal and emotionally charged environment of torture the idea that a code of ethics will sustain a person of weak character is unsupportable.[28] That it will cause a person who has no moral qualms about being involved with torture to think twice is also unsupportable. Certainly ordinary people can do extraordinarily brave things at times, but regulators cannot depend on that.

Can it be said *primum non nocere* has the status of natural law?[29] If it were a natural law, one would expect to see medically trained persons, especially M.Ds., willing to undergo sacrifices to fulfill their deeply felt moral urge to help people. It would be an inborn element of their character. But the medical profession as a group maintains an economic, political and legal monopoly on the practice of medicine that is hardly altruistic. The legal monopoly is closely associated with high social status and authority. To qualify as a natural law norm one would expect those desires to fail, to see physicians satisfied with making $30,000 or $40,000 year as long as they were fulfilling the "natural" law of healing people. Some, perhaps many, medical doctors fit this model.[30] But to admit this is to admit medical education is not related to the medical virtue of the graduate. If self-regulation is based on a virtuous profession, and there is no guarantee of such, then also admitted is the possibility of regulating the profession based on medicine as technical skill, not an outdated and impossible social contract in which M.Ds regulate themselves and most other health professionals in consideration of their virtuous dedication to the health of the populace, i.e., on the basis of their Parsonian character.

This is not an issue of professionalism, if by that is meant some persons have technical skills that require extensive education to learn, that confer significant power to affect a person's life or property, and that inherently imply a relationship

[28] The Stanford Prison Experiment, conducted for the Office of Naval Research to understand psychological dimensions of prisons, demonstrates how the power of the state disturbs untrained minds in positions of authority. *See* Stanford Prison Experiment web site, http://www.prisonexp.org. *But see*, Robert Macauley, *The Hippocratic Underground: Civil Disobedience and Health Care Reform*, 35:1 Hastings Center Report 38 (2005) (arguing doctors can, have and should continue to take the law into their own hands in the face of injustice); Haavi Morriem, Matthew Wynia and Chalmers Clark, *Letters to the Editor (in response to the Macauley article, id.)*, 35:4 Hastings Center Report 4 (2005). *See also*, American Medical Association, *Opinion 1.02, The Relation of Law and Ethics*, Code of Medical Ethics, Current Opinions (2002) ("In general, when physicians believe a law is unjust, they should work to change the law. In exceptional circumstances of unjust laws, ethical responsibilities should supersede legal obligations.").

[29] This entire essay is a discussion of the "do no harm" principle as positive law, the general conclusion being its status as positive law is only weakly embodied in the laws against torture and CID.

[30] *See, e.g.*, Fritzroy Sterling, *DEATH PENALTY: Increasingly, Doctors Refuse to Do Harm*, Inter Press Service News Agency (July 31, 2006).

of trust between the expert and the client. That is the legal model of professionalism, or that of the financial expert. If we assume that there is something special about medical professionalism, that it involves a special relationship because it deals with a person's body and mind, their most intimate experiences, then given the fact many medical graduates do not enter into such intimate relationships, it is clear that medicine is, in a significant way, really two professions, one personal and one impersonal.

In the discourse on doctor duties the principle of *primum non nocere* has no legal effect other than as implemented in state regulation of doctors. On the other hand it has strong rhetorical value as an ethical norm of venerable lineage. Rhetorically it refers to at least four distinct ethical duties: the general duty to use medical knowledge to heal people; the actual duty to avoid harming the patient; the related duty of loyalty to the patient; and the duty of confidentiality of knowledge of the patient's medical condition. In the discourse on torture the phrase is used synonymously with "medical ethics" and in that sense it can be seen as a proxy for the Hippocratic Oath, for the ten principles of the American Medical Association's (AMA) *Code of Ethics*, or for some other ethical code.

Let us look at the duty or duties of "medical ethics" more closely. In particular, when and how does the oath become attached to the person or doctor, when do the duties "take?" Is it acquired by the doctor during her medical training, when she has donned the white coat, or has achieved minimal competence in a minimal set of medical techniques and the acquired basic training in medicine; or when she formally recites the oath, when she graduates from medical school, when she passes her boards, when she is licensed to practice, or when she gets a job? Does the oath refer to a set of human virtues, or are they medical virtues? If it is a human virtue, it is obtained through education at some point, or it falls under the discussion of natural law above.[31] If it is a medical virtue, it must be obtained during medical education. But, is there anything about the medical education that morally requires that knowledge of the human mind/body be used to heal people? The answer must be no, because the knowledge is freely available to anyone who wants it, and there are many very well-trained in medicine who do not use their knowledge for healing.

Does the duty extend to other living things, such as animals and plants? If the duty originates in respect for human life that comes from knowledge of the living organism, then an argument can be made the commitment actually originates in the respect for life because all living things have life in common. On this argument, even though doctors are trained in human life, their intimate and close relationship with the ends of life require them morally to extend the same respect to all life. This would raise issues of whether doctors should be vegetarians, for example, or trained in the new domain of animal rights in which it is clear that it is impossible to

[31] See Fritz Allhoff, "Physician Involvement in Hostile Interrogations," *Cambridge Quarterly of Healthcare Ethics* 15 (2006): 392–402 (reprinted in this volume) for an argument that medicine is not inherently normative.

distinguish between some animals and some humans except by morphology. Since these conclusions are not part of the package of being a doctor, they are not considered part of the duty, thereby indicating the duty has inconsistencies with regard to respect for life and that it includes elements of being socially constructed. Thus there is an element of artificiality about the duty.

It appears then, assuming a duty or set of duties is identified, to individuals and perhaps to society, it is not possible to determine in general when or how they attach to the doctor, in the sense of becoming a virtue, an element of the doctor's character. I beg the question of whether the ethical duty can be adopted by an intellectual process, such as mere recitation of an oath. I trust it is obvious this is not the case. It is clear, however, that once a doctor-patient relationship is established certain legal duties do attach to the relationship. The doctor is supposed to be loyal to the patient vis-à-vis other interests, especially the doctor's own interests, and the doctor is not supposed to do anything under any circumstances to harm the patient. The duty ends upon the ending of the doctor-patient relationship or the death of either of them. These legal duties are embodiments of ethical duties (morals) as positive law, so we are not amiss in construing them as ethical duties. But it is important to note the duties do not have concrete existence outside of that special relationship as constrained by positive law. If the relationship does not naturally exist, do the duties naturally exist?

In this analysis we are looking at HCPs who work for science and drug companies, prisons or the military. We have seen that a condition of working as an employee or conscriptee in those positions involves the doctor giving his primary loyalty to his employer. If this is the case, do the doctors abrogate their oath upon accepting employment in one of these positions? It is clear that minimally they abrogate some of the duty, but I would argue that abrogating any of it is abrogation of the entire duty.

Is it possible for an employee-doctor to enter into a doctor-patient relationship with any patient? If the defining characteristic of the doctor-patient relationship is the activation of the duties, and the doctor no longer has full control of those duties or the full duty to give to the patient, the employee-doctor cannot enter into a doctor-patient relationship. He can enter perhaps into a partial doctor-patient relationship, but what does that mean?

Duties are associated with rights. If the doctor has the duty, who has the right, and what are the features of the right? In the ordinary doctor-patient relationship the patient would have the right if the HCP had the duty. But if the employer has some of the right, assuming there is a dual loyalty, which part of the right do they have? Obviously, the idea of splitting a right such as this into parts makes little sense. Could it be that the employer gets certain rights and the patient other rights, out of a total rights package? What if the employer controls the patient's autonomy? Does the patient ever have autonomy in these situations? No doctor-patient relationship can be formed without autonomy, so even under the most liberal circumstances for the formation of the doctor-patient relationship, the patient who is also a torture victim cannot enter into a doctor-patient relationship, as they have no control over their body.

Can the duty be waived? Obviously the employer waives it on behalf of the patient when the employer tells the doctor to treat the patient. Can the patient waive it? If it is a function of the medical education, it cannot be waived by a patient. Since the torturer removes the rights of the victim, does this imply the duty of the HCP employee is removed at the same time? Since the duty is general and associated with the social authority and role of the HCP does it ever give rise to a legal right in the patient (in the absence of a legal relationship)?

The doctor could argue that she never gives the duty up to the employer, but retains it for any sick person she will tend to. She then has to jump the hurdle of forming a doctor-patient relationship with the tortured person. What if the person seen is unconscious every time he is seen? What if the employer order medical care to be delivered but the injured person refuses? What if the employer will harm the doctor if the doctor does not deliver medical care? Or, as mentioned above, what if the potential patient has no autonomy. This argument by the doctor fails.

I argue the doctor becomes the moral agent of the employer upon accepting employment, and that the foregoing analysis demonstrates how fuzzy the idea of the principle *primum non nocere* is in the circumstance of torture. It is impossible for the doctor to have an ordinary doctor-patient relationship in the torture environment, therefore I question whether it should be assumed in any ethical code or regulation, unless it can be said the doctor has the duty to himself or herself. But the essence of "medical ethics" is altruism, and if there is a self-regarding element in it, it is minimal and of no import other than that the doctor should stay healthy in order to help others.[32]

Traditional responses to these issues are grounded in the health care paradigm of the late 19th century and legal paradigms of the late 20th century, and beg the question of whether a physician can legally use their training as the agent of a harmful principal. They assume the doctor *cannot*, but this no longer holds, if it ever did.

I agree though, with the idea there is something related to medical education that confers on the doctor special knowledge. This special knowledge itself must be regulated regardless of the location of the knowledge or the circumstances of its use. Specific regulation, not fuzzy ethical principles, should follow the doctor's skills regardless of employment.

We should recognize the gulf between medicine as a healing profession and medicine as a technology of the body/mind, and legislate accordingly. Doctors are legally bound only to the code of conduct promulgated by their licensing authority, which in the US is each state. Thus an appropriate response to disproportionalities between education, licensing, employment, and applicable norms should both occur at the level of the licensing entity and at the federal level.

---

[32] Just as the authors of the Belmont Report find a duty in all people to be research subjects, so too could a duty be found in all physicians to sacrifice themselves for their patients. Department of Health, Education and Welfare, *The Belmont Report: Ethical Principles and Guidelines for the Protection of Human Subjects of Research*, in ETHICS AND REGULATORY ASPECTS OF CLINICAL RESEARCH: READINGS AND COMMENTARY, 33–38, ¶16 (eds. Ezekiel Emanuel, Robert A. Crouch, John D. Arras, Jonathan D. Moreno, and Christine Grady, 2003).

5 Conforming Medical Licensure to Training and Employment

In the next two sections, I propose two independent regulatory approaches to two independent, but related problems. One approach specifically addresses the problems I raise by prohibiting involvement in torture by HCPs. The other approach is more structural and addresses not only the torture problem, but the general class of problems illustrated by the torture problem. I address the general approach first, and end with a discussion of the specific approach.

A law should be enacted that says HCPs that are given independent scopes of practice to practice medicine (broadly speaking) should be separately qualified before they can be employed in prisons, medical research or the military.[33] I call this Class II employment.[34] This can be done by either a state or federal regulatory scheme.

A federal regulation is easier in some ways because otherwise the regulation, which is intended to cover employment that is often inter-state, international and inter-jurisdictional, would have to be enacted by each state to be effective. Furthermore, since it is intended to cover military employment, a federal statute makes more sense and would be more effective. The jurisprudence of federalism reserves the right to regulate the profession and practice of medicine to the states, but since we are here distinguishing between the practice of medicine and the use of the medical training and degree for non-physician employment, or employment in strong dual-loyalty positions, federal jurisdiction could be posited on the national and international character of the employment.

The mechanism of regulation would be the establishment of a separate licensing authority for HCPs who work in prisons, as researchers or in other defined strong dual-loyalty environments. Licensing requirements should be a rigorous minimum education, licensure in the basic discipline, and a certification exam based on the education. The curriculum could be adopted by existing training programs, lengthening time spent at the institution for those intending to get the additional qualification.

The existing license should be limited to employment in which the physician would engage only in the one-on-one, familiar doctor-patient relationship that is

---

[33] Although I do not explicitly justify the extension of the proposed regulation to prison and research M.Ds, I assert the dual-loyalty situations they face are analogous to and have equivalent value as those faced by military M.D. All three positions are associated with torture. The prison is the locus of torture, and non-consensual medical treatment or experimentation was the subject of the Medical Trials at Nuremberg, and are prohibited as torture in the ICCPR, art. 7. *See, e.g.*, Annas and Grodin, *Legacies of Nuremberg, supra* note 24.

[34] *See, e.g.*, Gregg Bloche and Jonathan Marks, *When Doctors Go To War*, 352:1 New Eng. J. Med. 3 (2005) (reporting that physicians involved with torture at Guantanamo understood "physicians serving in these roles [involving torture] do not act as physicians and are therefore not bound by patient-oriented ethics."). For a philosophically oriented argument supporting this idea, *see* Fritz Allhof, *Physician Involvement in Hostile Interrogations*, 15:4 Cambridge Quarterly of Healthcare Ethics 392 (2006).

currently contemplated in both training and codes of conduct. I call this Class I employment. Doctors would be required to disclose their licensing status and it should include a separate and distinctive title.

There would be no dual-loyalty problems for doctors who hold a Class II license because their loyalty would be to their institution. Negligence law should be adjusted accordingly so in the event of negligence on the part of the HCP, the institution, or both, there is a theory of responsibility and a responsible party. With regard to the person receiving health care, the institution would owe them the primary responsibility of respect, and the other ethical duties properly owed to a potentially vulnerable person. There would be a clear line between Class I and Class II HCPs. Class II HCPs could treat sick people, but no doctor-patient relationship would result, at least not in the same sense as between a Class I physician and a client or patient. In essence, this scheme recognizes "corporate medicine" and uses it as an enforcement mechanism for the ethical principle of *primum non nocere* in situations in which the principle as ethical principles or state-based law cannot reach.

6 Making a Weak Ethical Principle Strong

Codes of medical ethics are numerous, inconsistent and weak.[35] Just because a norm can be articulated does not give it power. For actors who have assumed the tremendous authority of the sovereign or other great economic and political power law without an enforcement mechanism is not law. That is the Bush Administration's justification for ignoring public international law. Such actors see ethics codes and international law as the norms of the weak. When doctors work in these environments they become the moral and legal agents of their handlers. Codes of ethics are not relevant as norms in those situations, so regulation is needed.[36]

A law should be enacted that criminalizes torture and cruel, inhuman and degrading treatment by any HCP. It should establish a presumption that if an interrogation requires HCPs, then it consists of torture. This statute, as opposed to the one described in the first approach, is probably better conceived as a state-based project because it increases the likelihood of prosecutions for violations.

Each state in the US should enact a statute that applies to all health care providers, and other recipients of state privileges, who are, or have ever been, registered, certified or licensed by that state, who have ever applied for privileges in that state, or who have been trained in medical schools or other educational institutions in that state. It should attach to the health care provider or licensee regardless of when they received their state privilege or education, and it should remain attached whether

---

[35] *See, e.g.*, Baruch Brody et al., MEDICAL ETHICS: ANALYSIS OF THE ISSUES RAISED BY THE CODES, OPINIONS AND STATEMENTS 75–102, 127–160, 529–558 (2001).

[36] For articles that, taken together, demonstrate this point, *see* the December 25, 2005 issue of The Nation (to which the AMA directed their letter to the editor stating its policy on torture). *See*, AMA, *Letter*, *id.*

the privilege is active or not. Many regulatory schemes, such as medical practice acts, exempt health care providers in the uniformed services or Public Health Service if they do not maintain an office for private practice in the state. For the purposes of this statute, those exemptions should not exist. All health care providers that reside in the state for more than a few days, regardless of whether in transit or not, should be covered. The law should criminalize, with severe penalties, torture and cruel, inhuman and degrading treatment as those terms are defined in the Convention Against Torture and Other Cruel Inhuman and Degrading Treatment or Punishment (not the US reservations),[37] regardless of when and where it occurred. It should cover planning torture and being present when torture is conducted, and it should mandate that if the HCP is asked to treat a torture/CID victim, or has knowledge of torture/CID, regardless of when it happened, they are to report the incident, and failure to report, or misreporting, is covered by the same severe penalties. Retribution for reporting should also be criminalized. Treatment of a torture/CID victim should not be criminalized.[38] This would, in essence, create a system of state-based universal jurisdiction over HCP in the US that have contact with any state that has adopted the regulatory scheme. The Federation of State Medical Boards should be encouraged to draft a policy reflecting this plan accompanied by model legislation.

The virtue of this approach is that it embodies the morality of the vague "medical ethics" that HCPs are supposed to follow. It can also be used for related problems, such as refusing to carry out the death penalty.

Torture and CID are already criminalized, but the existing statutes do not distinguish or address the issue of the role of the HCP, and the reach of existing criminal laws is not clear. By locating this regulatory scheme in the 50 states there is a greater chance a violator will be brought to justice, since in all likelihood there will be multiple jurisdictions involved each of which can make its own decisions about whether to prosecute. With a federal statute the decision to prosecute on a matter like this will be made in Washington by political appointees who have a stake in the matter. It may also be easier to get effective legislation passed at the state level.

A statutory defense could be part of the statute. If an HCP can establish beyond a high evidentiary standard that their first exposure to the torture/CID was unforeseen and that he or she complied with the reporting mandate as soon as was practicable and removed themselves from the environment at the first opportunity there could be a rebutable presumption of lack of culpability.

The Federation of Boards of Medical Examiners (FBME) and the American Medical Association, both of which exercise tremendous influence in state regulation of HCPs, should draft appropriate policies recognizing this regulatory lacuna, and the FBME should draft model legislation for the employment based

---

[37] CONVENTION AGAINST TORTURE, *supra* note 6.

[38] *See, e.g.*, Steven P. Cohen, *Doctors Should Play Role in Prisoner Interrogation*, Baltimore Sun Editorial (February 14, 2006) (military doctor argues it is beneficial to have physicians involved at all stages of interrogation).

licensing scheme. State licensing authorities, the federation of boards of medical examiners and the AMA would be encouraged to educate the public about the new licensing scheme.

Since the most compelling moral issue the scheme is designed for, interrogation, torture and CID, is an international problem, the World Health Organization, the Council for International Organizations of Medical Sciences, the World Medical Association and medical associations of other countries should be encouraged to adopt this classification and certification scheme, and to widely publicize it.

However, resistance can be anticipated. It is possible the AMA and local associations of M.Ds will fight this restriction of their existing scope of practice, as there already is in existence a robust system for lobbying against expansions of non-M.D. scopes of practice. However, there is no policy based on public safety or welfare to justify the opposition.

7 Conclusion

Medically trained persons involved in interrogations are subject to strong national security laws and weak professional laws and ethical norms. Medical training does not guarantee internalization of Hippocratic norms, and early 20th century regulatory schemes do not comprehend contemporary institutional pressures on individual physicians. Instead of leaving well-intentioned medically trained persons to work in ethically complex dual-loyalty situations, I propose enacting regulatory schemes that solve the moral problems for them. The proposed schemes incorporate the morality of the Hippocratic Oath into the institutional laws and culture in which strong dual-loyalty problems occur. Not all M.Ds. are physicians anymore, and this is an important and dangerous enough distinction to require regulation.

Part III
Physicians and Weapons Development

Is Medicine a Pacifist Vocation or Should Doctors Help Build Bombs?[1]

Michael L. Gross

1 Introduction

Ever since World War I, pacifists have found refuge in medicine. What is it about medicine that is so alluring to those who make nonviolence their creed? And, if pacifists are drawn to medicine in time of war, perhaps medicine has a natural affinity for pacifism? Is medicine a pacifist profession? Must doctors always avoid harming others or may they help build bombs?

Historically, weapons technology asked little of medicine so that military surgeons could ignore both questions and adhere to their "vocational pacifism" without seriously affecting military capabilities. But modern warfare is quickly forcing changes. Increasingly, military and political leaders are turning to a range of weapons, some lethal and some non-lethal, that require the knowledge peculiar to the practice of medicine. Medicine may shun weapons development, as many might prefer, but only by embracing pacifism. Pacifism, however, is not a doctrine that medicine can support with any degree of cogency or enthusiasm. As a result, the medical community must seriously ask itself whether it may take up arms in its *professional* capacity and use medical expertise to build weapons that harm others. Briefly addressed by the Red Cross in 1996, questions about "the medical profession and the effects of weapons" were soon set aside and remain unanswered.[2]

2 Pacifism and Medicine: The Appeal of *Noncombatant* Military Medical Service

It is difficult to distance pacifism from medicine. When American Quaker pacifists faced conscription in 1917, their first thought was to establish an ambulance unit modeled on the Friends Ambulance Unit that Quakers had operated with great

[1] This chapter is adapted from Michael L. Gross, *Bioethics and Armed Conflict: Moral Dilemmas of Medicine and War* (Cambridge, MA: MIT, 2006), Chapters 8 and 9. Used with permission.

[2] International Committee of the Red Cross, "The Medical Profession and the Effects of Weapons," (Geneva: International Committee of the Red Cross), publication ref. 0668, 1996.

F. Allhoff (ed.), *Physicians at War: The Dual-Loyalties Challenge.*

success in Britain since the beginning of the war. Warming rapidly to the idea, Adventist pacifists launched the Cadet Medical Corps prior to America's entry into World War II to allow young Adventists to fulfill their civic duty without violating the biblical precept that absolutely forbids killing. Nor was the idea lost upon policy makers. Making room for conscripts who cannot, by reason of conscience, bear arms and serve in any capacity that might compel them to kill or harm others, military officials are, to this day, prepared to offer conscientious objectors "service in the *medical* department of any of the Armed Forces, wherever performed."[3]

Two core beliefs characterize pacifism:

1. *Anti-war-ism*: The belief that war is absolutely wrong[4]
2. *Nonmaleficence*: The belief that one "cannot conscientiously engage in any activity or perform any function contributing to the destruction of human life"[5]

These are two distinct principles. The first espouses an unconditional opposition to war in any form, the second to the role one must play during armed conflict. Individuals weigh these principles differently. Refusing to compromise on either principle, some pacifists suffer imprisonment, while the vast majority of "absolute" pacifists during World War II, for example, chose alternative public service to work in civilian agricultural camps and perform essential national service without joining and supporting the military. Others, however, were willing to compromise in the face of German aggression and sought ways to fulfill their military and moral duties simultaneously. They would support war but practice nonmaleficence. In doing so, they chose *noncombatant* military service and in nearly every case this translated into medical service in the US Army's Medical Department, the Royal Army Medical Corp or the Friends Ambulance Unit.

The obvious appeal lies in the symmetry between the nonmaleficence of pacifism and the nonmaleficence of medicine. As some pacifists set aside their anti-war-ism, they considered themselves "conscientious supporters" of war. They would back their nation's war effort but refuse to bear arms. It is a strange and marginal worldview but astonishingly close to one typically associated with the practice of medicine during armed conflict. Consider the following testimony:

---

[3] US Department of Defense, *Conscientious Objectors* (Washington, DC: Department of Defense, Directive Number 1300.6, August 20, 1971, certified as current, November 21, 2003), paragraph 3.3 ("Non-combatant service"). In World War I and the beginning of World War II, noncombatant military service included service in the medical, quartermaster, and engineering corp. In January 1943, noncombatant military service was restricted exclusively to the medical department.

[4] See Jenny Teichman, *Pacifism and the Just War: A Study in Applied Philosophy* (Oxford: Blackwell, 1986), 4.

[5] Rufus D. Bowman, *The Church of the Brethren and War 1708–1941* (Elgin, IL: Brethren Publishing House, 1944), 208. The Church of the Brethren declared these beliefs in January 1918. However, they also typify the pacifism associated with the Mennonites and Quakers. See Peter Brock and Nigel Young, *Pacifism in the Twentieth Century* (Syracuse: Syracuse University Press, 1999); Cynthia Eller, *Conscientious Objectors and the Second World War: Moral and Religious Arguments in Support of Pacifism* (New York: Praeger, 1991).

He will participate in any service, in the military service or out of it, which will contribute to the saving of human life.... [But is prevented] from engaging in any act which contributes to destroying or injuring human life, in the military service or out of it, in war or in peace ...[6]

"He" sounds like a physician but is, in fact, an Adventist pacifist. Adventists did not embrace anti-war-ism but did adhere to the principle of nonmaleficence following their literal and absolute belief in the 6th Commandment. This belief led them to seek noncombatant military positions and during World War II, nearly half of the 25,000 noncombatant medics were Adventists. Their numbers were not trivial but their perspective is decidedly idiosyncratic, and it would be disconcerting if medicine could not articulate its own version of nonmaleficence and general support for war in less than universally acceptable terms. But, it is not easy. Can anyone coherently embrace the principle of nonmaleficence but reject anti-war-ism? Most pacifists, whether secular or religious, cannot. They find the entire idea of "noncombatant military service" disingenuous and make no room for any cogent argument that might reconcile support for war and the duty to do no harm.

The argument is quite simple. Addressing the question, "Can a nonresistant nurse serve in the Army?" H.S. Bender, Chairman of the Peace Problems Committee for the Mennonites during World War II, states categorically that she cannot. "The army nurse," writes Bender, "is a regular member of the army, ... identifies herself with the organization which prosecutes the war, and takes her share of moral responsibility for the military operations of the army of which she is part.... The army nurse is essential to the operations of the army. Without nurses, the army could not continue to fight."[7] The same is true, of course, for medics, physicians and other male military medical personnel.

Handbooks advising secular conscientious objectors are no less circumspect:

[S]ome men are actually inducted into the medical service thinking that medics are instruments of mercy apart from the Army and its primary objectives. This erroneous conclusion can lead to serious personal difficulties. True, the medics save lives and ease suffering, sometimes in a manner which takes real heroism. But the medic is a soldier, and the ultimate objective of medics is to win battles.[8]

The argument of each critic is the same: any military role, combatant or noncombatant, inevitably violates the principle of nonmaleficence as military operations, of which one is an integral part, harm others. Nor are medical personnel in any

[6] General Conference Committee 1940, Seventh Day Adventist, General Conference Committee, September 1940, Carlyle B. Haynes, editor, *Studies in Denominational Principles of Noncombatancy and Governmental Relations* (Washington, DC: Seventh Day Adventist War Service Commission, 1943), 22–24, cited in Peter. Brock and Nigel Young, *Pacifism in the Twentieth Century* (Syracuse: Syracuse University Press, 1999), 177.

[7] H.S. Bender, "Can a Nonresistant Nurse Serve in the Army?" *Mennonursing* 1.1 (1947): 7.

[8] Arlo Tatum, *Handbook for Conscientious Objectors*, 10th ed. (Philadelphia, PA: Central Committee for Conscientious Objectors, 1970), 87–88; Robert A. Seeley, *Advice for Conscientious Objectors in the Armed Forces*, 5th ed. (Philadelphia, PA: Central Committee for Conscientious Objectors, 1998), 36.

way neutral or above the fray. Quite the contrary, medical care is an adjunct of war; it does not speak to easing the pain and suffering of individual soldiers as an end in itself, but of conserving manpower, maintaining military capabilities and preventing, as one military manual put it, "adverse effects of unevacuated casualties on combat efficiency by ... providing adequate medical care and rapid evacuation."[9]

If those conscientiously committed to the principle of nonmaleficence cannot square their duty to avoid harming others with support for war, can medicine manage it? If it can, military medical personnel must ask themselves how they might support the business of war; if they cannot they must either embrace pacifism and eschew war, or reject nonmaleficence and answer the call to arms by contributing their expertise to the development of modern weaponry.

3 Medicine and Pacifism: The Appeal of Vocational Pacifism

Perhaps "vocational pacifism" best characterizes the practice of medicine during war. Historically, the idea is associated with the clergy[10]:

> Clerics and bishops are forbidden to take up arms, not as though it were a sin, but because such an action is incompatible with their state .... certain occupations are so inconsistent with one another that they cannot be fittingly exercised at the same time.[11]

Substitute 'physicians' for 'clerics and bishops' and few would quarrel with paraphrasing Aquinas to describe the vocational pacifism of the medical profession. While neither clerics nor doctors oppose war, their vocations are the only two that successfully resist the state's call to arms with an appeal to nonmaleficence while, at the same time, reject anti-war-ism. How can they defend war *and* profess to do no harm?

The argument proceeds in three steps, each articulating a distinct principle:

1. *The Principle of Just War.* Nations have an obligation to their citizens to resist aggression by force of arms insofar as armed violence is necessary, does not bring more harm than good, and takes reasonable care to protect the welfare of noncombatants. These are the familiar principles of just war. Just war, by this argument, repudiates absolute anti-war-ism, and allows most individuals, including physicians, to support war under certain circumstances.

---

[9] Army Field Manual FM 4–02.6, 2002; FM 8–10–1, 1951.

[10] Vocational pacifism is also associated with the pacifism of the historic peace churches—Quakers, Mennonites and Brethren—who recognize a unique obligation or vocation to "bear witness" to nonviolence. I limit the discussion here, however, the pacifism of a particular professional vocation such as priests and doctors.

[11] Thomas Aquinas, *Summa theologiae* 2–2, q. 40, a 2 (translator, Fathers of the English Dominican Province, (New York: Benziger, 1947), cited in Kenneth W. Kemp, "Personal Pacifism," *Theological Studies* 56 (1995): 21–38, here page 23.

2. *The Principle of Collective Responsibility*. The state's obligation to defend its citizens is a collective undertaking. While a political community may incur an obligation to wage a just war, this obligation does not extend to each and every member of the community. Some are exempt if their participation undermines collective action (old men and children, perhaps) or if they have more useful things to do than harm others. It is therefore not presumptuous nor hypocritical that clerics and physicians eschew harm to others while encouraging or aiding their compatriots to kill during a just war.
3. *The Principle of Medical Necessity*. The practice of medicine is necessary to wage war successfully. Some observers suggest that clerics may abstain from violence during war because they are "uniquely situated to help victims of violence."[12] The same is true for physicians. In addition, the practice of medicine is necessary to wage peace successfully and any deviation from the principle of nonmaleficence irreparably undermines the integrity of medicine and the benefits it can bring to humankind.

There are no difficulties with the first two principles. Once satisfied that a war is just and certain vocations may have more important jobs to do than to bear arms, one moves to weigh the necessity of medicine during war. Although the principle of medical necessity is sound, it is important to see that actions satisfying medical necessity are contingent. Its implications, therefore, are neither straightforward nor obvious.

Ordinarily, practicing medicine with an eye toward never doing harm is of inestimable value to a nation waging war. The goal of military medicine is to preserve a nation's military capability. Sound medical practice accomplishes this by protecting soldiers from disease, instilling proper hygiene, and evacuating and treating the wounded. However, one can also imagine a different set of circumstances. If the principle of just war allows nations to defend themselves by force of arms and the successful deployment of arms requires medical expertise, then the principle of nonmaleficence may not serve medical necessity if it impairs the development the means necessary to wage a just war.

4 Military Arms and Medical Necessity

Clerics, bishops and religious pacifists are exempt from bearing arms because their participation in armed conflict *as combatants* is not necessary. Pacifists, in particular, pose a thorny problem for a democratic polity that finds itself compelled by its very principles to show tolerance for diverse ethical and religious viewpoints that would, should significant numbers espouse the same view, otherwise undermine the state.

[12] Kenneth W. Kemp, "Personal Pacifism," *Theological Studies* 56 (1995): 21–38.

Military officials are less perturbed precisely because the numbers of pacifists are small and manpower is fungible. Drafting conscientious objectors into medical service releases others for combat duty. There were never too many pacifists that officials could not afford to be magnanimous and avoid forcing pacifists to test their commitment to nonmaleficence by obligating them to bear arms.

Physicians are not so easy to deal with precisely because their duty *as combatants* is sometimes necessary. While in the overwhelming majority of cases, there is no reason to question the necessary role that medical nonmaleficence plays in just war, two strategic and/or tactical military options that can cause significant harm currently require medical expertise: chemical and biological deterrence and non-lethal weapons. Although current international law bans the development of chemical and biological weapons, a significant minority of nations have not ratified the ban, leaving them free to develop chemical or biological weapons for deterrent purposes. Moreover, the conventions leave room for the development of certain non-lethal chemical weapons for law enforcement and for use in "military operations other than war", as well as acoustical or optical non-lethal weapons that also cause varying degrees of injury.

4.1 Chemical and Biological Deterrence

The nations party to the Middle East conflict—Israel, Syria, Egypt and Jordan—have neither ratified the 1972 Biological Weapons Convention (BWC) nor the 1993 Chemical Weapons Convention (CWC) that generally ban the development and stockpiling of unconventional weapons. While Israel maintains the resources to develop nuclear weapons, the other nations of the Mideast must choose the "poor man's" option as they attempt to deter a nuclear threat with chemical or biological weapons.[13] While nuclear weapons programs get along very well without medical expertise, the same cannot be said for the development of chemical or biological weapons. This turns the principle of medical necessity on its head. In the geopolitics of the Mideast, physicians must help build unconventional weapons and repudiate their duty to do no harm in order to satisfy the principle of just war and to deter their enemies from aggression.

There are several ways to reason through this argument, but all bring medicine to question its absolute commitment to nonmaleficence during a just war. One avenue denies that a physician building a biological or chemical deterrent capability violates the principle of nonmaleficence. Nonmaleficence requires, at a minimum, intentional harm. Deterrence may demand neither. At best, deterrence only *threatens* harm in certain, contingent circumstances (a first strike, for example). Many may leave it at that, convinced that while the threat or intent to harm innocents is morally wrong,

[13] Eitan Barak, "Where Do We Go from Here? Implementation of the Chemical Weapons Convention in the Middle East in the Post-Saddam era," *Security Studies* 13 (2003): 106–155.

it pales before the benefits of successful deterrence. Deterrence, in other words, saves lives, a fact that the Cold War proved quite convincingly. Others, however, dismiss the claim that intent is at all necessary to transmit a credible threat. Political leaders may bluff or remain uncertain of how they will act in the future.

These arguments are neither novel nor particularly contentious but are indispensable if we accept the ethics of *nuclear* deterrence.[14] They apply with equal force to the ethics of chemical deterrence. Nor are they farfetched; in retrospect, chemical deterrence was one of the important achievements of World War II.[15] Each side laid massive stores of chemical weapons, and while the Allies maintained a public policy of "no first strike," there is no evidence of any well-planned blueprint to deploy these weapons. Stockpiling alone, together with moderate levels of distrust did the trick. Intentional harm was also conspicuously absent, for example, when President Reagan allowed the US to manufacture binary chemical weapons (those that combine ingredients in flight to produce nerve gas) in the 1980s as nothing more than a bargaining chip to induce the Soviets to end their own CBW program. And, he succeeded. The weapons were soon destroyed, no one was harmed, national security was enhanced and no one really knew if Reagan intended to begin bombing in 5 minutes. Any physician accepting these arguments may participate in the development of a chemical deterrent capability without violating the principle of nonmaleficence prohibiting intentional harm.

Intentional harm, however, emphatically informs the idea of "supreme emergency," those unique circumstances that permit a political community to violate the principles of just war by inflicting horrific injury to combatants and noncombatant alike if faced with genocide.[16] Supreme emergencies demand rigid criteria and there are few compelling examples. To egregiously violate the principle of noncombatant immunity a community must face a grave threat that only extreme means can avert. Neither the indignity nor the hardship of surrender nor the likelihood of significant military casualties allow a belligerent to obliterate an enemy's civilian population. Because the gravity of a threat is often in the eyes of the beholder and the effectiveness of indiscriminately bombing civilian populations is often questionable, the criteria of supreme emergency are difficult to apply in practice.[17] This leaves it detractors to shun any sweeping breach of noncombatant immunity based on broad

---

[14] Russell Hardin, "Symposium on Ethics and Nuclear Deterrence," *Ethics* 95.3 (1985).

[15] John Ellis van Courtland Moon, "Chemical Weapons and Deterrence: The World War II Experience," *International Security* 8.4 (1984): 3–35; Stockholm International Peace Research Institute, "The Non-use of CB Weapons During World War II" in *The Problem of Chemical and Biological Warfare, Volume 1: The Rise of CB Weapons* (Stockholm International Peace Research Institute; New York: Humanities, 1971), 294–335.

[16] Daniel Statman, "Moral Tragedies, Supreme Emergencies and National-Defence," *Journal of Applied Philosophy* 23.3 (2006): 311–322; Daniel Statman, "Supreme Emergencies Revisited," *Ethics* 117 (October 2006): 58–79.

[17] George H. Quester, "The Psychological Effects of Bombing Civilian Populations: Wars of the Past," in Betty Glad, ed., *The Psychological Dimensions of War* (Newbury Park, CA: Sage, 1990), 201–235.

calculations of utility. But whether the extreme means necessitated by a supreme emergency are morally justified or simply a tragic choice between two evils, one must consider the possibility that physicians may face the call to arms. Just as one may seriously ponder the obligation of a Jewish scientist to manufacture a weapon of mass destruction to end the Holocaust, one cannot ignore the obligation of a Kurdish doctor, for example, to use his medical expertise to help build a chemical weapon to injure and kill Iraqi civilians if it would have prevent the same threat that Saddam Hussein posed to his own people during his dictatorship.

4.2 *Non-lethal Weapons*

Unlike weapons of deterrence, non-lethal weapons are developed with the explicit purpose of harming others and are now emerging as an appealing and feasible option for military planners contemplating counterinsurgency warfare during asymmetrical warfare.[18] Unable to bring devastating firepower upon militant forces fighting in built-up civilian areas, policy makers are warming to a weapon that allows them to quell insurgencies or fight terror without permanently harming noncombatants.[19] Non-lethal weapons employ optical, acoustical, millimeter wave devices, and chemical agents to cause disorientation, tactile discomfort, severe nausea or temporary unconsciousness to incapacitate opposing forces and minimize collateral harm to noncombatants.[20] Nonlethal acoustical and energy wave weapons are designed to repulse crowds and thereby avoid direct contact with hostile forces. Chemical agents, on the other hand, can temporarily incapacitate an enemy to allow troops to overwhelm and disarm combatants. In both cases, non-lethal weapons provide a "force continuum" allowing a wide range of options between using high explosives and doing nothing when faced with "low intensity" military threats.

---

[18] John P. Alexander, "An Overview of the Future of Nonlethal Weapons," *Medicine, Conflict and Survival* 17 (2001): 180–193; Nick Lewer and Steven Schofield, *Nonlethal Weapons: A Fatal Attraction?* (London: Zed Books, 1997).

[19] National Research Council, *An Assessment of Nonlethal Weapons Science and Technology*, Committee for an Assessment of Nonlethal Weapons Science and Technology, Naval Studies Board Division on Engineering and Physical Sciences (Washington, DC: The National Academies Press, 2003).

[20] Neil Davison, "The Development of 'Nonlethal' Weapons During the 1990's, Occasional Paper No. 2," *Bradford Nonlethal Weapons Research Project (BNLWRP)* (Bradford: Department of Peace Studies, University of Bradford, March 2007). See, for example, John P. Alexander, *Future War: Nonlethal Weapons in the Twenty First Century* (New York: Thomas Dunn Books, 1999); Margaret Coppernoll, "The Nonlethal Weapons Debate," *Naval War College Review* 52.2 (1990): 112–131; Malcolm Dando, *A New Form of Warfare: The Rise of Nonlethal Weapons*, (London: Brassey's, 1996); Nick Lewer and Neil Davison, "Nonlethal Technologies—An Overview," *Disarmament* 1 (1995), 36–51; and Lewer and Schofield, *Nonlethal Weapons: A Fatal Attraction?*

All of these weapons cause some degree of harm and all require some level of medical expertise as they are developed and tested. At the same time, nonlethal weapons may also be lethal. The chemical concentration of many agents that incapacitate most people may kill others, while reviving the injured may require special medical facilities that are not always available. This is one of the lessons learned when the Russians used calmatives to free hostages from a theater in Moscow in 2002. During the rescue effort, 130 of the 850 hostages died.[21] There are no assurances that non-lethal weapons will always cause less harm than conventional weapons. On the contrary, some fear that non-lethal weapon will function as a "force-multiplier" to increase the lethality of conventional weapons. The Russians did not capture incapacitated terrorists, but killed them. During the Vietnam War, the US Army used irritants and tear gas to flush North Vietnamese soldiers from tunnels and then, once exposed, shelled them with high explosives. Physicians developing nonlethal weapons must be aware of these implications.

Beyond the question of harm non-lethal weapons pose also lies a legal minefield.[22] The Chemical Weapons Convention (1993) prohibits the use of chemical weapons in armed conflict but does not extend to "law enforcement, including domestic riot control purposes (article II.9 (d)).[23] To control domestic riots, law enforcement agents may use, and nations may develop, "riot control agents (RCA)." RCAs encompass "any chemical which can produce rapidly in humans' sensory irritation or disabling physical effects which disappear within a short time following termination of exposure."[24] In light of these restrictions, the place of calmatives remains controversial. Some policy analysts exclude calmatives from armed conflict *and* law enforcement because they are not RCAs. For others, however, calmatives are either a form of RCA (because its incapacitating effects are fleeting) or are permitted by the CWC under a broad interpretation which "does not support restricting Article II.9(d) to toxic chemicals that are [only] RCAs."[25] Given this wide range of

---

[21] Monterey Institute of International Studies, The Chemical and Biological Weapons Nonproliferation Program, Center for Nonproliferation Studies, "The Moscow Theater Hostage Crisis: Incapacitants and Chemical Warfare," http://cns.miis.edu/pubs/week/02110b.htm, cited 4 June 2007.

[22] David P. Fidler, "The International Legal Implications of 'Nonlethal' Weapons," *Michigan Journal of International Law* 21.1 (1999): 51–100; David P. Fidler, "Nonlethal Weapons and International Law." *Medicine Conflict and Survival* 17 (2001), 194–206.

[23] *Convention on the Prohibition of the Development, Production, Stockpiling and Use of Chemical Weapons and on Their Destruction*, 1993, http://www.opcw.org/docs/cwc_eng.pdf, cited 4 June 2007.

[24] Convention on the Prohibition of the Development, Production, Stockpiling and Use of Chemical Weapons and on Their Destruction, Article II (7), 1993, http://www.opcw.org/docs/cwc_eng.pdf, cited 4 June 2007.

[25] Monterey Institute of International Studies, "The Moscow Theater Hostage Crisis: Incapacitants and Chemical Warfare"; David P. Fidler, "The Meaning of Moscow: "Nonlethal" Weapons an International Law in the Early 21st Century," *International Review of the Red Cross* 87.859 (2005), 525–552, here 535–536.

interpretations, many agree that the Russians did not violate the CWC as they fought to enforce the law against terrorists in central Moscow.[26]

At the same time, the scope of "law enforcement" today includes the fight against terror and a range of nebulously defined "military operations other than war." The CWC, for example, allows occupying military forces (such as the US in Iraq) or UN authorized peacekeeping forces to use chemical agents to enforce the law, preserve public order and protect their security forces.[27] The official US position is more expansive. Executive order 11850 (1975) allows US forces to use RCAs in some combat operations including rescue missions and "in situations in which civilians are used to mask or screen attacks."[28] Although the CWC prohibits the use of "toxic" weapons in armed combat, there is no universal understanding that all forms of neural inhibitors, gastrointestinal convulsives, neuropharmacological agents, calmative agents, disassociative hallucinogens and sedatives are necessarily toxic chemicals.[29] In this vein, the US National Research Council endorsed calmatives and other chemical non-lethal weapons that "offer the theoretical possibility of peacefully incapacitating combatants/agitators, reducing the need for the violence that is frequently associated with many of the current methods."[30]

In the very near future, nonlethal weapons will form an important part of the arsenal that Western and UN forces rely on as they intervene militarily to restore peace, fight terror, provide humanitarian aid or remove despots from power. Serbia, Croatia, Rwanda, Somalia, Afghanistan, Iraq and Darfur are, were or should be testing grounds for the justice of humanitarian intervention. Although these conflicts are not wars of "self-defense" as traditionally understood, there is growing recognition that the international community bears responsibility for protecting human rights and restraining despotic and genocidal regimes by force

---

[26] Mark Wheelis, "Will the New Biology Lead to New Weapons?" *Arms Control Today* (July/August 2004), http://www.armscontrol.org/act/2004_07–08/Wheelis.asp?print#sidebarnotes3, cited 4 June 2007.

[27] See Fidler, "The Meaning of Moscow," 540–547.

[28] "Executive Order 11850, Renunciation of Certain Uses in War of Chemical Herbicides and Riot Control Agents," http://www.fas.org/bwc/eo11850.htm, cited 4 June 2007.

[29] Coppernoll, "The Nonlethal Weapons Debate," 122.

[30] National Research Council, *An Assessment of Nonlethal Weapons Science and Technology*, Committee for an Assessment of Nonlethal Weapons Science and Technology Naval Studies Board Division on Engineering and Physical Sciences (Washington, DC: The National Academies Press, 2003), 81; Joan Lakoski et al., *The Advantages and Limitations of Calmatives for Use as a Nonlethal Technique* (Hershey, PA: College of Medicine/State College, PA: Applied Research Laboratory, Pennsylvania State University, 2000). Donald Rumsfeld, former US Secretary of Defense, complained that the CWC straitjacketed US forces: "In many instances, our forces are allowed to shoot somebody and kill them, but they're not allowed to use a nonlethal riot-control agent.... There are times when the use of nonlethal riot agents is perfectly appropriate, although legal constraints make for 'a very awkward situation'" Brad Knickerbocker, "The Fuzzy Ethics of Nonlethal Weapons," *The Christian Science Monitor* (February 14, 2003), http://www.csmonitor.com/2003/0214/p02s01-usmi.html, cited 4 June 2007.

of arms.[31] In these cases, non-lethal weapons may be advantageous, and it is their peculiar nature that most cannot be constructed without medical expertise. Should physicians develop these weapons if necessary for international law enforcement?

4.3 *The Role of Physicians*

Some observers are unequivocal about the role of physicians in weapons development:

> The development of this new generation of ["non-lethal"] weapons incorporates knowledge from the remarkable advances made in medical science; two examples are calmatives and eye attack lasers .... *The medical community must guard against use of its knowledge for the purposes of weapon development.*[32]

In the context of the theoretical structure just outlined, Coupland's appeal cannot get off the ground unless he can argue that weapons development violates the criterion of just war or medical necessity. Some non-lethal weapons violate the principle of just war by causing "unnecessary suffering and superfluous injury." There are very few laws in war that regulate how combatants may harm one another but one of the most enduring is the prohibition on weapons that go beyond disabling an enemy and, in addition, inflict horrendous wounds that "uselessly aggravate the sufferings of disabled men."[33] This understanding led the international community to ban blinding optical lasers and take a strong stand against land mines.[34]

For international jurists, as well as medical workers, however the problem of unambiguously defining unnecessary suffering and superfluous injury with regard to other nonlethal weapons systems remains. Coupland took up this challenge in 1996 by listing several criteria for superfluous injury and unnecessary suffering. These include weapons that cause:

---

[31] Barcelona Report of the Study Group on Europe's Security Capabilities, 2004, *A Human Security Doctrine for Europe*, http://www.lse.ac.uk/Depts/global/Human%20Security%20Report%20Full.pdf, cited 4 June 2007.

[32] Robin. M. Coupland, " 'Nonlethal Weapons': Precipitating a New Arms Race." *BMJ*, 1997, 315:72 (12 July), emphasis added.

[33] Declaration Renouncing the Use, in Time of War, of Explosive Projectiles Under 400 Grammes Weight. Saint Petersburg, 29 November/11 December 1868.

[34] CCW, Protocol II, 1980. *Protocol on Prohibitions or Restrictions on the Use of Mines, Booby-Traps and Other Devices* (Protocol II to the *Convention on Prohibitions or Restrictions on the Use of Certain Conventional Weapons Which May be Deemed to be Excessively Injurious or to Have Indiscriminate Effects* (CCW), Geneva, 10 October 1980). Geneva, 10 October 1980.

CCW, Protocol IV, 1995. *Protocol on Blinding Laser Weapons* (Protocol IV to the *Convention on Prohibitions or Restrictions on the Use of Certain Conventional Weapons Which May be Deemed to be Excessively Injurious or to Have Indiscriminate Effects* (CCW), Geneva, 10 October 1980), 13 October 1995.

1. A field mortality of more than 25% or hospital mortality of more than 5%
2. Effects for which there is no "well recognized and proved treatment"
3. Specific disease, abnormal physiological/psychological state or specific and permanent disability or specific disfigurement[35]

"Most people," writes Coupland, consider warfare waged with weapons developed in laboratories by biomedical scientists unacceptable ... the primary effect [of weapons] should not be to target a specific part of the human anatomy, physiology or biochemistry."[36]

How do these criteria affect the development of nonlethal weapons? Do nonlethal weapons violate the injunction against superfluous injury and unnecessary suffering? First, nonlethal weapons do not kill 25% in the field as high explosives do. Nor is there no recognized or proven treatment. The injuries that nonlethals weapons cause is both treatable and preventable by a wide array by of protective devices such as masks, suits, and antidotes. Morbidity and mortality were never objections to chemical weapons. Even in World War I the mortality rate of poison gas (3%) was far less than that caused by high explosives (25%). Instead, the suffering associated with nonlethal weapons, particularly chemical weapons is not suffering *per se* but their ability to attack on the human anatomy in a way that many find insidious.

Whether weapons that "target a specific part of the human anatomy or physiology" constitutes superfluous injury and unnecessary suffering is, perhaps, a question for sociologists rather than philosophers or physicians. On one level, nonlethal weapons do not meet any reasonable criteria for unnecessary suffering. Nevertheless, there is a fear their use may create a slippery slope and lead nations to cross the line between lethal and nonlethal weapons. But this claim is, as yet, unproven. At another level, however, there is a deep seated fear about any weapon—chemical, optical or acoustical—that targets human anatomy. It may stem from a age-old repugnance to killing anyone by poison. Or it may be, as Martin van Creveld surmised, that the distinction between chemical and other weapons exists solely in "man's mind;" a "cultural" aversion to choking people to death or incapacitation. Or, it may be linked to "shamanism" and the fear of investing physicians with the power to destroy or harm life as well as saving it. Regardless of how we think of the harm that nonlethal weapons may bring, it will be difficult to deny them a place on the battlefield as long as they ultimately cause fewer casualties and prove more useful to prosecute asymmetrical wars of humanitarian intervention than many weapons systems currently allow.

---

[35] Robin M. Coupland, *The Red Cross Wound Classification*, 2nd ed. (Geneva: International Committee of the Red Cross, 1991); Robin M. Coupland, "The Effect of Weapons: Defining Superfluous Injury and Unnecessary Suffering," *Medicine and Global Survival* 3 (1996): A1; Robin M. Coupland, "Abhorrent Weapons and 'Superfluous Injury or Unnecessary Suffering': from Field Surgery to Law," *British Medical Journal* 315 (1997): 1450–1452.

[36] Robin M. Coupland, "The Effect of Weapons: Defining Superfluous Injury and Unnecessary Suffering," *Medicine and Global Survival* 3, 1996: A1.

As a result, the debate surrounding the place of nonlethal weapons continues unabated. Nevertheless, the important point to recognize is that a physician's commitment to nonmaleficence is subject to medical necessity. In the vast majority of cases, the practice of medicine and with it the great good it brings to mankind requires medical practitioners to avoid doing harm to others. War, however, may upset this thinking. Medicine is not a pacifist vocation. Physicians, unlike clerics and pacifists, but like other citizens, cannot commit themselves to an unconditional principle of nonmaleficence. Michael Frisina, writing for the US Army's textbook on military medical ethics (2003) advises military medical personnel that "medical professionals ought to stay in the business of healing and not hurting, which includes not participating in or contributing to weapons research and development."[37] This declaration, however, requires a caveat. Insofar as medical expertise is not necessary to prosecute a just war, physicians should indeed stay in the business of healing. When their expertise is necessary, however, they may, and indeed must, aid those developing weapons. These may be nonlethal weapons that are designed to cause minimal harm but may also include weapons of mass destruction when built for deterrent purposes. Doctors may build bombs, just as we all may, if necessary to safeguard the welfare of the political community.

5 Medicine, War and Community Welfare

The relationship between medicine and the welfare of the community is important to understand. Medical practitioners do not answer a higher calling that transcends the material interests of their community. Quite the contrary, medicine is a professional calling subordinate to the welfare of the community that bestows upon it its obligations and privileges. When David Thomasma and Edmund Pelligrino refer to medicine's "sacred trust" or "covenant," they do not mean, I hope, a covenant akin to the one binding God and the ancient Hebrews, but one that binds physicians and the community.[38] Most often, the medical interests of the community translate into the interests of its individual patients and here medicine finds its vocation and imperative to do no harm. But not always; during war the interests of the community may move from individual health care to collective interests. Communities have interests of their own that sometimes complement but sometimes conflict with those of their members. These interests reflect the "super-personality" of the community and highlight a shared ethos or way of life that nations and their citizens fight for during war. During war the duties of the medical practitioner, like any

---

[37] Michael E. Frisina, "Medical Ethics in Military Biomedical Research," in Thomas E. Beam, and Linette R. Sparacino, eds., *Military Medical Ethics*, vol. 2 (Textbooks of Military Medicine series; Washington, DC: Borden Institute, 2003).

[38] David C. Thomasma and Edmund D. Pellegrino, *The Virtues in Medical Practice* (Oxford: Oxford University Press, 1993).

member of the community within which he or she lives, are often shaped by collective welfare. In fact, it is precisely because the community sanctions the medical profession's privileged access to medical knowledge that physicians must use their knowledge in the service of their community. Ordinarily this demands overriding attention to beneficence and scrupulous attention to their duty to do no harm. However, during armed conflict communal interests change. The health related interests of individual patients gives way to the welfare of political community. Nonmaleficence may then yield to active participation in a just war and require physicians to take up arms in their professional capacity.

When doctors are called upon to aid a nation's war effort by taking up arms in their professional capacity it is impossible to ignore the legacy of Nazi Germany. Here, too, physicians offered their professional services to the state during war in a way that brought death and devastation to others. The Nazi doctors, however, trumpeted medical necessity without ever examining the justice of the war they were fighting. The abject failure to consider the ends and means of German aggression was not only a problem for Nazi doctors but for anyone who gladly took up the Nazi cause. Nevertheless, we are often perturbed by the behavior of physicians because we expect their professional duties to come to the fore and temper, if not override, their duty to the state in time of war. We expect the professional obligations of the physician, and perhaps the clergy, to stand as a bulwark against inhumanity during armed conflict. In this sense, perhaps, physicians like the clergy, must above all "bear witness" to their vocational pacifism and the principle of nonmaleficence that informs medicine and categorically reject any attempt on the part of the state to involve medical professionals directly in the sordid business of war. While this may illustrate the idea of a "higher calling" that some have in mind when they picture the practice of medicine, I find the claim difficult to accept. Medicine is not a minority morality. Members of the medical profession have the same duty, no more and no less than any of us, to respect the laws of decency and humanity. Their professional duties to do not commit physicians to pacifism. Rather, members of the medical community share the obligation of every responsible citizen to subject the actions of state to close scrutiny. This demands their unconditional aid when wars are just, but vociferous resistance when they are not.

References

Alexander, John P. 1999. *Future War: Nonlethal Weapons in the Twenty First Century*. New York: Thomas Dunn Books.

Alexander, John P. 2001. An Overview of the Future of Nonlethal Weapons. *Medicine, Conflict and Survival* 17: 180–193.

Army Field Manual. 1951. FM 4-02.6, 2002; FM 8-10-1.

Barak, Eitan. 2003. Where Do We Go from Here? Implementation of the Chemical Weapons Convention in the Middle East in the Post-Saddam Era. *Security Studies* 13: 106–155.

Barcelona Report of the Study Group on Europe's Security Capabilities. 2004. *A Human Security Doctrine for Europe*. http://www.lse.ac.uk/Depts/global/Human%20Security%20Report%20Full.pdf. Cited 4 June 2007.

Beam, Thomas E. and Linette R. Sparacino, eds. 2003. *Military Medical Ethics*, vols. 1–2 (*Textbooks of Military Medicine* series). Washington, DC: Office of the Surgeon General, Department of the Army, and Borden Institute).

Bender, H.S. 1947. Can a Nonresistant Nurse Serve in the Army? *Mennonursing* 1.1: 7.

Bowman, Rufus D. 1944. *The Church of the Brethren and War 1708–1941*. Elgin, IL: Brethren Publishing House.

Brock, Peter and Nigel Young. 1999. *Pacifism in the Twentieth Century*. Syracuse: Syracuse University Press.

CCW, Protocol IV, 1995. *Protocol on Blinding Laser Weapons* (Protocol IV to the *Convention on Prohibitions or Restrictions on the Use of Certain Conventional Weapons Which May be Deemed to be Excessively Injurious or to Have Indiscriminate Effects*). Geneva (10 October 1980, 13 October 1995).

CCW, Protocol II, 1980. *Protocol on Prohibitions or Restrictions on the Use of Mines, Booby-Traps and Other Devices* (Protocol II to the *Convention on Prohibitions or Restrictions on the Use of Certain Conventional Weapons Which May be Deemed to be Excessively Injurious or to Have Indiscriminate Effects*). Geneva (10 October 1980).

Convention on the Prohibition of the Development, Production, Stockpiling and Use of Chemical Weapons and on Their Destruction. 1993. http://www.opcw.org/docs/cwc_eng.pdf. Cited 4 June 2007.

Coppernoll, Margaret. 1990. The Nonlethal Weapons Debate. *Naval War College Review* 52.2: 112–131.

Coupland, Robin M. 1997. Abhorrent Weapons and 'Superfluous Injury or Unnecessary Suffering': From Field Surgery to Law. *British Medical Journal* 315: 1450–1452.

Coupland, Robin M. 1997. Nonlethal Weapons: Precipitating a New Arms Race. *BMJ* 315: 72 (12 July).

Coupland, Robin M. 1991. *The Red Cross Wound Classification*, 2nd ed. Geneva: International Committee of the Red Cross.

Coupland, Robin M. 1996. The Effect of Weapons: Defining Superfluous Injury and Unnecessary Suffering. *Medicine and Global Survival* 3: A1

Dando, Malcolm. 1996. *A New Form of Warfare: The Rise of Nonlethal Weapons*. London: Brassey's.

Davison, Neil. 2007. The Development of 'Nonlethal' Weapons During the 1990's, Occasional Paper No. 2. *Bradford Nonlethal Weapons Research Project (BNLWRP)*. Bradford: Department of Peace Studies, University of Bradford, March 2007.

Declaration Renouncing the Use, in Time of War, of Explosive Projectiles Under 400 Grammes Weight. Saint Petersburg, 29 November/11 December 1868.

Eller, Cynthia. 1991. *Conscientious Objectors and the Second World War: Moral and Religious Arguments in Support of Pacifism*. New York: Praeger.

Executive Order 11850. *Renunciation of Certain Uses in War of Chemical Herbicides and Riot Control Agents*. http://www.fas.org/bwc/eo11850.htm. Cited 4 June 2007.

Fidler, David P. 2005. The Meaning of Moscow: "Nonlethal" Weapons an International Law in the Early 21st Century. *International Review of the Red Cross* 87.859: 525–552.

Fidler, David P. 2001. Nonlethal Weapons and International Law. *Medicine Conflict and Survival* 17: 194–206.

Fidler, David P. 1999. The International Legal Implications of 'Nonlethal' Weapons. *Michigan Journal of International Law* 21.1: 51–100.

Gross, Michael L. 2006. *Bioethics and Armed Conflict: Moral Dilemmas of Medicine and War*. Cambridge, MA: MIT.

Hardin, Russell. 1985. Symposium on Ethics and Nuclear Deterrence. *Ethics* 95.3.

International Committee of the Red Cross. 1996. *The Medical Profession and the Effects of Weapons*. Geneva: International Committee of the Red Cross, Publication ref. 0668.

Kemp, Kenneth W. 1995. Personal Pacifism. *Theological Studies* 56: 21–38.

Knickerbocker, Brad. 2003. The Fuzzy Ethics of Nonlethal Weapons. *The Christian Science Monitor* (February 14, 2003). http://www.csmonitor.com/2003/0214/p02s01-usmi.html. Cited 4 June 2007.

Lakoski. Joan, et al. 2000. *The Advantages and Limitations of Calmatives for Use as a Nonlethal Technique*. Hershey, PA: College of Medicine/State College, PA: Applied Research Laboratory, Pennsylvania State University.

Lewer, Nick and Steven Schofield. 1997. *Nonlethal Weapons: A Fatal Attraction?* London: Zed Books.

Lewer, Nick and Neil Davison. 1995. Nonlethal Technologies—An Overview. *Disarmament* 1: 36–51.

Monterey Institute of International Studies. 2002. The Chemical and Biological Weapons Nonproliferation Program, Center for Nonproliferation Studies. *The Moscow Theater Hostage Crisis: Incapacitants and Chemical Warfare*. http://cns.miis.edu/pubs/week/02110b.htm. Cited 4 June 2007.

National Research Council. 2003. *An Assessment of Nonlethal Weapons Science and Technology*, Committee for an Assessment of Nonlethal Weapons Science and Technology, Naval Studies Board Division on Engineering and Physical Sciences. Washington, DC: The National Academies Press.

Quester, George H. 1990. The Psychological Effects of Bombing Civilian Populations: Wars of the Past. In *The Psychological Dimensions of War*, ed. Betty Glad, 201–235. Newbury Park, CA: Sage.

Seeley, Robert A. 1998. *Advice for Conscientious Objectors in the Armed Forces*, 5th ed. Philadelphia, PA: Central Committee for Conscientious Objectors.

Statman, Daniel. 2006. Moral Tragedies, Supreme Emergencies and National-Defence. *Journal of Applied Philosophy* 23.3: 311–322.

Statman, Daniel. 2006. Supreme Emergencies Revisited. *Ethics* 117: 58–79.

Stockholm International Peace Research Institute. 1971. The Non-use of CB Weapons During World War II. In *The Problem of Chemical and Biological Warfare, Volume 1: The Rise of CB Weapons*, 294–335. Stockholm International Peace Research Institute. New York: Humanities Press.

Tatum, Arlo. 1970. *Handbook for Conscientious Objectors*, 10th ed. Philadelphia, PA: Central Committee for Conscientious Objectors.

Teichman, Jenny. 1986. *Pacifism and the Just War: A Study in Applied Philosophy*. Oxford: Blackwell.

Thomasma, David C. and Edmund D. Pellegrino. 1993. *The Virtues in Medical Practice*. Oxford: Oxford University Press.

US Department of Defense. 1971. *Conscientious Objectors*. Washington, DC: Department of Defense, Directive Number 1300.6, August 20, 1971, certified as current, November 21, 2003, paragraph 3.3 ("Non-combatant service").

van Courtland Moon, John Ellis. 1984. Chemical Weapons and Deterrence: The World War II Experience. *International Security* 8.4: 3–35.

Wheelis, Mark. 2004. Will the New Biology Lead to New Weapons? *Arms Control Today* (July/August 2004). http://www.armscontrol.org/act/2004_07–08/Wheelis.asp?print#sidebarnotes3. Cited 4 June 2007.

The Case Against Doctor Involvement in Weapons Design and Development

Vivienne Nathanson

1 Introduction

Medicine and medical practitioners face a wide variety of challenges in a world where the knowledge and skills of physicians can be of use in contexts far removed from medicine itself. A key part of this work and knowledge environment is the way in which society and physicians themselves regard this skill and knowledge set, and how open or closed they are to its use outside a traditional medical setting.

Some of the examples of such challenges are well addressed elsewhere in this volume. Others, especially those that may challenge many physicians in everyday clinical practice, are addressed elsewhere. Dual loyalties generally are not always seen as the most interesting ethical matters, and they attract less public interest than the challenges of dealing with new technology, "cutting edge" medical science or beginning and end of life issues. Indeed a trawl of print and broadcast media would find enormous collections of reporting on matters such as "face transplants" but nothing on dual loyalties.

There are few areas of medicine where dual loyalties are as sharply seen as in the potential for physician involvement in weapons development. The essential conflict here is not between two "employers" as it is in army or prison medicine, or indeed in certain aspects of public health ethics where the conflict is between the individual and the collective, but is about the question of the use of medical knowledge and skills. Simply put, the question is whether it is ever legitimate to use medical knowledge for a purpose which has no direct relationship to healing and reduction of suffering. The dual loyalties are between the ethos of medicine and the will of an individual to use his/her knowledge "outside the box" of conventional clinical medicine.

As with other highly contentious areas of medicine there are arguments for and against. While it is possible to present these in a balanced manner there are also emotional reasons behind many of the arguments. Opposition to doctor involvement in weapons and weapons system design is classified as pacifism, or relegated to a decision based upon one of the Tom Beauchamp and James Childress's "four principles" (Gross 2006). It is, in fact, far more profound. Opposition comes from many facets summarized by being action contrary to the core ethos of medicine itself.

F. Allhoff (ed.), *Physicians at War: The Dual-Loyalties Challenge.*

Is medicine essentially a pacifist profession? The simple answer is no, the history of medicine is littered with individuals and groups who have served in the military and rendered huge service to them, healing the injured and generally saving lives. In some circumstances (e.g., plastic surgeons and burns-injured RAF pilots), the techniques developed have gone on to be of enormous value to civilian patients injured and ill in a manner unconnected to fighting.

Even where the physicians "only" patients are the war-injured, their work is not contrary to the ethos of medicine nor is it contrary to a basic pacifist tenet. Nobody wants war. It would be wrong to suggest that professional armies want wars. They want to be in a position to be as good as they can be in the event of war but prefer and expect that their excellence and professionalism is a deterrent to factors leading to a war. Ensuring that the medical response to a war is equally excellent can also be seen as part of the prevention/deterrence model. Even if that were not the case it is simple humanity—caring and compassion in terms of core values—extended to war injured that motivates the military physician. Society does not deny soldiers the right to compassionate care; pacifists refusing to become soldiers during war time conscription became ambulance drivers and part of the military care service demonstrating that health care giving is always an acceptable activity.

One major reason given by those who wish to encourage or enable the involvement of physicians in this work is that new weapons systems designed by doctors might be less awful than current or other future alternatives. Others see a medical degree as simply another type of scientific training and see no bar to the application of that knowledge greater than, for example, the application of pure mathematics or another science (e.g., Allhoff 2006; reprinted in this volume). Is medicine, and therefore the holders of medical training, somehow different? If it is different, what are the reasons?

One matter that requires discussion is the basic values and beliefs that are held by all or most doctors, perhaps especially as they enter this profession. Without this examination it is impossible to justify the assertion that this work would be contrary to the ethos of medicine.

Medicine has long been described as a vocation or calling rather than a simple career choice. Even in today's world where many are uncomfortable with such concepts there is considerable support. Work by the British Medical Association and others (1994) demonstrated that older doctors and young doctors all agreed that there were core values or principles. The only difference in the lists that emerged from the two groups was that younger doctors included in their definition of "commitment" a commitment to being a whole person, to having a life outside of medicine, not least as a balancing tool to make one a better and more resilient doctor.

The profession's ancient virtues distilled over time remain doctors' greatest asset. They include: competence; caring; commitment; integrity; compassion; responsibility; confidentiality; spirit of enquiry; and advocacy.

A survey of UK doctors (British Medical Association 1994) not only confirmed this list but also put the value in this order. Many other values were also identified—such as empathy, humility altruism and humanity. What was most remarkable was the consistency of opinion across all groups of physicians. The commentaries were about the sense of responsibility to patients and to the public, and about the need for an agreed overriding ethos for all the profession.

It follows from this that doctors are likely to have many elements of their non-religious beliefs system—or values—in common. Some writers say that medicine attracts pacifists. This is not the case. Medicine attracts people with a value system that is founded on reducing human suffering, healing individuals and communities, and recognizing that we are all one people. The values acquired along with the technical skills and knowledge of a practicing physician re-enforce these values.

This is not to say that all physicians have exactly the same beliefs. Doctors adhere to a wide variety of religious and political beliefs, which can, in and of themselves, take individuals down widely varying paths. But the underpinning values are the same.

What does this mean for doctors as weapons designers? Weapons design is not about helping humanity, or about using the arts and sciences of medicine to aid people and alleviate human suffering. It is about increasing the power of one state or non-state actor against others. It is about state, not individual, security.

Some would argue that the purpose of weapons development is to produce less medically horrific weapons. Making this argument flies in the face of the history and politics of organized weapons deployment. Weapons are developed to be more efficient at their essential purpose—removing obstacles from he way of an advancing military force. Those objects may be buildings, defensive objects, or men.

When are weapons used? Weapons are used in every country of the world in a wide variety of situations. This includes weapons used in sports and pastimes (e.g., hunting) as well as weapons designed primarily for use against human either in aggression and for defense. But however varied the circumstance the main focus of those developing weapons is for war, other types of conflict and "policing" situations. This is simply because this is the largest market; it delivers the potential for multibillion dollars of sales. Money matters, especially when developing a new product for a market many would already see as fairly saturated. Clearly this does not stop any such development from leaking into other areas—sports, self protection—but these relatively regulated markets are not the key driver of development.

The one area outside the military in which new weapons development would readily find a market is law enforcement. Here the demands are similar to those in many conflict situations, albeit the rights of individuals to kill others are usually more strictly limited. Essentially both law enforcement and the military seek weapons that would allow them to end hostage situations without harming the hostages and whether those situations arise in civilian life or in the midst of armed conflict.

Those who use weapons, and those who live in societies where they are commonly used have some understanding of the effects of the most frequently used weapons, although they may not know how this effect can be modified by the situation in which they are used. Battlefield conditions in particular are scarcely ideal for obtaining the maximum effect. Even those with experience in the use of projectile (and to a less extent exploding) weapons usually have little experience of assessing the medical effects. In developed nations there are many misperceptions about weapons effects including amongst physicians. The expectation is often that the injury is either immediately lethal or relatively trivial. A key message for emergency room and military surgeons is the effect of energy distribution from a projectile on human tissue.

2 Why Might Physicians' Knowledge and Skills Be Sought?

The history of weapons development includes the production of systems that allow one person to injure or kill another at increasing distance. As Dave Grossman (1996) has shown while man is a violent animal, capable of brutality to his own species, the majority find it difficult to deliberately and in cold blood harm another person. Armies train soldiers to overcome this reluctance, but evidence from major conflicts is that only a small minority of combatants take a life. The development of weapons occurs in parallel to the development of psychological tools to encourage reluctance to harm others. The use of technology to distance one soldier from the other encourages a depersonalization of the enemy, and thus an ability to take his life. But even this does not always make it easy for soldiers to kill without anger.

Generals do not want their soldiers reluctant to kill, but nor do they want them angry and out of control. So medical techniques, especially psychological conditioning, are part of the weapons arsenal used by modern armies. While these techniques are not weapons developments per se, they are key to the way in which weapons are used. There are complex issues relating to the involvement of doctors in training soldiers to kill without compunction. There is a clear need for physicians to understand the complex psychology of killing by soldiers, or they cannot help those who are traumatized by what they have seen or done.

The weapons that soldiers use are primarily projectile and exploding/blast weapons. Although those outside the military assume very high lethality for such weapons the only substantial research—performed by the International Committee of the Red Cross (Grossman 1996) recording the injuries of thousands of consecutive patients in war zone hospitals—demonstrates a lethality that is remarkably consistent at around 16%. Indeed the ICRC has argued (SIrUS 1997) that this is such a standard that weapons which might have far higher lethality may be unacceptable under the laws of war. While many disagree with this concept there is general agreement that the ICRC documentation of injury highlights a consistency that is relevant when measuring the effect of new weapons, as required under law. Some of the aims of the project were not achieved but the most important aim—of reinforcing the need for an expert medical input to the assessment of new weapons—was clearly won.

Lethality is not the only relevant matter when assessing the legal acceptability of a weapon Governments are required to assess whether the weapons cause injuries that are superfluous to or suffering that is unnecessary when weighed against the military necessity for their use. If such measurements are to be made there is a clear case for involving physicians.

When physicians contribute they should do so using their medical expertise about the physical and psychological effects of the weapon. When some governments developed, manufactured and deployed blinding laser weapons it was clear that the view taken about the injury caused by these weapons did not consider the full medical evidence of the harm caused by sudden and irreversible blinding. The concept behind the weapon appears to have included the notion that physical pain requiring surgery and perhaps leading to death was the outcome to be avoided and that anything else was "better".

Developed on the basis that blinding was less traumatic than penetrating projectile injuries, and particularly less likely to be fatal, the assessment clearly underestimated the psychological impact. These were to be battlefield weapons, and therefore deployed predominantly against young men. Permanent blinding would end the careers of those working as professional soldiers and further seriously limit their opportunities for employment outside the military. In many countries, blindness can make survival questionable. In addition, blindness renders activities of daily living difficult, and in the short term seriously limits social intercourse. Newly blinded young adults often suffer severe depression and may develop long-term incapacitating mental health problems. Where were these facts in the assessment of the level of suffering caused? The intervention of medical experts and experts on living with blindness reversed the policy and blinding lased weapons are now banned under international humanitarian law (the laws of war).

There is no evidence that design by physicians produces weapons that are "better" in this way. Indeed it is unlikely there could be such evidence. Before we consider the effects that might be part of a better weapon we must first consider the reason for use of weapons.

Weapons are used in war to remove soldiers of the enemy who are threatening your defense or your advance. To be effective they should remove the maximum number and, if possible, there should be minimal effect on the surroundings. Weapons that wound leaving victims urgently in need of medical attention are especially useful as the process of evacuation from the battlefield removes a number of combatants from action as well as removing the injured individual.

Is this a case for medical involvement in the development of weapons? That is, if doctors had been involved would the eventual weapons produced using new scientific developments have been in some way better? Less traumatic? Legally and morally more acceptable?

One key to discussion is that this is an example of a weapon based upon medical knowledge. It is medical and scientific work that developed lasers and studied their impact on the retina. Medical lasers are used for a variety of ophthalmic treatments and surgery. Medical knowledge has developed additionally in response to the need for regulation on the use of lasers in industry to prevent accidental blinding of workers. All of these elements of knowledge came together to produce a blinding laser weapons that would quickly and effectively target the retina without collaterally damaging material. Those involved in the development presumably did not think of the short term or longer consequences on individuals, merely of the technical challenge of producing the weapon.

The scientists, medical and other types of expert, worked in a technical vacuum omitting any holistic consideration of the effect of use of their weapon. Indeed many of those writing about their work on new weapons technologies have the same tunnel vision seeing the means to certain ends but not putting that end (an effective weapon) into a broader social context. The legitimate use of weapons in war or police actions ends, and the post wounding effects of the weapons become the predominant features. In terms of blinding, some young men would have preferred their odds on targeting with projectile weapons.

In an ideal world, then, the major role of doctors would be to abort the development, manufacture, deployment and use of weapons with medically unacceptable consequences. Sadly physicians are rarely quick or effective at taking part in such debate. Nor, indeed, do states party to the Geneva Conventions involve physicians widely in assessing the impact of future weapons against the requirements that they do not cause superfluous injury or unnecessary suffering. Nor are physicians as effective as anti-weapons lobbyists as might be expected given their education, status, media access and public credibility. The global campaign that has led the majority of countries to stop using anti-personnel landmines was led by public activists rather than health professionals. This is not meant to disregard the role of physicians and others, not least through the International Committee of the Red Cross, who produced much of the technical data that explained the effect of the weapons, and the life threatening injuries they caused (International Committee of the Red Cross 1996). Physicians groups—such as IPPNW—are often influential but the greatest success is with physicians as part of a broader public movement.

But in the anti-landmines campaign physicians did not readily find a place in the debate which they could occupy and use to protect public and individual health. That place exists, and health care professionals need to gain confidence in using their skills in this way.

3 Social Acceptability

Society generally and politicians specifically have learned from the anti-personnel landmines case that public opinion once activated does not readily get set aside. In the landmines case the international intergovernmental meeting was blocked by pressure from a limited number of countries from producing an effective ban. But the public pressure led to one government (Canada) setting up an alternative process to develop a ban, and many other countries joining them. While the process was far from perfect the outcome was a rapidly achieved and far reaching international instrument clearly demonstrating that governments are prepared to listen to public opinion, and to ignore the wishes of a powerful minority.

The other side of social acceptability gets to the heart of the question: how would society feel if its physicians are using their skills and knowledge to develop weapons? If society can be seen to have a view, a supplementary question needs to be asked about whether there is any evidence that attitudes to doctors could be effected, positively or negatively.

The answers to these questions are interesting, but reflect limited evidence. Society wants its wars won, won quickly with minimum casualties and a sustainable peace to follow. This is quite clear from global analysis of attitudes after the two world wars. Indeed recent analysis of public response to the war in Iraq suggests that even supporters of the war are disappointed by the lack of preparation for victory or of attention to post-war reconstruction.

Physicians are as likely to be patriots as any other member of society. They may see their involvement as contributing to national security. They may choose not to judge their involvement by medical ethical norms, but by the responsibility the feel as citizens.

4 Solferino and After

War is, inevitably a brutal and bloody business. Throughout history civilizations have bowed to its inevitability but attempted to erect limits to the brutality and to agree rules. The use of toxins and poisons has happened over many centuries but is one example where a series of civilizations have established rules to limit their use. In this way the Geneva Convention of 1925 and more recently the conventions on Chemical Weapons and on Biological and Toxin Weapons are our modern equivalent. As with previous examples they are far from perfect and equally far from being perfectly observed. They reflect a public horror of the use of such weapons, emanating from knowledge about he effects of the extensive use of toxins in the 1914–1918 war. Whatever other abuses were perpetuated between 1939 and 1945 these did not include battlefield use of toxins and chemical weapons. War is subject to limits—the laws of war—meant to specifically protect against unlimited brutality.

After the battle of Solferino, the level of suffering seen led to the development of the International Committee of the Red Cross and through it to formalized agreements to limit the brutality of war, and eventually to the development of the Geneva Conventions and the Conventions on Chemical and Biological Weapons. While not perfect (predominantly because of the difficulty of enforcement) these rules are important principles that few states openly violate. Coupland (1999) has called this the "Solferino Cycle"—understanding of increasing brutality leading to essentially voluntary agreements to limit across all parties the use of certain weapons or weapons groups.

Any examination of recent political history clearly shows that governments have demonstrated a wish to use powerful new scientific knowledge and skills to develop weapons to achieve their political aims. Infamously the Apartheid regime in South Africa sought ethnic weapons to be deployed against those with black skins—a weapon which would have clearly contravened the Biological and toxin weapons or chemical weapons conventions. The Russian government used drugs as a weapon to end the Moscow theatre siege—arguable a weapon banned under the

Chemical weapons convention. Conventions have less force that they should as government choose to ignore them. Medical science could be seen to be complicit in breaking down conventions designed and agrees to reduce the brutality of war.

5 Ethical Analysis

There are a wide variety of systems of ethics analysis. Using Beauchamp and Childress's four principles one must address: beneficence, non-malfeasance, autonomy and justice.

In each case it is necessary to examine both sides or parties and the balance of effect on each. It is not sufficient to examine the principle non-malfeasance without also examining the other; the conclusion should relate to the balance between conclusions on all four.

If one equates beneficence with doing good then the question is whether and how physician involvement with weapons production, development design and deployment does good. It may well do good for the physician: it offers him/her an employment opportunity and a chance to develop and use specific skills and knowledge. It allows them to act autonomously—if they wish to use these skills and this knowledge in this way—and to profit from their use.

Against that they well be producing "good" to society—if one equates government will with societal will—and acting in a way which is certainly legal and acceptable for "lay" or non-medical scientists. The evidence that by using physicians to design weapons we will produce weapons which are less awful is clearly untrue; effective weapons are essentially always awful. If they do not produce harm they are not effective, and there is no evidence that medical knowledge somehow produces "cleaner" weapons; blinding lasers are an example of how doctors can get it seriously wrong.

Weapons always do harm; it is the essential element of their nature. If we accept—and most do—that there is such a thing as a just war (the arguments are usually about whether a particular conflict fits the definition not whether the definition is be accepted) then the question of doing harm must be about the nature of the harm, its level against the good done and other factors. Looking at laser weapons they are effective in taking a group of people off the battle field (the injured soldier and several colleagues to get him to safety) but the damage done in permanently blinding exceeds the military advantage (or good) obtained.

While autonomy or self-determination is seen by many to be an overriding principle, that is of the highest importance, it is not absolute or unlimited. Again countervailing questions must be dealt with. If in acting autonomously we impinge on the freedoms others have a right to enjoy then our own autonomy should be limited.

A doctor might autonomously wish to use his skills and knowledge to develop weapons. But in doing so he has a direct and an indirect impact on other doctors. There is evidence that the trust patients have in anesthetics and in anesthetic practitioners was compromised by the use of anesthetic agents in the Moscow theatre siege (Nathanson 2007). The trust in medical research is undermined when evidence of research for non-medical reasons surfaces. Trust in the essential good of doctors was seriously undermined by evidence of the work of Josef Mengele, Wouter Basson, and others. Even in the era of free and valid consent to medical testing and treatment a large element of trust is essential to the patient doctor relationship: such evidence as there is shows that medical involvement in weapons development undermines that trust. This trust is so important that any reasonable conjecture that it could be undermined by a specific action makes it imperative that the right of that individual to act in that way is curtailed.

Justice is probably essentially neutral in terms of this argument, except if the suggestion is to produce weapons that specifically inequitably target one group, when again the examination would come firmly down on the side of not allowing medical knowledge or skills to be used.

Many would describe the overall objective of medicine, *primum non nocere* or, above all, do no harm. Producing weapons, weapons systems, weapons deployment, etc. must always do harm. If the overall ethos of medicine is about the acquiring of skills and knowledge and the use of those same skills and knowledge to help humanity then its use for weapons development is contrary to that ethos.

Public health and wellbeing are often cited as reasons for medical involvement. Whether this is because doctors would somehow lessen the harm, or make victory quicker, the arguments are rendered invalid both because history and science do not bear them out and because this involvement is contrary to the ethos of medicine.

Physicians have a major public health role to play. It is essential they engage in dialogue with government and other planners to deal with the consequences and aftermath of conflict and of systematic weapons use. Military planners consider how best to get a rapid victory. They will often plan to minimize the damage to infrastructure, but they will often also plan to use massive aerial bombardment (Ulman and Wade 1996). This inevitably leads to International evidence is tat they are far less effective at considering the public health effects of their actions and things that must be done to ameliorate the harms produced. Doctors, especially public health experts, know what health harms are produced by the physical disruptions caused by explosive weapons, and which must be repaired first to minimize public health harms.

The fundamental ethos of medicine is the use of knowledge and skills to alleviate human suffering. Medical ethics debate considers how physicians carry out this function, and balance the potential conflicts between the rights of individuals and those of society. Beauchamp and Childress's principles are one way of assessing this balance.

Those who support physician involvement in developing weapons cite different means of reducing human suffering to back up their belief. In theory, physicians could develop new ways of harming, disabling or killing others that do not entail the pain and possible disability consequent on the use of conventional weapons. Evidence from the development of new weapons internationally is that physician involvement does not produce such weapons: most planners and designers believe that such weapons are beyond current or reasonably foreseeable science.

Weapons research is carried out for a variety of reasons, including increasing the effectiveness of the weapon, but also so that defenses against the weapon can be improved. Physicians are inevitably involved in this; they explore and categorize weapons effects better to design defense and treatment options. Although this knowledge is useful for weapons designers that is not its principle purpose and thus this work is clearly ethical.

Moving beyond this to identify technology, techniques and mechanisms to improve the effectiveness of weapons is a move into the area of unacceptable activity.

6 Conclusion

It is all too easy to argue that doctors should devise weapons. If they do so the weapons will benefit from the medical knowledge and somehow be more humane, less painful, better. But this is not based upon sound science or sound ethics and may even be a real slippery slope argument. Medical knowledge could be used to make torture "better" or to improve executions. But such use of medical knowledge is and always shall be an abuse; these actions are not about improving health, wellbeing and welfare for individuals or communities, but about aiding security services, policing and other actions which are not about health and health care.

Arguing that decreasing insecurity improves health may be accurate but is irrelevant. Doctors can and indeed must be involved in planning for the aftermath of war and in treating those who are ill—physically or psychologically—because of conflict. They must also consider the conditions in which the population—on their patients or service users—and have a moral responsibility to make governments aware of the dangers to health of different courses of action.

Medicine is not about pacifism although doctors may be come pacifists as their personal knowledge of the effects of war develops. Their place in the "Solferino cycle" is of explaining to experts outside the field of health just how damaging armed conflict is on the health welfare and wellbeing of individuals and of societies. They also have a role in negotiating for a proper process for planning the aftermath of war or other conflict. But they cannot remain doctors and be involved in developing weapons and weapons systems; that is an abuse of their knowledge, skills and privileged place in society.

References

Allhoff, Fritz. 2006. Physician Involvement in Hostile Interrogation. *Cambridge Quarterly of Healthcare Ethics* 15.2: 392–402.

British Medical Association. 1994. *Core Values for the Medical Professional in the 21st Century.* Report of a conference held on 3–4 November. General Medical Council and others.

British Medical Association. 1994. *Core Values.* Survey report.

Coupland, Robin M. 1999. The Effects of Weapons and the Solferino Cycle. *British Medical Journal* 319: 864–865.
Coupland, Robin M. and Peter Herby. 1999. Review of the Legality of Weapons: A New Approach—the SIrUS Project. *International Review of the Red Cross* 835 (Sept): 583–592.
Gross, Michael L. 2006. *Bioethics and Armed Conflict: Moral Dilemmas of Medicine and War*. Cambridge, MA: MIT.
Grossman, Dave. 1996. *On Killing: The Psychological Cost of Learning to Kill in War and Society*. New York: Little Brown.
International Committee of the Red Cross. 1996. *The Medical Profession and the Effects of Weapons*. Report of a symposium. http://www.icrc.org/WEB/ENG/siteeng0.nsf/htmlall/ p0668?OpenDocument&style=Custo_Final.4&View=defaultBody2. Cited 1 June 2007.
Nathanson, Vivienne, ed. 2007. *The Use of Drugs as Weapons: The Concerns and Responsibilities of Healthcare Professionals*. London: British Medical Association.
The SIrUS Project. 1997. *Towards a Definition of Which Weapons Cause Superfluous Injury or Unnecessary Suffering*. International Committee of the Red Cross.
Ulman, Harlan K. and James P. Wade. 1996. *Shock and Awe: Achieving Rapid Dominance*. Washington, DC: National Defense University, Institute for Strategic Studies.

Armed Conflict and Value Conflict: Case Studies in Biological Weapons[1]

Michael J. Selgelid

1 Introduction

This paper provides ethical analysis of two case studies arising in the context of biological weapons. The first concerns what is commonly known as "the dual-use dilemma", which arises when knowledge gleaned from scientific research can be used for both good and bad purposes. Scientific discoveries that constitute important advances in science and medicine, for example, may sometimes facilitate biological weapons development. For well-intentioned researchers, this creates difficult choices about whether or not to publish findings that could be used for harmful purposes by malevolent actors. Society or the government must likewise make tough choices about whether and/or how to regulate dual-use research and the dissemination of information that results from such research. For both individual scientists and the government, the dual-use dilemma poses a conflict between the protection of security, on the one hand, and the promotion of science and medicine, on the other. In the context of governmental regulation, the protection of security may also conflict with the protection of liberties such as academic freedom and freedom of speech.

The second case study considers conflicting values associated with public health care measures that might be called for in the actual event of a bioterrorist attack with a contagious infectious disease. In such a scenario, coercive (and potentially harmful) measures such as quarantine may be required in order to protect public health. Health workers and policy makers would then be faced with a conflict between the (more libertarian or deontological) aim to protect the rights and well-being of individual patients, on the one hand, and the (more utilitarian) aim to promote the greater good of society on the other.

In both case studies, I conclude that we should seek balance between the values at stake rather than attributing absolute priority to—or having overriding loyalty towards—one value or another. I offer specific policy recommendations for striking such a balance in practice.

---

[1] I thank the Brocher Foundation in Hermance, and the Institute for Biomedical Ethics at the University of Geneva, in Switzerland, for hosting me as a visiting researcher during the period this paper was written.

F. Allhoff (ed.), *Physicians at War: The Dual-Loyalties Challenge.*

2 Dual-Use Research[2]

2.1 *Ethics and Genetics*

Given all of the attention to ethical, legal and social issues (ELSI) associated with genetics, it is ironic that so little bioethics discourse has focused on the implications of genetic science with respect to biological weapons development. The lack of attention to this topic is partly revealed by the fact that, despite all the links that are drawn between genetics and atomic weapons, Robert Cooke-Deegan's canonical history of the Human Genome Project—*The Gene Wars*,[3] which explicitly includes coverage of the politics and ethical debate surrounding the new genetics, and which even includes a chapter titled "Genes and the Bomb"—never mentions (discussion or debate about) the biological weapons implications of genetics. It is commonly said that the power of genetics is comparable to the power of atomic physics, and that we need more ethical discussion and reflection about the former than the latter received when the first atomic bombs were made and used—the idea being that more socially responsible decisions about science should be made in genetics than were made in the context of nuclear energy. The usual topics of ELSI genetics discourse, however, reveal that the power of genetics with regard to weapons development is not what those concerned with the ethics of genetics usually have in mind.

Another link between genetics and atomic weapons is that important origins of the Human Genome Project are found in the US Department of Energy—and the Los Alamos labs where the first atomic bombs were made. Such organizations were interested in genetics partly because they wanted to learn about radiation's effects on genes. Given these organizations' explicit concern with (albeit nuclear) weapons of mass destruction—not to mention these organizations' governmental and military affiliations—one expects that those involved would have recognized and thought about the weapons potential of the genetics revolution very early on. The absence of biological weapons discussion in Cooke-Deegan's history, however, is telling.

One wonders if it was a mere oversight (on the part of key historical actors) that there has not already been more academic and public discussion about the weapons implications of genetics. Rather than drawing cynical conclusions about conspiracy, for now I merely highlight this lacuna as a historical curiosity. Proper historical investigation and analysis (beyond the scope of this paper) is required to explain it.

Further evidence, aside from Cooke-Deegan's book, that such a gap exists is provided by the ELSI genetics literature more generally. Initial controversy surrounded the worry that recombinant DNA might pose environmental hazards. More

---

[2] The following discussion of dual-use draws heavily from Michael J. Selgelid, "A Tale of Two Studies: Ethics, Bioterrorism, and the Censorship of Science," *Hastings Center Report* 37.3 (2007): 35–43.

[3] Robert Cooke-Deegan, *The Gene Wars: Science, Politics, and the Human Genome* (New York: Norton, 1994). The discussion that follows is not meant to critique Cooke-Deegan's work.

recent debate has focused on things like genetic determinism, genetic testing, discrimination by employers and insurance companies, selective reproduction, genetic enhancement, cloning, stem cell research, DNA fingerprinting, and the patenting of DNA sequences. That these have to date been *the* standard topics is quickly revealed by examination of titles, tables of contents, and indexes of texts concerned with ethical, legal, and social implications of genetics. At the time of this writing (in 2007), a huge number of journal articles and books on ethics and genetics have been written; but these include little if any discussion of genetics' potential role in weapons-making.

Though hardly discussed among bioethicists, meanwhile, the weapons implications of genetics could turn out to be *the* most serious consequence of the genetics revolution. This is implied by what is said in an unclassified CIA document titled "The Darker Bioweapons Future":

> A panel of life sciences experts convened for the Strategic Assessments Group by the National Academy of Sciences concluded that advances in biotechnology ... have the potential to create a much more dangerous biological warfare (BW) threat. The panel noted [that t]he effects of some of these [genetically] engineered biological agents could be worse than any disease known to man.[4]

This is no small claim, and it originates from eminent scientists rather than the CIA itself.

2.2 *The Bioweapons Threat*

Why do experts take the biological weapons threat so seriously?

Biological weapons have a long history including, among other things, ancient Greeks and Romans poisoning enemy wells with carrion; Tartars catapulting plague victims' bodies over enemy walls on the Crimean Peninsula during the 14th century; the British Army's provision of smallpox-laden blankets to American Indians in the 1800s; Germany's use of anthrax against livestock during the First World War; and Japan's bombing of China with plague during the Second World War. More recent incidents include activities of cult organizations such as the Rajneeshee which poisoned salad bars in The Dalles (Oregon) with *Salmonella* in 1984; and Aum Shinrikyo, which launched a number of (unsuccessful) anthrax attacks in Japan during the 1990s.[5] Last but not least were the anthrax attacks that killed five people in the US, shortly after the events of 11 September 2001. History reveals that humans can be all-to-willing to use biological weapons.

---

[4] Central Intelligence Agency, "The Darker Bioweapons Future," 3 November 2003, http://www.fas.org/irp/cia/product/bw1103.pdf, cited 4 June 2007.

[5] See Judith Miller, Stephen Engelberg, and William Broad, *Germs: The Ultimate Weapon* (London: Simon & Schuster, 2001).

A second concern relates to proliferation. Until its collapse in the early 1990s, the former Soviet Union ran an enormous illegal biological weapons program employing 60,000 workers.[6] Known as "Biopreparat", this program had the capacity to produce hundreds (or, in some cases, thousands) of tons of anthrax, plague, smallpox, Marburg virus, and numerous other biological weapons agents.[7] Soviet scientists also attempted to create novel pathogens for weapons purposes. One project aimed at development of a "chimera" hybrid between smallpox and Ebola; the goal was a microbe as contagious as the former and as deadly as the latter. The program allegedly successfully developed vaccine-resistant strains of anthrax and drug-resistant strains of anthrax, glanders, and plague.[8] The whereabouts of most of the scientists who worked for this program are now unknown. Also unknown is what happened to the vast supply of Soviet bioweapons stocks. Not to mention the instability that followed collapse of the Soviet empire, proliferation is a serious concern given that biological weapons agents are so small, especially in comparison with nuclear weapons.

A final reason for fear about biological weapons—illustrated by the story of Biopreparat and also by the CIA claim above—is that recent scientific progress may revolutionize biological weapons-making. This is partly because of the "dual-use" aspect of biomedical science: the very same developments that may lead to advancements in medicine—e.g., genetic sequencing and genetic engineering—can also (often enough) lead to advancements in biological weapons-making. This problem is compounded by the fact that there is a long history of complete openness and the free sharing of information in the life sciences. Potentially dangerous information is routinely published in the life science literature. Biology here contrasts sharply with physics, where there is a long tradition of secrecy—and where discoveries with nuclear weapons implications are automatically "born classified".[9]

2.3 Controversial Cases

Questions about how to regulate the conduct of "dual-use" research and the dissemination of information regarding potentially dangerous discoveries have thus become paramount in debates about biosecurity.[10] Much of the debate has focused

---

[6] Ken Alibek and Stephen Handelman, *Biohazard: The Chilling True Story of the Largest Covert Biological Weapons Program in the World—Told from the Inside be the Man Who Ran it* (New York: Delta, 1999).

[7] Miller et al., *Germs*.

[8] Alibek and Handelman, *Biohazard*.

[9] National Research Council, *Biotechnology Research in an Age of Terrorism* (Washington, DC: National Academies Press, 2004).

[10] Such debate has to date been dominated by science and security communities, rather than ethicists.

on a number of recently published studies. Australian scientists in Canberra, for example, used standard genetic engineering techniques to insert the IL-4 (interleukin) gene into the mousepox virus.[11] Their hope was that the altered virus would sterilize mice and thus provide means of pest control. They accidentally discovered, however, that they had produced a superstrain of mousepox in the process. The altered virus killed both mice that were naturally resistant to, and mice that had been vaccinated against, ordinary strains of mousepox (which is a close cousin of smallpox). They published their results in the *Journal of Virology* in 2001. In a second study, American researchers at the State University of New York (SUNY) at Stony Brook artificially synthesized a "live" polio virus from scratch. They strung together commercial available strands of DNA, purchased over the Internet, in correspondence with the map of the RNA polio genome, which is published on the Internet. The addition of protein resulted in a live virus that paralyzed and killed mice. *Science* published the study in 2002.[12] A third study, published in *Science* in 2005,[13] used similar techniques of genetic engineering and synthetic biology to reconstruct the 1918 flu virus, which killed between 20 and 100 million people. In all three of these cases, the published studies included description of materials and methods used.

All three studies lead to complaint by critics who claimed that publishing studies like these both alerts bioterrorists to new possible ways of producing biological weapons and, worse, actually provides them with explicit instructions—"recipes", "roadmaps", or "blueprints"—for doing so.[14] The mousepox technique, for example, might provide means for production of vaccine-resistant smallpox. This would be serious because there is no treatment for smallpox; vaccine is our only defense against it. Even ordinary smallpox already tops lists of feared biological weapons agents. Smallpox is believed to have killed more people than any other infectious disease in history. In the 20th century alone, it killed between 300 and 500 million people—three times more than were killed by all the wars of that period.[15] An implication of the polio study is that it may allow bioterrorists to construct dangerous pathogens that they might not otherwise have access to. There are fears that the technique could be used to construct smallpox or Ebola, for example. The flu study,

[11] Ronald J. Jackson, Alistair J. Ramsay, Carina D. Christensen, Sandra Beaton, Diana F. Hall, and Ian A. Ramshaw, "Expression of Mouse Interleukin-4 by a Recombinant Ectromelia Virus Suppresses Cytolytic Lymphocyte Responses and Overcomes Genetic Resistance to Mousepox," *Journal of Virology* 75.3 (2001): 1205–1210.

[12] Jeronimo Cello, Aniko V. Paul, and Eckard Wimmer, "Chemical Synthesis of Poliovirus cDNA: Generation of Infectious Virus in the Absence of Natural Template," *Science* 297 (2002): 1016–1018.

[13] Jocelyn Kaiser, "Resurrected Influenza Virus Yields Secrets of Deadly 1918 Pandemic," *Science* 310 (2005): 28–29.

[14] The three examples discussed above have been among the most high-profile cases; but they are by no means the only studies that have aroused this kind of controversy in recent years.

[15] Michael B. A. Oldstone, *Viruses, Plagues, and History* (New York: Oxford University Press, 1998).

finally, might enable aspiring bioterrorists to construct and unleash the virus responsible for one of the worst epidemics in human history.

In all three cases, the scientists and editors involved defended their actions. Although they understood the potential dangers, they argued that the benefits outweighed the risks of publication. In the mousepox and polio studies, for example, they claimed it was important to alert the scientific community that new possibilities for bioweapons development had been discovered. The scientific community, they claimed, needs to be aware of these possibilities in order to recognize the importance of developing protections—e.g., new treatments and vaccines—against them. In the case of the 1918 flu reconstruction, the public health imperative of studying the virus was said to outweigh risks of bioterrorism, especially in light of current concerns about H5N1 (avian influenza)—and because it is just a matter of time until the next naturally occurring major flu pandemic will strike (regardless of what happens with H5N1). This study may facilitate development of new treatments and vaccines that would not be possible if key scientific achievements are kept secret.

In response to the complaint that at least the materials and methods sections of the articles should have been altered or omitted, defenders of publication appealed to the importance of open communication in science. Scientific methodology requires replication and verification of others' findings—but this would not be possible if detailed description of materials and methods are not provided in published studies. Scientific progress would be compromised if this kind of information is withheld from publication.

2.4 Policy

Despite all the controversy about whether or not these and other studies should have been published, there is now widespread agreement that dual-use research poses important dangers that must be addressed. In the aftermath of the mousepox and polio studies—and the events surrounding September 11, which heightened fears about terrorism—a great amount of dialogue regarding dual-use research ensued between scientists, editors, and security experts.[16] Outcomes include a number of important statements, reports, and guidelines. Another outcome was the formation of the National Science Advisory Board for Biosecurity (NSABB) in the US in 2004.

In 2003 a joint "Statement on Scientific Publication and Security" of the "Journal Editors and Authors Group" was simultaneously published by *Science, Nature*, the *Proceedings of the National Academy of Sciences*, and the American Society for Microbiology journals. It addition to reiterating the importance of "publishing manuscripts ... in sufficient detail to permit reproducibility" and the importance of sometimes publishing studies with bioweapons implications in order

[16] Much of this dialogue took place in advance of the above-mentioned flu publication.

to facilitate biodefense preparations, it states that journals will implement policy to screen manuscripts that raise security issues, and that editors will reject or modify—i.e., censor—manuscripts when "the potential harm of publication outweighs the potential societal benefits."[17]

Though the censorship of science should not be taken lightly, we should all agree that censorship may sometimes be appropriate. There are at least imaginable cases where publication could be disastrous. If scientists discover a cheap and easy way of making smallpox—or some new microbe just as contagious, deadly, and untreatable—then instructions for doing so is surely not information we would want in the public domain. I imagine and hope that almost no one disagrees with this.

For those who agree that censorship would—imaginably at least—sometimes be called for, a more difficult question is what the process of censorship should be. Should the government decide what gets censored, for example, or should we rely on voluntary self-governance of the scientific community? Scientific progress matters, but security matters too; and neither goal should be given absolute priority over the other. It is safe to say that a consensus has emerged that a system is wanted for striking a balance between these two kinds of goals.[18] In a landmark treatise on dual-use research widely known as "The Fink Report", the US National Research Council has taken the stance that this balance should be achieved through reliance on voluntary self-governance of the scientific community—its concern being that governmental control over what gets published in science would stall important areas of scientific research.[19]

In resonance with much of what is said by the NRC, the Council on Ethical and Judicial Affairs (CEJA) of the American Medical Association (AMA) apparently claims that scientists are, furthermore, in the best position to judge which discoveries should or should not be published. In discussion of new AMA "Guidelines to Prevent Malevolent Use of Biomedical Research", CEJA claims that:

> Although this is an undoubtedly complicated undertaking, physician-researchers, who possess profound knowledge of their research and of human health and disease, are arguably in the best position to assess the potential for and the ramifications of misapplications of their research.[20]

If correct, this might provide additional support for the idea that voluntary self-governance of the scientific community would provide appropriate means to control what gets published in science.

---

[17] Journal Editors and Authors Group, "Uncensored Exchange of Scientific Results," *Proceedings of the National Academy of Sciences* 100.4 (18 February 2003): 1464, www.pnas.org/cgi/doi/10.1073/pnas.0630491100, cited 4 June 2007.

[18] See National Science Advisory Board for Biosecurity (NSABB), http://biosecurity-board.gov, cited 4 June 2007.

[19] National Research Council, *Biotechnology Research in an Age of Terrorism.*

[20] Shane K. Green, Sara Taub, Karine Morin, and Daniel Higginson for the Council on Ethical and Judicial Affairs of the American Medical Association, "Guidelines to Prevent Malevolent Use of Biomedical Research," *Cambridge Quarterly of Healthcare Ethics* 15 (2006): 435.

NRC guidelines, meanwhile, have apparently been followed and (with the possible exception of federally-funded research subject to classification)[21] the status quo in the US involves reliance upon voluntary self-governance. The NSABB was established in 2004 to "provide advice and guidance to the federal government"[22] regarding dual-use research. The establishment of this advisory board followed a recommendation of the NRC. Though part of its role has been to review scientific papers raising security issues, referral of cases to the NSABB is voluntary and its conclusions (about the advisability of publication in any given case) are not legally binding. The *Science* paper on the 1918 flu reconstruction was sent to the NSABB for review in 2005. Though NSABB members unanimously agreed that the paper should be published, *Science* editor-in-chief Donald Kennedy subsequently wrote that, unless the paper was classified, the magazine would have published it "even if the NSABB had voted otherwise".[23]

2.5 A Balanced Solution

Conflicting values surround questions about communication of dual-use information. A system involving minimal governmental restriction may be best at promoting liberty and the advancement of science—but this may have costs in terms of security. A more restrictive system, on the other hand, may promote security, but this would have costs in terms of liberty and scientific advance.[24] As there is no good reason to give absolute priority to the promotion of liberty and scientific advance over security, or vice versa, the censorship process should aim to strike a balance between both kinds of values without being biased towards either. Decision-makers, furthermore, should have sufficient expertise to evaluate the extent to which both kinds of values are threatened and/or likely to be promoted by their choices.

The scientific community is right to be wary about governmental censorship. Given what they do for a living, it is not unlikely that bureaucrats and security

---

[21] Classification of biological research is not an option except when the research is federally funded. This contrasts with nuclear research with weapons implications, where discoveries are automatically "born" classified whether or not funded by the US government. See National Research Council, *Biotechnology Research in an Age of Terrorism*.

[22] See NSABB, http://biosecurity-board.gov, cited 4 June 2007.

[23] Donald Kennedy, "Better Never Than Late," *Science* 310 (2005): 195.

[24] For further consideration of policy options, see Seumas Miller and Michael J. Selgelid, *Ethical and Philosophical Implications of the Dual-Use Dilemma in the Biological Sciences* (Canberra, Australia: Centre for Applied Philosophy and Public Ethics [CAPPE], The Australian National University, and Charles Sturt University, 2006). That project resulted from a CAPPE consultation with the Australian Department of Prime Minister and Cabinet, National Security and Technology Unit. It involved collaboration with Antony Della-Porta, Christian Enemark, Peter Kerr, and Ian Ramshaw. An excerpt from the report is included in this volume. My thinking about the dual-use dilemma has benefited from participation in that project.

experts would be biased in favor of security values over scientific values. There is also reason to doubt that governmental decision makers will always have sufficient expertise to judge the scientific importance of publishing studies they might want to censor. An additional worry about the censorship of science by government is that this would be one more step down the path of liberty infringement in the name of the war on terrorism—and that governmental censorship would threaten academic freedom and freedom of speech more generally.

The current reliance on voluntary self-governance of the scientific community, however, is unacceptable as well. Just as bureaucrats are likely to be biased in favor of security protection over scientific progress, scientists are likely to be biased in favor of the promotion of science over security. Another problem with voluntary self-governance is that clear conflicts of interest will occur. Because career advancement in academia requires a strong publication record, individual scientists will have self-interested reasons for publishing their work even when security risks arise. Just as bureaucrats may lack sufficient expertise to judge the scientific importance of publication, finally, scientists will generally lack expertise for judging the security risks of publication. Scientists simply are not usually security experts. Most have had little or no training whatsoever in security studies. Scientists might be best able to evaluate the scientific implications of their discoveries, but *security* implications are something different. Scientists might be best able to determine the likelihood, for example, that the mousepox technique could be used to produce to vaccine-resistant smallpox—and they might be best able to determine what the public health implications of a smallpox attack would be. But scientists do not have any special knowledge or skill to determine what the security implications of a smallpox attack would be.

Last, but not least, scientists are sometimes systematically denied information crucial to risk assessment. Rather than a mere hypothetical possibility, this is true for one of the cases that has been central to biosecurity debates about censorship—i.e., the mousepox study.[25] The risk of that publication (partly) depends on the likelihood that would-be bioterrorists have access to the smallpox virus. In order to employ the mousepox genetic engineering technique on smallpox, a bioterrorist must possess the smallpox virus to begin with. All of the world's samples of smallpox are, however, officially supposed to be safe-and-secure at the Centers for Disease Control and Prevention in Atlanta and at a similar facility in the former Soviet Union. It is possible that there has been proliferation from Soviet weapons stocks of smallpox, but any details about this are classified information that scientists generally lack access to. Scientists are thus denied information essential to estimating the risk of the mousepox publication. In the crucial case of the mousepox study, the AMA suggestion that scientists are "in the best position to assess the potential for and the ramifications of misapplications of their research"[26] should thus be flatly rejected.

[25] This point, however, was apparently unnoticed by the main parties to the debate in question.

[26] Green et al., "Guidelines to Prevent Malevolent Use."

What would be a better solution? We want a decision body that embodies both security and science *values* (without being biased towards either) and security and science *expertise* (to a sufficiently high degree). This might be achieved by providing decision making authority to a mixed panel of experts, all of whom are granted high-level security clearance. Such a panel could be constituted by members half of whom work for government and half of whom are civilians, and half of whom are security experts and half of whom are scientists. Twenty-five percent of members would be governmental security experts, 25% would be governmental scientists, 25% would be civilian security experts, and 25% would be civilian scientists.[27] Members of each group could be nominated by salient organizations they represent. Governmental members could be nominated by the Department of Health and Human Services, the Department of Homeland Security, the Department of Defense, and/or the CIA. Civilian members could be nominated by the National Academies, and so on. To avoid inclusion of biased members with extreme values and narrow expertise, each organization could be given veto power over the nominations of other groups' members. Referral of research that meets criteria specified by the panel would be required—e.g., via implementation of a binding code of scientific conduct—and the decisions of the panel would be required by law.

Though I have here sketched a domestic solution,[28] the dangers of dual-use research are global in nature—and so an international solution is ultimately needed. As with other global public goods problems,[29] international governance may ultimately be required to solve this problem. In the absence of international government, an international treaty could require that a system along the lines of that described above is implemented within signatory states and/or that an international panel along the lines of that described above is established and given regulatory authority over what gets published within signatory states.

3 Coercive Social Distancing: Isolation and Quarantine

Above we considered value conflict arising in the context of research with weapons implications. Value conflict may likewise arise in the actual event of a biological attack with a contagious infectious disease.[30] Depending on the disease and the extent to which it is contagious and deadly, standard public health care measures for containing the outbreak may involve coercive measures such as isolation or

---

[27] Selgelid, "A Tale of Two Studies." I here suggest these four categories for the sake of simplicity. A better panel would include some ethicists!

[28] My main purpose has been to reject NRC recommendations regarding voluntary self-governance and to argue that the status quo in the US in unacceptable.

[29] Both scientific knowledge and security can plausibly be considered global public goods.

[30] The following discussion of social distancing draws heavily from Michael Selgelid, "Ethics of Infectious Disease Control," in *The Encyclopedia of Public Health*, ed. H. Kristian Heggenhougen (Amsterdam, The Netherlands: Elsevier, forthcoming).

quarantine of infected individuals, those suspected to be infected, and/or those who have been exposed. In this case, the goal to promote the greater good of society in the way of public health (and security) may conflict with the goal to protect the rights and liberties of individuals. Mandatory confinement would conflict with the right to freedom of movement; and quarantine may conflict with the most basic right of all—i.e., the right to life. The quarantine of an airplane containing passengers with a contagious deadly disease, for example, may lead to the infection—and death—of previously uninfected passengers who are confined in close proximity with those who are infected.

Does this mean that coercive social distancing measures such as isolation and quarantine would be unethical or wrong? Not necessarily. We should again seek to strike a balance between conflicting goods in the context in question. Individual rights and liberties matter. We should not ride roughshod over individuals in the name of public health. This would involve utilitarian thinking that most philosophers, policy makers, and ordinary citizens reject upon reflection. The goal to promote (utility in the way of) public health matters, but it should not be given absolute priority.

Individual rights and liberties, however, should not be given absolute priority either. If a catastrophic epidemic would result from the maximal protection of individual rights and liberties, then individual rights and liberties must be compromised. Even arch-libertarian Robert Nozick hints that we may need to violate "side-constraints" (i.e., human rights) when this is necessary to avoid "catastrophic moral horror".[31] Though it should be considered an extreme or exceptional measure, there is no reason to in principle rule out quarantine altogether, even if it sometimes ends up killing innocent people, just as there is no ethical reason to rule out participation in (just) war—which also inevitably involves compromise of innocent individuals' rights, including the right to life. If quarantine, despite its costs to individuals held in confinement, is required to enable prevention or minimization of what would otherwise be an enormous public health (and security) disaster, then it may be considered an acceptable and necessary, though unfortunate, means of responding to a bioterrorist attack.

The ethical questions, then, are: who should have ultimate authority to impose quarantine[32] and how can quarantine decisions be made in a responsible, rational, well-informed, balanced manner? Principles regarding the ethical acceptability of quarantine should arguably include the following. First, an extreme measure such as this should not be employed unless there are compelling reasons to believe that it would be an effective means of controlling disease in the circumstances under consideration. While authors such as George Annas deny that quarantine actually works,[33] this is of course an empirical question. We should avoid making and/or

---

[31] Robert Nozick, *Anarchy, State, and Utopia* (New York: Basis Books, 1974), 30n.

[32] Answers to this first question are beyond the scope of this paper, but see Lawrence O. Gostin et al., "Model State Emergency Health Powers Act" (21 December 2001), http://www.publichealthlaw.net/MSEHPA/MSEHPA2.pdf, cited 4 June 2007.

[33] George J. Annas, *American Bioethics: Crossing Human Rights and Health Law Boundaries* (New York: Oxford University Press, 2005).

accepting sweeping empirical claims in the absence of empirical evidence. There are historical cases—such as that of American Samoa during the 1918–1919 flu pandemic—where coercive social distancing measures appear to have been highly effective.[34] The evidence for or against the effectiveness of quarantine warrants further study. Given the difficulty of conducting controlled studies in the context of quarantine, however, it will not be easy to conclusively demonstrate whether or not quarantine would be effective in any given circumstance, and greater uncertainty will arise in the case of unknown novel pathogens. There is an ethical imperative, in any case, that researchers with relevant expertise further examine this issue as best they can; relevant information is required for solving ethical/policy questions as well as questions that are more purely concerned with public health science.

Second, mandatory quarantine should not be employed unless it is actually required. If alternative, less restrictive means are available to achieve the same ends regarding public health protection, then these should be employed instead. If voluntary quarantine, for example, would likely be just as effective as mandatory quarantine, then the latter should not be imposed. Mandatory quarantine should only be used as a last resort.[35]

Third, an extreme measure such as quarantine should not be imposed unless consequences of failing to do so would be great. It would be wrong to think that rights violations and the imposition of harms on individuals are justified whenever this would lead to a net payoff for society as a whole. The maximal promotion of public health should not be the sole goal of ethical public health policy. Ethical public health policy should aim to balance the goal to promote public health with other legitimate aims such as respecting the rights and protecting the well-being of individuals. Some have argued that perhaps less public health justification would be required for the imposition of quarantine in the event of a bioterrorist attack in comparison with a naturally occurring outbreak of an infectious disease—because the goal to fight the evil of terrorism provides additional justification in the former circumstance.[36] This plausible idea warrants further discussion. The stakes would in any case still need to be high, all things considered, in order for draconian liberty infringing measures to be legitimate.

Fourth, for quarantine to be ethically acceptable, it must be implemented in an equitable manner. It would be unjust, that is, if quarantine is used (as it often has been in the past) in a discriminatory fashion against those who are already socially

---

[34] Alfred W. Crosby, *Americas Forgotten Pandemic: The Influenza of 1918*, 2nd ed. (Cambridge: Cambridge University Press, 2003). The important case of American Samoa reveals that we should reject the often heard claim that measures like quarantine would/could only have an early and minor role in the event of a major flu pandemic. That might be true in places like the US, but demographic context matters here—and islands, at least, are a different story.

[35] Lawrence O. Gostin, "Public Health Strategies for Pandemic Influenza," *JAMA* 295 (2006): 1700–1704.

[36] Evan S. Michelson, "Individual Freedom or Collective Welfare? An Analysis of Quarantine as Response to Global Infectious Disease," In *Ethics and Infectious Disease*, eds. Michael J. Selgelid, Margaret P. Battin, and Charles B. Smith (Oxford: Blackwell, 2006).

marginalized or disempowered. One could argue that the grounds for imposing quarantine must be strongest when those being considered for confinement are members of the worst-off groups in society. Just as research ethics guidelines give special protection to those who are vulnerable, that is, quarantine guidelines should arguably do the same.

Fifth, quarantine, if implemented, should be made as minimally burdensome as possible. Insofar as is feasible, those confined should be provided with basic necessities such as food, water, comfort, and healthcare. A sixth, and related, point is that those who suffer quarantine for the benefit of society should be compensated in return. It would be wrong if confined individuals are expected to themselves suffer a disproportionate amount of the burden required for the protection of society as a whole. The burdens associated with epidemic disease are shared more fairly if those who make sacrifices by succumbing to quarantine are provided with compensation for doing so. If there are limited amounts of medicine and vaccine available, for example, then those who have been quarantined may deserve special priority when allocation decisions about medical resources are made. Those confined will also deserve financial compensation for inconvenience, missed work, and so on. In addition to compensating coerced victims for harms/losses suffered, it might be appropriate to provide them with additional (financial) rewards. If a net social dividend results from liberty infringement, then part of this should be allocated to those who make this possible by succumbing to coercion. This is a matter of reciprocity.[37] A benefit of putting a compensation/reward scheme into place is that this would likely enhance trust in—and thus cooperation with—the public health system.[38] It is widely acknowledged that trust is important for public health systems to succeed.

The best way to address anticipated potential conflict between the goal to promote public health and the goal to respect individual rights and liberties would be to bypass the conflict altogether—by avoiding situations were quarantine would be necessary to public health protection. Greater availability of wide-spectrum vaccines and anti-infective treatments[39] would make quarantine less necessary in general. The need to confine people would arise less often if we were better able to vaccinate and treat people. It is well known that the pharmaceutical industry, however, has largely neglected anti-infective research and development (R&D) in comparison with more profitable areas of drug development (e.g., of lifestyle drugs and drugs for chronic disease). Increased governmental financing of R&D for vaccines and anti-infective treatments could promote both public health protection (against bioterrorism and naturally occurring outbreaks of disease) and the protection of individual liberties at the very same time.

---

[37] University of Toronto Joint Centre for Bioethics, Pandemic Influenza Working Group, "Stand on Guard for Thee: Ethical Considerations in Preparedness Planning for Pandemic Influenza" (2005), http://www.utoronto.ca/jcb/home/documents/pandemic.pdf, cited 4 June 2007.

[38] Theresa Ly. "Pandemic and Public Health Controls: Towards an Equitable Compensation System," forthcoming.

[39] Such as antibiotics and antivirals.

4 Conclusion

I have shown how conflicting values arise in two different contexts involving biological weapons: dual-use research with weapons implications, and the use of coercive social distancing measures in the event of a bioterrorist attack. In both cases I argue that, rather than attributing absolute priority to one value or another, we should aim to strike a balance between the conflicting values at stake. In both cases I provide specific policy recommendations for striking such a balance in practice. In the case of dual-use research, I argue against NRC recommendations regarding voluntary self-governance of the scientific community regarding matters of censorship—and that the current status quo in the US is unacceptable. In the case of coercive social distancing measures, I enumerate principles to be followed when making decisions about isolation and quarantine—and I argue that the need to employ such measures would arise less often if the government provided more funding for R&D of vaccines and anti-infective treatments.

References

Alibek, Ken and Stephen Handelman. 1999. *Biohazard: The Chilling True Story of the Largest Covert Biological Weapons Program in the World—Told from the Inside be the Man Who Ran it*. New York: Delta.

Annas, George J. 2005. *American Bioethics: Crossing Human Rights and Health Law Boundaries*. New York: Oxford University Press.

Cello, Jeronimo et al. 2002. Chemical Synthesis of Poliovirus cDNA: Generation of Infectious Virus in the Absence of Natural Template. *Science* 297: 1016–1018.

Central Intelligence Agency. 2003. *The Darker Bioweapons Future*. 3 November 2003. http://www.fas.org/irp/cia/product/bw1103.pdf. Cited 4 June 2007.

Cooke-Deegan, Robert. 1994. *The Gene Wars: Science, Politics, and the Human Genome*. New York: Norton.

Crosby, Alfred W. 2003. *Americas Forgotten Pandemic: The Influenza of 1918*, 2nd ed. Cambridge: Cambridge University Press.

Gostin, Lawrence O. 2006. Public Health Strategies for Pandemic Influenza. *JAMA* 295: 1700–1704.

Gostin, Lawrence O. et al. 2001. *Model State Emergency Health Powers Act*. 21 December 2001. http://www.publichealthlaw.net/MSEHPA/MSEHPA2.pdf. Cited 4 June 2007.

Green, Shane K. et al. for the Council on Ethical and Judicial Affairs of the American Medical Association. 2006. Guidelines to Prevent Malevolent Use of Biomedical Research. *Cambridge Quarterly of Healthcare Ethics* 15: 435.

Jackson, Ronald J. et al. 2001. Expression of Mouse Interleukin-4 by a Recombinant Ectromelia Virus Suppresses Cytolytic Lymphocyte Responses and Overcomes Genetic Resistance to Mousepox. *Journal of Virology* 75.3: 1205–1210.

Journal Editors and Authors Group. 2003. Uncensored Exchange of Scientific Results. *Proceedings of the National Academy of Sciences of the United States of America* 100.4: 1464. www.pnas.org/cgi/doi/10.1073/pnas.0630491100. Cited 4 June 2007.

Kaiser, Jocelyn. 2005. Resurrected Influenza Virus Yields Secrets of Deadly 1918 Pandemic. *Science* 310: 28–29.

Kennedy, Donald. 2005. Better Never Than Late. *Science* 310(2005): 195.

Ly, Theresa. Forthcoming. *Pandemic and Public Health Controls: Towards an Equitable Compensation System.*

Michelson, Evan S. 2006. Individual Freedom or Collective Welfare? An Analysis of Quarantine as Response to Global Infectious Disease. In *Ethics and Infectious Disease*, eds. Michael J. Selgelid, Margaret P. Battin and Charles B. Smith. Oxford: Blackwell.

Miller, Judith et al. 2001. *Germs: The Ultimate Weapon.* London: Simon & Schuster.

Miller, Seumas and Michael J. Selgelid. 2006. *Ethical and Philosophical Implications of the Dual-Use Dilemma in the Biological Sciences.* Canberra, Australia: Centre for Applied Philosophy and Public Ethics (CAPPE), The Australian National University and Charles Sturt University.

National Research Council. 2004. *Biotechnology Research in an Age of Terrorism.* Washington, DC: National Academies Press.

National Science Advisory Board for Biosecurity (NSABB), http://biosecurity-board.gov. Cited 4 June 2007.

Nozick, Robert. 1974. *Anarchy, State, and Utopia.* New York: Basic Books.

Oldstone, Michael B. A. 1998. *Viruses, Plagues, and History.* New York: Oxford University Press.

Selgelid, Michael J. 2007. A Tale of Two Studies: Ethics, Bioterrorism, and the Censorship of Science. *Hastings Center Report* 37.3: 35–43.

Selgelid, Michael. Forthcoming. Ethics of Infectious Disease Control. In *The Encyclopedia of Public Health*, ed. H. Kristian Heggenhougen. Amsterdam, The Netherlands: Elsevier.

University of Toronto Joint Centre for Bioethics, Pandemic Influenza Working Group. 2005. *Stand on Guard for Thee: Ethical Considerations in Preparedness Planning for Pandemic Influenza.* http://www.utoronto.ca/jcb/home/documents/pandemic.pdf. Cited 4 June 2007.

Ethics and the Dual-Use Dilemma in the Life Sciences[1,2]

Seumas Miller and Michael J. Selgelid

[...]

1 Introduction

1.1 What Is the Dual-Use Dilemma?

The "dual-use dilemma" arises in the context of research in the biological and other sciences as a consequence of the fact that one and the same piece of scientific research sometimes has the potential to be used for evil as well as for good. Consider as an example of this kind of dilemma recent research on the mousepox virus.[3] On the one hand, the research program on the mousepox virus should have been pursued since it may well have led to a genetically engineered sterility treatment that would have helped combat periodic plagues of mice in Australia. On the other hand, this research project should not have been pursued since it led to the

[1] The following selection has been excerpted from a complete report prepared by the Centre for Applied Philosophy and Public Ethics (CAPPE) for the Australian Department of Prime Minister and Cabinet, National Security Science and Technology Unit. The full citation for that report reads as: Seumas Miller and Michael Selgelid, *Ethical and Philosophical Consideration of the Dual-Use Dilemma in the Biological Sciences* (Canberra, Australia: Centre for Applied Philosophy and Public Ethics [An Australian Research Council funded Special Research Centre], Australian National University and Charles Sturt University, 2006). Contributors to the report included Antony Della-Porta, Christian Enemark, Peter Kerr, and Ian Ramshaw. The excerpt has been reformatted for consistency with the other essays in this volume.

[2] I would like to thank Seumas Miller and, especially, Michael Selgelid for bringing my attention to this report and for making recommendations about which of its elements would be appropriate for this volume.

[3] Ronald J. Jackson et al., "Expression of Mouse Interleukin-4 by a Recombinant Ectromelia Virus Suppresses Cytolytic Lymphocyte Responses and Overcomes Genetic Resistance to Mousepox," *Journal of Virology* 75.3 (2001): 1205–1210.

creation of a highly virulent strain of mousepox and the possibility of the creation—by, say, a terrorist group contemplating a biological attack—of a highly virulent strain of smallpox able to overcome available vaccines.

A dual-use dilemma is an *ethical* dilemma, and an ethical dilemma for the *researcher* (and for those who have the power or authority to assist or impede the researcher's work, e.g., governments). It is an *ethical* dilemma since it is about promoting good in the context of the potential for also causing harm, e.g. the promotion of health in the context of providing the wherewithal for the killing of innocents. It is an ethical dilemma *for the researcher* not because he or she is aiming at anything other than a good outcome; typically, the researcher intends no harm, but only good. Rather, the dilemma arises for the researcher because of the potential actions of *others*. Malevolent non-researchers might steal dangerous biological agents produced by the researcher; alternatively, *other* researchers—or at least their governments or leadership—might use the results of the original researcher's work for malevolent purposes. The malevolent purposes in question include bio-terrorism, bio-warfare and blackmail for financial gain.

In the recent and not so recent past, a number of governments have sought to develop weapons of mass destruction (WMDs), including biological weapons, and in some cases have actually used them, e.g., the use of mustard gas by the German and British armies in World War I, the dropping of atomic bombs on Hiroshima and Nagasaki by the US air force in World War II, the existence of a large-scale biological weapons program in the Soviet Union from 1946 to 1992, and the use of chemical agents against the Kurds by Saddam Hussein's regime in 1988.

In the aftermath of the 11 September 2001 attacks in the US, bio-terrorism is widely considered to be a real threat, especially to populations in western countries. Moreover, it is seen as a greater threat from non-state terrorist groups than, say, nuclear WMDs, given the availability of the materials and technical knowledge necessary to produce the relevant biological agents and the feasibility of weaponization. This is not to say that there are not obstacles for would-be bioterrorists, including the dangers to themselves in handling pathogens. But it is to say that there is a non-negligible bio-terrorist threat, and it is likely to increase rather than decrease. It should be noted that a small number of animal, human and plant pathogens are readily obtainable from nature and that it is possible that bioterrorists with some microbiological training could use these to inflict causalities or economic damage.

In short, *some* research in the biological sciences has the potential for great harm, as well as great good and, unfortunately, there are any number of malevolent individuals, political and religious groups and governments ready, willing and (increasingly) able to use this research to cause harm rather than to do good. This is the larger context in which the dual-use dilemma in the biological sciences arises.

The expression 'dual-use dilemma' is in need of some conceptual unpacking. Here we need to introduce a number of sets of distinctions.

1. In relation to the *purposes* (or ends) of the research, we can distinguish the following conceptual axes: good/evil; military/non-military; and (within the category of military

purposes, the sub-categories of offensive/protective. Consider the aerosolization of a pathogen undertaken for a military purpose. The purpose in question might be offensive, e.g., bio-warfare; but it might simply be protective, e.g., to understand the nature and dangers of such aerosolization in order to prepare protections against an enemy known to be planning to deploy the aerosolised pathogen as a weapon.

The categories good/evil and military/non-military do not necessarily mirror one another. Some non-military purposes are, nevertheless, evil, e.g., the supplier of a vaccine releasing a pathogen to make large numbers of people sick in order that the sick buy the vaccine against the pathogen and, thereby, increase the supplier's profits. And some military purposes might be good, e.g., the above-mentioned research on the aerosolization of a pathogen undertaken for purely protective purposes in the context of a just war. The United States Project BioShield is an example of research aimed at providing "new tools to improve medical counter-measures protecting Americans against a chemical, biological, radiological or nuclear (CBRN) attack."[4] However, some of the protective research would probably yield results that could assist in the development and delivery of biological weapons.

2. Dual-use refers to two temporally and logically distinct "users" of the research: those who initially undertake the research (original users) and those who use the results of the work of these original researchers for some purpose other than that intended by the original researchers (secondary users). For example, the above-mentioned research on the aerosolization of a pathogen (conducted by the original users) might be used for offensive purposes by those fighting an unjust war (the secondary users).
3. In relation to the term 'use' we can distinguish: actually or potentially used in accordance with the purpose for which it was designed (design-purpose) and actually or potentially used for some purpose other than that for which it was specifically designed. Dual-use dilemmas can involve original researchers whose purpose is a design-purpose, e.g., demonstrate how to render a vaccine against a highly transmissible pathogen ineffective. This design-purpose can itself be in the service of a benevolent purpose of the original researchers, e.g., the purpose of enhancing the effectiveness of the vaccine. Alternatively, the achievement of this design-purpose could be used for a malevolent non-design purpose by secondary researchers, e.g., to render the vaccine ineffective in the context of spreading the pathogen in question.

   On the other hand, secondary users might build on the original research in such a way as to create, say, a new pathogen, e.g., a more virulent strain of smallpox as opposed to a more virulent strain of mousepox, in which case we might be inclined to say that they had a new *design*-purpose (albeit a malevolent one).

---

[4] US Department of Health and Human Services—Fact Sheet (21 July 2004), "HHS Fact Sheet Project Bioshield," http://www.hhs.gov/news/press/2004pres/20040721b.html, cited 27 June 2006.

4. In relation to the *outcomes* of the research, we can distinguish: intended outcomes; unintended but foreseen outcomes; and unforeseen and perhaps unable to have been foreseen outcomes. An example of an unintended outcome is an outbreak of smallpox resulting from inadequate safety procedures in a laboratory setting. However, such accidents are not instances of the dual-use dilemma. For something to be an instance of a dual-use dilemma, both outcomes (the two horns of the dual-use dilemma) need to be (actually or potentially) intended (or at least foreseen) by someone; there needs to be two sets of (actual or potential) *users*. Naturally, an outcome might be unintended and unforeseen (even unforeseeable) by the original researcher but, nevertheless, intended by the secondary user. Thus, scientists who preserve a small number of smallpox samples for pure research purposes in the context of a policy of mandatory destruction of samples might not intend or foresee that they might be used for malevolent purposes by others, e.g., weaponized.

The dual-use dilemma is obviously a dilemma for researchers, viz. those researchers involved in biological research that has the potential to be misused by bio-terrorists, criminal organisations and governments engaged in bio-warfare. But it is also a dilemma for the private and public institutions, including universities, that fund or otherwise enable research to be undertaken. The dilemma is made more acute for university-based researchers and for universities, given their commitments to such values as academic freedom and the unfettered dissemination of research findings; and for private companies, given their commitment to free-enterprise. More generally, it is a dilemma for the individual communities for whose benefit or, indeed, to whose potential detriment, the research is being conducted, and for the national governments who bear the moral and legal responsibility of ensuring that the security of their citizens is provided for. Finally, in the context of an increasingly interdependent set of nation-states—the so-called, global community—the dual-use dilemma has become a dilemma for international bodies such as the United Nations.

1.2 Biological Weapons Convention

Given the general threat to public health posed by transmissible pathogens, and given that biological agents can be used as WMDs in the hands of state actors, terrorist groups and criminal organisations, there is an imperative to strictly regulate the development, production, stockpiling, weaponization and use of pathogens. At the international level, a key instrument in this regard is the Biological Weapons Convention (BWC)—more precisely, *Convention on the Prohibition of the Development, Production and Stockpiling of Bacteriological (Biological) and Toxin Weapons and on Their Destruction*. (Signed at London, Moscow and Washington on 10 April 1972; Entered into force on 26 March 1975; Depositories—UK, USA and Soviet governments.) Australia is a signatory to the BWC.

The general aim to which the BWC is directed is, "for the sake of mankind, to exclude completely the possibility of bacteriological (biological) agents and toxins being used as weapons. Convinced that such use would be repugnant to the conscience of mankind and that no effort should be spared to minimise this risk".

In accordance with Article 1 of the BWC, "Each State Party to this Convention undertakes never in any circumstances to develop, produce, stockpile or otherwise acquire or retain:

1. Microbial or other biological agents, or toxins whatever their origin or method of production, of types and in quantities that have no justification for prophylactic, protective or other peaceful purposes
2. Weapons, equipment or means of delivery designed to use such agents or toxins for hostile purposes or in armed conflict"

While the BWC is an important step in relation to its stated aims of prohibiting and eliminating the possibility of using biological agents as weapons, it has a number of possible loopholes and lacunae.

The BWC evidently has requirements regarding technology transfers from prohibited to non-prohibited purposes and vice versa.[5] For example, technology transfers from non-prohibited purposes, e.g., prophylactic, to prohibited, e.g., military offensive, are prohibited under all circumstances.

However, the BWC does not make a formal distinction between civilian and military purposes. Indeed, in speaking of "protective purposes" (clause 1, above) the BWC seems to allow protective military purposes. This has the consequence that a technology transfer from civilian to military is allowable, if the latter purpose is protective and not offensive. But now an issue arises as to what counts as protective, as opposed to offensive. (See below for more on this issue.)

Moreover, the BWC does not provide for any robust verification processes, e.g., unlike the Chemical Weapons Convention (CWC) there is no international organisation or national authority to verify compliance with the BWC.

1.3 Aims and Scope of This Research Project[6]

In general terms, the aims and scope of this project are to provide a reasonably comprehensive array of (possibly competing) answers to the following questions (and to the further more specific questions to which these answers give rise):

---

[5] Jean Pascal Zanders, "Introduction", *Minerva* 40.1 (2002): 3–13.

[6] Some of these aims and scope refer to parts of the report that are not contained in this excerpt. This section has been include here to inform the reader as to the other topics that the report covers in case he/she would like to investigate them in the full report.

1. Morally impermissible research

   - What, if any, research in the biological sciences that does *not* give rise to a dual-use dilemma is morally impermissible, e.g., research undertaken for purely offensive military purposes?
   - What is the dual-use dilemma in the biological sciences, and in what categories of research does it arise, e.g., experimental research undertaken to assist in the combating of mice plagues that might in fact result in the development of a more virulent form of smallpox?
   - What are the moral and other considerations in play in these various categories of research that give rise to dual-use dilemmas, e.g., potential to save human life versus potential to destroy human life?
   - In the light of these considerations what, if any, research in the biological sciences that gives rise to a dual-use dilemma is morally impermissible?
   - Who is to decide what research, if any, in the biological sciences is morally impermissible, e.g., biosecurity committees?

2. Physical and regulatory conditions under which (permissible) experiments of concern ought to be undertaken:

   - In relation to the various categories of *prima facie* permissible research that, nevertheless, give rise to dual-use dilemmas, what are the safety and security—and associated regulatory—conditions under which this research ought to be undertaken, e.g., background checks and security clearance for research personnel?

3. Dissemination

   - What are the moral and other considerations in play in relation to the ownership rights (intellectual property) of permissible, safe and secure research in the biological sciences that, nevertheless, gives rise to dual-use dilemmas?
   - What are the moral and other considerations in play in relation to the dissemination of findings from permissible, safe and secure research in the biological sciences that, nevertheless, gives rise to dual-use dilemmas?
   - In relation to permissible, safe and secure research in the biological sciences that, nevertheless, gives rise to dual-use dilemmas what, if any, restrictions ought to be placed on its dissemination?
   - In relation to permissible, safe and secure research in the biological sciences that, nevertheless, gives rise to dual-use dilemmas who ought to decide what, if any, research findings ought not to be disseminated or ought to have restrictions placed on their dissemination?

Note that our primary concern in this report is with moral or ethical (we use the terms interchangeably) principles and values, as opposed to legal or, for that matter, regulatory rules. There is, of course, a close relationship between the moral and the legal. For instance, typically criminal laws, such as the laws against murder, assault and theft, "track" or follow antecedent moral principles; there is a law against murder, for example, precisely because we regard murder as *morally* wrong.

Nevertheless, the moral and the legal are conceptually distinct, and the distinction needs to be kept in mind in what follows. An important corollary of the existence of this moral/legal distinction is that it is not necessarily the case that every research practice rightly regarded as immoral or unethical should always be made unlawful.

2 Experiments of Concern

Human knowledge and understanding of the natural world is, presumably, both desirable in itself and a means to the provision of other human goods, such as health and longevity. Moreover, human freedom, including freedom of intellectual inquiry, is agreed on all hands to be an intrinsic human good. Accordingly, there is a presumption in favor of allowing research in the biological sciences, as there is in other areas of human knowledge. In short, research in the biological sciences is morally permissible, absent special considerations in relation to specific kinds of such research. What, if any, research in the biological sciences is morally impermissible?

Research in the biological sciences undertaken for the purpose of weaponizing biological agents so that they can be used to kill or cause illness in human populations is presumably morally impermissible, whether the research in question is undertaken by state actors (non-state) terrorist groups, criminal organisations or malevolent individuals. So much is proclaimed in the BWC, notwithstanding the fact that arguments have been used from time to time to justify the use of biological weapons in the context of a just war. It has been argued, for example, that some biological weapons are more "humane" than some conventional weapons. It is not within the scope of this report to discuss the moral complexities arising from the use of various forms of weaponry, albeit this is an important and somewhat neglected topic. However, we note that in so far as biological weapons are a species of WMD then there is a *general* moral objection to their use, namely, that inevitably they target civilian populations and not merely combatants. As such, they violate the so-called *jus in bello* condition of just war theory; the condition that, among other things, gives expression to the moral principle of civilian immunity in war.

An analogue of the moral principle of civilian immunity in conventional wars between nation-states is the moral principle not to deliberately target civilians that is adhered to by some—but obviously not all—*non-state* actors engaged in armed struggles. For example, for most if not all of its history the African National Congress (ANC) in its armed struggle against the apartheid government in South Africa adhered to this moral principle; military and police personnel were regarded by the ANC as legitimate targets but not ordinary civilians. On the other hand, terrorist groups such as al Qaeda obviously violate this moral principle, as would any terrorist group using biological weapons as WMDs. Naturally, terrorist groups might use "new generation" biological weapons that are able to target particular individuals, e.g., a biological weapon of assassination. However, use of such a biological weapon would not constitute use of a WMD.

In addition to the general concern that biological weapons may serve as weapons of mass destruction is the concern that their effects are generally-speaking hard to predict and control; this latter feature was a central rationale behind the BWC. The fact that biological weapons are relatively inexpensive and easy to produce (in comparison with other WMDs) also means that the potential for an arms race in the context of biological weapons is especially problematic.

At any rate, our assumption in this report is that research in the biological sciences undertaken for the ultimate purpose of using weaponized biological agents is in fact morally impermissible.

The moral problem that now arises concerns research in the biological sciences that is not undertaken *by the original researchers* for the ultimate purpose of using weaponized biological agents, but might be used by secondary researchers (or other users) for this impermissible purpose, i.e., the moral problem presented by so-called dual-use dilemmas.

As already noted, a particularly morally problematic species of the dual-use dilemma arises in the case of research undertaken to enable the assessment of the threat posed by the biological weapons (BW) of other nation-states (including nation-states who might seek to use BW as instruments of terror against civilian populations) or the biological agent focused projects of non-state terrorist groups. Such "threat assessment" research involves experimenting with the offensive applications of pathogens so as to determine appropriate counter-measures. In order to develop defenses against a putative BW agent, it is necessary to understand: the underlying mechanisms for pathogenicity, including infectivity and virulence; the way in which a micro-organism evades the human immune system or acquires resistance to antibiotics; and, the ways in which the agent may be dispersed, and its infectivity by each route. However, an understanding of these factors is also exactly what would be required for the development of BW.[7] An analogous point can be made in relation to non-state terrorist groups engaged in, for example, developing improvised equipment that could be used to grow a biological agent.

In relation to the dual-use dilemma in the biological sciences, the approach of the US National Research Council (NRC) in its 2004 report, *Biotechnology Research in an Age of Terrorism*, is to map the range of these dual-use dilemmas by identifying and taxonomizing a set of salient "experiments of concern". We accept this approach in the context of our attempt to isolate the morally permissible from the morally impermissible in relation to dual-use research in the biological sciences. Our first task, then, is to map the terrain of such dual-use dilemmas; hence, our recourse to experiments of concern.

According to the NRC report "experiments of concern" are those that would

1. Demonstrate how to render a vaccine ineffective
2. Confer resistance to therapeutically useful antibiotics or antiviral agents

[7] Jonathan King and Harlee Strauss, "The Hazards of Defensive Biological Warfare Programs," in *Preventing a Biological Arms Race*, ed. Susan Wright (Cambridge, MA: MIT, 1990), 123.

3. Enhance the virulence of a pathogen or render a non-pathogen virulent
4. Increase the transmissibility of a pathogen
5. Alter the host range of a pathogen
6. Enable the evasion of diagnosis and/or detection by established methods
7. Enable the weaponization of a biological agent or toxin[8]

Other possible categories are:

8. Genetic sequencing of pathogens
9. Synthesis of pathogenic micro-organisms
10. Any experiment with *variola virus* (smallpox)
11. Attempts to recover/revive past pathogens

[...]

3 The Ethics of Dual-Use Research

By definition, dual-use research is morally problematic. On the one hand, such research provides benefits (at least potentially); on the other hand, there is the risk of misuse by rogue states, terrorists groups and the like.

Broadly speaking, the most obvious benefits of research in the biological sciences of the kind in question are: the protection of human life and physical health against diseases (including novel ones), the protection of existing, and (more controversially) the provision of novel, food sources; and the protection of human populations against biological weapons.

By contrast, the potential burdens of such research are death and sickness caused by the use of biological agents as weapons in the hands of malevolent state actors, terrorist groups, criminal organisations and individuals.

More fine-grained analyses of the benefits and burdens of such research would elaborate on the additional kinds of benefit/burden and recipients/bearers thereof, e.g., the economic wealth accrued by large pharmaceutical corporations and their shareholders, the economic costs of expensive, unsuccessful (or only marginally beneficial) research programs in the biological sciences and, more generally, the dis/utility and in/justice of specific allocations of resources to, and the distribution of benefits and burdens from, different research programs in the biological sciences, e.g., the evident disutility of the large 1946–1992 Soviet biological weapons program.

Fine-grained ethical analyses of dual-use research in the biological sciences would seek to *quantify* actual and potential benefits and burdens, and actual and potential recipients/bearers of these benefits and burdens. These analyses would also identify a range of salient policy options. Each option would embody a set of trade-offs between present and future benefits and burdens, and recipients and

[8] National Research Council, *Biotechnology Research in an Age of Terrorism* (Washington, DC: National Academies of Science, 2004), 5.

bearers thereof. The construction of these options and the process of selection between them would consist in large part in the application of various ethical principles, including human rights principles—e.g., right to life, freedom of inquiry, and free speech—and principles of utility and of justice.

We are not (here) in a position to provide any such fine-grained ethical analysis, but will rather focus (somewhat simplistically) on a single ethical consideration, namely, human health (including human life) that gives rise to the dilemma; and do so without exploring questions of which human populations or how many individual humans have benefited/been burdened or are likely to benefit/be burdened, and so on. Viewed from this perspective the dual-use dilemma concerns human health (as a simple, unquantified human good), and the dilemma consists in the fact that research undertaken to promote human health might instead be used to destroy human health. As such, the dilemma gives rise to questions of security; what are reasonable and ethically justified forms and degrees of security in this context?

The security in question is a complex notion. It consists in part in the physical security of, for example, samples of biological agents against theft. Relatedly, security consists in part in the processes in place to ensure, for example, that the researchers themselves cannot, or will not, conduct research for malevolent purposes.

As we will see in the section following this one,[9] security in this sense also consists in part in restrictions that might be placed on the dissemination of research findings.

Thus far we have offered a somewhat static mode of analysis of the dual-use dilemma consisting of the quantification of harms and benefits, the identification of salient options, and the selection of an option on the basis of ethical principles. However, a more dynamic, indeed creative, mode of analysis is called for.

In the first place, options are not static because well-intentioned scientists, malevolent actors and security personnel are *responsive* to the problems that they confront, including the problems provided by other actors. The response of scientists to a pathogen with enhanced virulence might be the development of a new vaccine. The response of security personnel to a new bioterrorist threat might be an enhanced regulatory system. Accordingly, the mode of analysis of the dual-use dilemma must be dynamic in character.

In the second place, ethical dilemmas are not necessarily—or even typically—to be resolved by careful calibration of the differential ethical weight that attaches to the options provided for in the dilemma. Rather the dilemma must, if possible, be resolved by *designing* a new third or fourth option, i.e., by bypassing the dilemma. Consider the question of whether to disseminate dual-use research findings or not disseminate them: academic freedom versus security. Perhaps the solution is to find a third option, such as to disseminate them in a manner that will not enable the experiments in question to be replicated (other than by those with adequate security clearance and to the extent necessary for purposes of verification). This mode of analysis is *creative*. It lets us have our cake and eat it; it squares the ethical circle.

[9] Not included in this excerpt, but see the chapter in this volume by Selgelid.

Let us refer to this kind of ethical analysis as *designing-in ethics*. Naturally, this mode of analysis is not always applicable; but it is important to keep it in mind.

In the light of these considerations of health and security—and of this designing-in ethics mode of analysis—let us address the question of the moral permissibility of dual-use research, albeit in highly general terms. Here there appear to be three separable ethical questions. First, the ethical question as to whether or not a putative biological agent to be researched ought in fact to be eliminated (or, if already eliminated, not retrieved). Here the *possibility* of research is removed; no possibility of research because no biological agent to be researched. We have in mind the case of smallpox and the arguments in favor or against the elimination of all samples of smallpox. (We note that in the context of the recent possibility of genome mappings of biological agents, it may not matter so much whether the organism actually exists; since it might be possible to recreate it from the sequence alone.) Second, the ethical question (or questions) arising from dual-use research in relation to a biological agent whose present and/or future existence is taken as a given; there is no intention to eliminate or not retrieve or not bring into existence the biological agent in question. For example, research to determine whether or not avian influenza could trigger a human pandemic might lead to the creation of dangerous new strains that could be used by terrorists. Such research might include work intentionally undertaken to create novel pathogens or synthesising existing ones, albeit work whose ultimate purpose was to develop, say, a vaccine against these pathogens. Thirdly, the ethical question of whether to undertake dual-use research for the purpose of protection against weaponized pathogens, e.g., research into the aerosolization of pathogens.

Let us consider these ethical questions in order, beginning with the question of the elimination of pathogens. As already mentioned, the salient example here is smallpox. The "retentionists" focus on the possibility that smallpox might re-emerge in the future. They see potential sources for a return as including the corpses of smallpox victims preserved in Arctic permafrost, and samples of *variola* virus retained without WHO permission—inadvertently or deliberately—in laboratory freezers around the world. The former Soviet Union reportedly had enormous weapons stockpiles of the virus, for example, and their destruction has never been verified. There is also some concern that genetic mutation of the monkeypox virus, which causes symptoms clinically almost indistinguishable from smallpox, might make it more virulent and more transmissible, thus resembling the public health threat once posed by *variola*. Against these eventualities, it is thought prudent to study the smallpox virus in order to be better prepared. Another argument in favor of retention (and perhaps retrieval) is that basic research with live *variola* could yield new insights into the process of viral infection generally and the workings of the human immune system.[10]

---

[10]Joshua Micah Marshall, "Known Stocks of the Smallpox Virus Should Be Retained for Research," in *Biological Warfare: Opposing Viewpoints*, ed. William Dudley (Farmington Hills, MI: Greenhaven, 2004), 192–197; Jonathan B. Tucker, *Scourge: The Once and Future Threat of Smallpox* (New York: Atlantic Monthly Press, 2001), 171.

"Destructionists" have included many veterans of the smallpox eradication campaign, including D.A. Henderson and Frank Fenner. They argue that, because the DNA sequences of representative viral strains have been determined, there is no need to retain live *variola* in order to identify smallpox were it to reappear in the future. Moreover, they argue, live virus is not required to protect against a future outbreak because the smallpox vaccine—derived from the *vaccinia* virus—could be retained (or retrieved) and stockpiled just in case. There is also the argument that eliminating the remaining laboratory stocks of *variola*, and universally criminalizing mere possession of the virus, would strengthen the moral case against using smallpox as a biological weapon.[11]

The smallpox debate is essentially about balancing the desirability of retaining the virus for prospective research purposes against the uncertain risks associated with not destroying it. In an attempt to achieve this balance, the WHA in 1999 established a Variola Advisory Committee (VAC). At its last meeting in November 2004, the VAC recommended further experimentation on the live smallpox virus, including genetic modification. This proposal met with a cool reception when the WHA convened in May the following year. The WHO Director General, Lee Jong-Wook, rejected the recommendation to allow insertion of smallpox genes into related, less virulent poxviruses such as those that cause monkeypox and cowpox.[12] And the WHA urged the VAC to take extra steps to ensure laboratories had strong safety and security measures in place before smallpox research was carried out.[13] One good reason for such caution is that the deliberate release of modified smallpox virus or a poxvirus expressing smallpox genes could trigger a public health catastrophe.

Let us now consider the second ethical issue; it concerns dual-use research on presently existing or novel pathogens (where their present and/or future existence is accepted).

There are a number of types of experiment from our list of experiments of concern that are relevant to this question. However, the general problem here is the unintended (by the original researcher) untoward consequences of otherwise benign research. These consequences are threefold. First, there is an unintended dangerous biological research outcome, e.g., a pathogen with enhanced virulence or transmissibility or at least the knowledge of how to create such a pathogen. (As we have seen, there are some *intended* dangerous research outcomes, e.g., intentional creation of a vaccine resistant strains of a disease, undertaken for, say, prophylactic purposes, e.g., to test

---

[11] D.A. Henderson and Frank Fenner, "Recent Events and Observations Pertaining to Smallpox Virus Destruction in 2002," *Clinical Infectious Diseases* 33.7 (2001): 1057–1059; Tucker, *Scourge*, 170–171.

[12] World Health Organisation Media Release (20 May 2005), "Establishing Smallpox Vaccine Reserve," http://www.who.int/mediacentre/news/notes/2005/np_wha02/en/index.html, cited 10 June 2005.

[13] Lawrence Altman, "WHO Moves Toward Allowing Smallpox Gene Experiment," *New York Times* (21 May 2005): A6.

the adequacy of a vaccine, and which have no untoward consequences.) Whether or not such an unintended and untoward outcome is possible or likely is a scientific question, best answered by biological scientists.

Second, there is an outcome not intended by the original scientist but, nevertheless, intended by some malevolent state actor, non-state terrorist group, criminal organisation or individual, e.g., the weaponization (and use as a weapon) of the pathogen that has been unintentionally created. Whether or not this outcome is possible or likely—given, say, a pathogen has already been (unintentionally) created—is a security question, best answered by security experts (with input from relevant non-security specialists such as engineers).

Third, there is the ultimate outcome intended by the malevolent individual or organisation, namely, the public health outcome consequent on the biological attack. What the public health outcome of a given biological attack is likely to be, e.g. the extent of loss of life, is a public health question, best answered by public health experts or teams thereof (including biological scientists, medical personnel and weapons experts, but also those knowledgeable about public health resources and infrastructure).

The danger attendant upon a given dual-use research program can be crudely quantified by determining the probability, be it low, medium or high, of a given untoward outcome, and multiplying this probability by the (quantified) disvalue (or disutility) of that outcome, e.g., in terms of the numerical loss of human life. A more fine-gained ethical analysis would explore the variety of decision making/ risk-taking strategies—including the precautionary principle—that might be considered appropriate in this context. Presumably, dual-use research that has a high probability of resulting in substantial loss of human life ought not to be undertaken. On the other hand, the danger attendant upon dual-use research is not the only moral consideration in play. Another important moral consideration is the (intended) benefits of the research. Clearly trade-offs need to be made between the (intended) benefits of the research and its (unintended by researchers) potential untoward outcomes. Moreover, the process of arriving at suitable trade-offs is in large part a process of moral reasoning, including the weighing of one moral consideration against another. However, as noted above, it is important to bear in mind the possibility of creative solutions that bypass the dilemma; perhaps we do not need to make the trade-offs we initially think we need to make.

The general point to be made here is that in the context of the yet to be decided grey area of dual-use research marked off by the experiments of concern, there are a complex mix of scientific, security, public health and ethical considerations in play. Moreover, the process of moral reasoning involved will require trade-offs between ethical considerations and, hopefully, it will involve the provision of creative solutions that bypass the dilemma. The result will presumably be that some putative experiments of concern will be relegated to the impermissible category and others to the permissible category, albeit in the latter case under stringent conditions of safety and security.

Consider an experiment of concern involving enhancing the virulence of a pathogen. Susan Wright has argued, "[i]f there is no evidence of a threat posed by, say, a genetically engineered strain of cowpox that attacks the immune system, then there is no reasonable justification for developing such an organism. Arguably, to do so crosses the line between defense and offense."[14] No doubt, pace Wright, there needs to be some evidence of a threat. But this raises a number of questions: What counts as evidence?; How immediate is the threat?; Does the development of the more virulent pathogen constitute a greater threat than the original threat that it is supposed to protect against? Surely when a microbial threat exists only in a scientist's imagination, an experiment to create such a microbe is both unnecessary and overly risky.

There are a couple of additional points that should to be stressed here. One pertains to the process of moral reasoning. We have been speaking in broadly utilitarian and consequentialist terms, e.g., using notions of future benefits/burdens, quantified loss of life, disvalue and disutility. However, some would argue that this mode of reasoning is flawed (and not only by virtue of its inherently static character—see above). For example, consequentialist reasoning is arguably one-dimensional and fails to give sufficient weight to the intrinsic moral properties of current actions, e.g., perhaps human rights of current persons override future utility. Again, there are a range of moral considerations that are absent from our discussion thus far, e.g., the human right to free inquiry, intellectual property rights (both individual and collective). We do not have the space here to unravel all these moral complexities, or to develop and defend our own favored account of moral reasoning as it might apply to the dual-use dilemmas in question. Accordingly, we have simply sought to gesture at some of the moral considerations in play and at the general kind of process of moral reasoning that should take place.

Another point pertains to uncertainty. Proceeding in the manner of a risk assessor assumes that the probabilities of specific outcomes can realistically be determined; risk assessment is, presumably, more than mere guesswork. But the reliability of probability judgments in relation to outcomes from dual-use research in the biological sciences is, to say the least, open to question. Arguably, the possibility of the development of a vaccine-resistant strain of smallpox based on research undertaken on mousepox to develop a contraceptive for mice could not have been realistically predicted. This is, of course, not to say that attempts should not be made to foresee untoward outcomes; it is merely to caution against over-confidence in the results of such attempts. Moreover, because the actors involved in dual-use dilemmas are, as noted above, responsive to problems and to one another's actions, probability judgments need to take this into account. One way to do so is to analyze, for example, a security risk from bioterrorists in part in terms of a complex set of variables including the ability, opportunity and motivation of the bioterrorists, the likely intelligence possessed by, and the likely assessment made by, the terrorists, the capacity to respond to specific forms of bioterrorist attack, the likely movements of

---

[14] Susan Wright, November/December 2004, "Taking Biodefense Too Far," *Bulletin of the Atomic Scientists*, http://www.thebulletin.org/issues/2004/nd04/nd04wright.html, cited 1 November 2004.

innocent third parties at risk from specific security responses, the relevant moral principles, the rights and duties of the various actors involved, and so on.

However, what might be crucial here is the capacity to generate a creative response to the security problem thus analyzed. Perhaps a focus on reducing the opportunities available to bioterrorists by establishing a licensing system for laboratories using dual-use technologies is a case in point.

Our third ethical question arising from dual-use research pertains to weaponization. As already noted, a particularly morally problematic species of the dual-use dilemma arises in the case of R&D projects on biological weapons (BW). In order to develop defenses against a putative BW agent, it is necessary to understand the underlying mechanisms for pathogenicity and the ways in which the biological agent may be dispersed. However, an understanding of these factors is also exactly what would be required for the development of BW.

As stated above, our assumption in this report is that the weaponization of pathogens for offensive military purposes is morally impermissible. Moreover, in so far as military defense is understood to include using biological weapons against an attacker (whether the attack in question is a biological attack or not) then the weaponization of pathogens for defensive military purposes—in this sense of defense—is also morally impermissible. On the other hand, research that is defensive in the sense that it serves the purpose simply of enabling combatants and civilians to *protect* themselves against a biological attack by, for example, developing early warning indicators of the presence of aerosolized novel pathogens is *prima facie* morally permissible. Let us refer to such research as research undertaken for the purpose of *protection* (as opposed to military *defense*). The problem is that such research for protective purposes might itself involve, for example, the creation of a virulent and highly transmissible novel pathogen and the weaponization of it. As such, the weaponization of pathogens for protective purpose gives rise to a dual-use dilemma of a very acute kind.

The issue resolves itself into whether or not in practice the weaponization of pathogens for protective purposes can be distinguished from the weaponization of pathogens for offensive purposes (including defensive purposes in the above adumbrated sense of that term).

Presumably, if these two conceptually distinct activities are to be distinguished in practice then this is because there are *verifiable* differences in respect of: intention or purpose and/or physical properties of the weaponized pathogen.

In relation to the former, for example, if the intention is protection then the pathogen in question will be one that some identified malevolent state or terrorist group is known to have weaponized (or it is known that they are in the process of weaponizing the pathogen).[15]

In relation to the latter, for example, if the weaponized pathogen is possessed in large quantities, i.e., quantities appropriate for a military offensive but unnecessary

---

[15] Naturally, there are other evidentiary possibilities that might reach a reasonable threshold of justification in relation to protective research on weaponization, e.g., a high probability in relation to an easily weaponized readily available pathogen that some malevolent group or other is weaponizing this pathogen.

for research serving purely protective purposes, then it is a case of weaponization for offensive purposes. Also one might expect there to be some differences in the *results* of research involving weapons constructed in accordance with the design-purpose only of testing protections against an attack using that weapon from the *results* of research undertaken with the design-purpose of making a successful attack using that weapon, i.e., an attack against which the enemy is not protected. For example, in the case of the former the research result might be a protective vaccine, whereas in the case of the latter the research result might be a weaponized pathogen that is resistant to any vaccine.

Moreover, the *results* of such dual-use research on the weaponization of pathogens undertaken only for protective purposes, e.g., the vaccine mentioned above, might be more likely to be disseminated; after all, it is not only one's own civilians and combatants that ought to be protected from biological attack. Or at least one would expect, other things being equal, there to be less need for secrecy in relation to such relatively benign research and a willingness on the part of those engaged in it to be subject to verification checks.[16]

[...]

References

Altman, Lawrence. 2005. WHO Moves Toward Allowing Smallpox Gene Experiment. *New York Times* (21 May 2005): A6.

Jackson, Ronald J. et al. 2001. Expression of Mouse Interleukin-4 by a Recombinant Ectromelia Virus Suppresses Cytolytic Lymphocyte Responses and Overcomes Genetic Resistance to Mousepox. *Journal of Virology* 75.3 (2001): 1205–1210.

Henderson, D. A. and Frank Fenner. 2001. Recent Events and Observations Pertaining to Smallpox Virus Destruction in 2002. *Clinical Infectious Diseases* 33.7: 1057–1059.

King, Jonathan and Harlee Strauss. 1990. The Hazards of Defensive Biological Warfare Programs. In *Preventing a Biological Arms Race*, ed. Susan Wright, 123. Cambridge, MA: MIT.

Marshall, Joshua Micah. 2004. Known Stocks of the Smallpox Virus Should Be Retained for Research. In *Biological Warfare: Opposing Viewpoints*, ed. William Dudley, 192–197. Farmington Hills, MI: Greenhaven.

Miller, Seumas and Michael Selgelid. 2006. *Ethical and Philosophical Consideration of the Dual-Use Dilemma in the Biological Sciences*. Canberra: Centre for Applied Philosophy and Public Ethics (An Australian Research Council funded Special Research Centre), Australian National University and Charles Sturt University.

National Research Council. 2004. *Biotechnology Research in an Age of Terrorism*. Washington, DC: National Academies of Science.

Tucker, Jonathan B. 2001. *Scourge: The Once and Future Threat of Smallpox*. New York: Atlantic Monthly Press.

US Department of Health and Human Services. 21 July 2004. Fact Sheet. *HHS Fact Sheet Project Bioshield*. http://www.hhs.gov/news/press/2004pres/20040721b.html. Cited 27 June 2006.

[16] Naturally, other things might not be equal. We might be concerned that if a malevolent state knew what our defensive capabilities were they would be more likely to develop new ways to overcome them.

World Health Organisation Media Release. 20 May 2005. *Establishing Smallpox Vaccine Reserve*. http://www.who.int/mediacentre/news/notes/2005/np_wha02/ en/index.html. Cited 10 June 2005.

Wright, Susan. November/December 2004. Taking Biodefense Too Far.*Bulletin of the Atomic Scientists*. http://www.thebulletin.org/issues/2004/nd04/nd04wright.html. Cited 1 November 2004.

Zanders, Jean Pascal. 2002. Introduction. *Minerva* 40.1: 3–13.

Part IV
Physicians on the Battlefield

Triage Priorities and Military Physicians[1]

Marcus P. Adams

1 Introduction

When resources are limited, physicians are faced with the difficult decision of having to choose to prioritize the care of some patients over others. Triage is the principled manner by which physicians make these decisions. Civilian physicians in emergency room settings must triage patients when necessary, especially when faced with an acute influx of individuals needing care. Unlike their civilian counterparts, military physicians appear to face unique difficulties when standard triage methods conflict with current military objectives. As a result, it seems that military physicians are forced to choose between two competing loyalties—the goals of the chain of command and the wellbeing of their patients.

In this paper, I will first outline briefly the general triage practices that are common in both civilian and military contexts. The triage procedures which are of current interest, of course, are not these general practices that both civilian and military triage procedures share; rather, of primary interest are those procedures which military commanders mandate during severe battle conditions. In these extreme situations, military protocol mandates the reversal of normal triage procedures, with the least wounded being treated first so that they can rapidly return to the battlefield. It is during these times that tension between two competing loyalties seems to occur.

After discussing the battle conditions under which these triage procedures are recommended, I will argue on the grounds that military commanders possess fiduciary obligations that these triage procedures during extreme battle conditions are not only morally permissible but, moreover, that in certain cases they are required so that military commanders may fulfill their obligations. Furthermore, I will contend that, given seemingly subtle differences between the civilian patient-physician relationship and the relationship into which military physicians enter with those

[1] I would like to thank Fritz Allhoff and Shannon Bernard-Adams for their feedback and criticisms of this paper. I have benefited immensely from their comments and suggestions.

needing medical attention, there are instances in which it is appropriate for the military physician to act in accordance with the chain of command's desires and not enter into this relationship. We should perhaps view the military physician in these circumstances as acting in a different role than the civilian physician, i.e., acting to maintain the strength of the fighting force. In other words, the relationship into which military physicians and the wounded that are in need of treatment enter is dissimilar enough to warrant the difference in care priorities during extreme battle conditions.

2 Triage as a Principled Decision Procedure

The term 'triage' itself has no ethical implications.[2] In its early uses it simply referred to the sorting or culling of goods into different categories according to quality, e.g., coffee and wool.[3] The early uses of the term in agricultural contexts provide a background for the use of 'triage' in medical contexts today—patients are sorted, not according to quality, but according to their medical condition or according to some other priority. This is the only aspect that medical triage appears to share with the term 'triage' in its early use. For example, triage of a product such as wool involves none of the outside influences that seem to impact medical triage, e.g., shortage of supplies or physicians. Additionally, concerns in medical triage over the impartiality of the "sorter" are not shared with triage in its agricultural use. With medical triage, sorting is just the first step of the process; ethical dilemmas come after the sorting process is complete when decisions about whom to treat first must be made.

Before examining the similarities between military and civilian triage procedures, it would be beneficial to note first that most triage contexts do not involve a *dire* shortage of resources.[4] Most civilian hospitals in the US and other established countries staff enough physicians to handle basic care needs and, as a result, triage

[2] Some argue that the term 'triage' has an implicit utilitarian connotation and prefer to use what they believe are more neutral terms. See, for example, John F. Kilner, *Who Lives? Who Dies?* (New Haven, CT: Yale University Press, 1990), xi. I will use 'triage' throughout the paper since it is the more widely used term. Any ethical implications that the term appears to possess are an artifact of discourse.

[3] "Triage, n.[1]," *The Oxford English Dictionary*, 2nd ed. 1989, OED Online (Oxford: Oxford University Press), http://dictionary.oed.com/cgi/entry/50257397, cited 8 March 2007.

[4] I will only be examining triage procedures relating to incoming patients with acute (not chronic) injuries or diseases. Many other situations require triage, e.g., the allocation of organs to those in need of transplants or the priority of treatment for chronic conditions such as kidney dialysis, but these will not be the focus of my discussion of general triage procedures. I am using the term 'dire' to denote a situation in which patients will die as a result of the priority for care they are given. Most of the time in general contexts someone will not die, all else being equal, due to the care priorities given after the sorting process.

is chiefly employed to prioritize the care of some patients over others in a manner which responsibly allocates resources. These triage methods have an implicit egalitarian goal, namely, attending first to the care of the individuals most in need of medical attention.[5] In other words, it would be impossible for a hospital to have a one-to-one patient-physician ratio, so triage priorities are set to regulate the distribution of resources. Under these care levels, those most in need of medical attention are assisted first.[6] The same follows for the majority of military treatment facilities, whether on the battlefield or not.

Military medicine and its use of triage, at least the type practiced outside of extreme battle conditions, shares much in common with this sort of civilian triage. Most triage procedures in both contexts prioritize the wellbeing of individual patients, without concern for some larger overall goal.[7] When there are sufficient medical resources or even a slight scarcity, patients with the most severe injuries or illnesses are treated first, and those with less severe conditions wait until medical personnel are able to treat them. Most have experienced this triage procedure when visiting an emergency room; if an illness is not considered "severe" there may be a wait of several hours before a doctor administers treatment. This system of prioritizing patient wellbeing when the level of resources is sufficient (or at least not dire) seems so intuitively appropriate in these contexts that I will not argue for it. The difficulty in these procedures, however, lies in deciding what exactly counts as "most severe." At first glance, this decision appears to be impacted by a variety of elements.

There are numerous competing factors that appear to surround general triage practices. Here are just a few: the staffing level of physicians and nurses, the availability of medical supplies and medicine, and the number of beds available in a given treatment site. These will all vary from facility to facility, but the one aspect of general triage decision making which ought to remain constant whether resources

---

[5] James F. Childress ("Triage in Response to a Bioterrorist Attack," in *In the Wake of Terror*, J.D. Moreno, ed. [Cambridge, MA: MIT, 2003], 77–93, here 80) argues that triage is fundamentally utilitarian, with the only distinction being between medical utility (what I am here calling an egalitarian concern) and social utility. For this discussion, I will operate under the assumption that triage based only medical concerns is egalitarian since it places priority on an individual's medical needs.

[6] Of course, there are varying levels of triage for different situations. Triage during ordinary E.R. intake is quite different than E.R. intake after a disastrous plane crash with 50 victims needing immediate care. The point here is just that in ordinary situations where the level of care is sufficient to prevent patient death (perhaps not sufficient to give the best quality of life to each person, though) the triage procedure employed is generally egalitarian and gives first priority to those most in need of care.

[7] This prioritization of the treatment for those most in need of medical care even occurs in ICU admissions practices where resources in civilian contexts are often scarce. Patients who are less in need of ICU care often turned away. See, for example, Robert Baker and Martin Strosberg, "Triage and Equality: An Historical Reassessment of Utilitarian Analyses of Triage," *Kennedy Institute of Ethics Journal* 2.2 (1992): 103–123, esp. 106–110.

are sufficient or slightly scarce is that individual patient well-being should be the highest priority. Therefore, the decision over what is considered "most severe" will often involve a detailed assessment when multiple patients require care. This medical decision is mapped out well for practitioners in various triage guidebooks.[8] When there is no dire shortage of resources there will be a level of priority assigned by the individual assessing the incoming patients, but there will most likely not be a significant risk that lives will be lost due to patients waiting for treatment.

In general, there are three primary categories in both military and civilian triage procedures into which patients are placed once they have been evaluated: those who will live without medical care and require only minor treatment; those who will die whether or not they receive medical care; and those who will die if they do not receive medical care.[9] These categories, since only dependent on medical diagnosis, are not the direct cause of ethical dilemmas. There may be debate, of course, at the borders of each category about which medical conditions merit placement into one or the other. For example, say patient A has a condition that is viewed as life-threatening and patient B has a condition viewed as close to life-threatening (how close is close?). The individual assessing the two patients assigns a probability of survival and then treats each of the patients accordingly, with the person more in need of care being treated first. Perhaps A has a 20–25% chance of survival and B has a 30–35% chance of survival.

These issues surrounding which patient is placed into which group are, however, medical and diagnostic dilemmas and not ethical ones. Ethical dilemmas arise, rather, in how each of these categories is given priority in terms of treatment. In general practice, military and civilian procedures give priority to the last group of patients, i.e., those who will die if they do not receive treatment. Ethical dilemmas seem to arise when, during battle conditions that commanders believe warrant it, military physicians must reverse triage procedures[10] and give priority to the first group, i.e., patients who will live without medical care and who only require minor treatment. In the next section, I will discuss military guidelines relating to three levels of battle conditions and the triage procedure used for each.

[8] For examples of triage guidebooks, see Polly G. Zimmerman and Robert D. Herr, *Triage Nursing Secrets* (St. Louis, MO: Mosby Elsevier, 2006); and Thomas E. Bowen and Ronald F. Bellamy, eds., *Emergency War Surgery* (Second Revision of NATO Handbook; Washington, DC: Department of Defense, 1988).

[9] These broad categories are generally expanded into, perhaps, five categories or more (see, for example, Bowen and Bellamy, *Emergency War Surgery*). Since the primary focus of this paper is the ethical issues surrounding military medical triage and not the medical aspect involved in evaluating patients, these three general categories are adequate.

[10] Hereafter, I will refer to this as a "triage reversal" because the group that receives priority in terms of medical care under this triage model is the group that normally receives care last.

3 Military Triage and Battle Conditions

As mentioned above, many military triage practices model the egalitarian triage practices used in most civilian contexts.[11] If a soldier requires medical treatment while on a tour of duty or while stationed at a base, his or her individual medical needs will be the primary factor taken into account. Sometimes, however, medical resources are not sufficient to prevent the death of those in need of care, so decisions must be made about who will be treated first (and likely live) and who will be denied care or have care postponed (and likely die). These are difficult decisions that no one would ever desire to make, but they must be made when resources are insufficient (in these cases, it is not often whether or not some will die, but rather how many and which ones). Before discussing the ethical dilemmas surrounding military triage, it is first important to consider various levels of battle conditions and the triage procedures which are recommended during each. Here I will highlight the triage procedures the US military employs, but much of what is said could also apply to countries in NATO and to other developed nations.

Rather than relying on a single principle to guide the decision of which group of wounded soldiers should receive care first, some distinguish battle conditions and the objectives of the chain of command during these battle conditions as relevant.[12] The appeal of a "one-size-fits-all" triage prioritization system seems fairly obvious. Having a triage procedure that operates on one primary principle for deciding whom resources should be devoted to first would seem to simplify matters. The opposite, in fact, appears to be the case.

One such example is Gerald Winslow's study on triage where he argues against triage guided by utilitarian principles and seeks to develop an overall egalitarian principle to serve as the foundation for triage procedures. Throughout the book, Winslow critiques the use of utilitarian principles, but in the end allows for at least some aspects outside of the medical needs of individual patients to enter into triage prioritizing. For example, Winslow argues that those operating under a Rawlsian view would most likely favor egalitarian principles, but that they would also allow for the possibility that those with special skills (e.g., doctors) might be treated first in mass-casualty situations.[13] This would clearly violate the egalitarian principles for which Winslow argues. Here Winslow is careful to not label such an exception to his egalitarian views as utilitarian; instead, he claims that this is a way of coming "... as close as possible to equal treatment in the long run" and not any sort of maximizing principle.[14]

[11] See, for example, Bowen and Bellamy, *Emergency War Surgery*, part 3, Chapter 2.

[12] See, for example, Thomas E. Beam, "Medical Ethics on the Battlefield: The Crucible of Military Medical Ethics," Chapter 13 in *Military Medical Ethics*, vol. 2, Dave E. Lounsbury, ed., Office of the Surgeon General of the Army, http://www.bordeninstitute.army.mil/published_volumes/ethicsVol 2/Ethics-ch-13.pdf, cited 17 March 2007, 381–384.

[13] Gerald R. Winslow, *Triage and Justice* (Los Angeles, CA: University of California Press, 1982), 152–153.

[14] Ibid., 153. Just after this sentence, though, Winslow admits that while this strategy, which he states rests on the "difference principle" he discusses, "may produce identical strategies" to a utilitarian model, he claims that they each "clearly exemplify different perspectives" (ibid.).

Whatever the case may be, Winslow's concession to the admissibility (and perhaps necessity) of a principle other than an overall egalitarian principle muddies the water a great deal. Since in a given situation one must evaluate whether it is appropriate to act contrary to what appears to be an egalitarian need, it seems that this addition risks collapse into utilitarianism, or at least into a general triage procedure that mostly follows egalitarian values but allows utility to be considered in special circumstances. Whether or not this is the case, it appears that rather than attempting to find a "one-size-fits-all" triage model for use by military physicians, it would be better to explicitly separate cases in which egalitarian models are to be preferred from cases in which utilitarian models or other models might be appropriate.[15]

In one such model that separates cases where utilitarian concerns should drive the priority assigned to each group after the initial triage sorting, Thomas Beam describes three battle conditions which current military guidelines have established as relevant to triage procedures; each of these uses a different triage model. These levels of battle conditions are as follows: non-austere battle conditions, austere battle conditions and extreme battle conditions.[16] The first battle condition, the non-austere, is the battle condition most common for the US military,[17] and in it patients are treated according to egalitarian triage priorities. In this setting, as described above, there is no dire shortage of resources and physicians are able to consider individual patients' welfare above all other external or overall concerns.

In the second type of battle conditions, the austere battle conditions, Beam argues that physicians should act to save as many soldiers as possible. This triage model, Beam claims, is utilitarian in emphasis, and the primary good sought is saving as many lives as possible. As a result, those who will be most easily treated receive priority (e.g., those with only superficial or minor wounds), and the care of those requiring more attention is delayed. This is analogous to the approach taken in many civilian mass-casualty scenarios. Here Beam argues the good achieved by using this triage method seems clear: maximizing the number of total lives that are saved. Whether one should appeal to utilitarian concerns to justify such a triage prioritization in a military context will be discussed in more detail in §4.

One ambiguity that might arise from this second level of battle conditions and the triage procedure corresponding to it is the question about what exactly counts as a "life saved." Is the *quantity* of life the primary concern? In other words, should only the number of soldiers who live after treatment count as the good achieved by changing which group receives treatment first? Or, should physicians work to also

---

[15] Michael L. Gross (*Bioethics and Armed Conflict* [Cambridge, MA: MIT, 2006]) argues along similar lines regarding military triage. Here Gross notes that British soldiers have distinguished between mass-casualty triage and conventional triage (ibid., 144–148), noting that mass-casualty triage appeals to principles of "salvage" and "utility."

[16] Beam, "Medical Ethics on the Battlefield: The Crucible of Military Medical Ethics," 381.

[17] Ibid. Here Beam notes the following: "This is the model that is most frequently seen and that occurred throughout the Persian Gulf War for most units, including American hospitals for Iraqi POWs."

improve the *quality* of the lives those they are treating will lead? This would involve a goal beyond just having a high quantity of soldiers who live after treatment. For example, imagine an instance where a soldier has been in contact with an explosive mine and needs to have her leg amputated. Should a physician work *primarily* to save her life, e.g., perhaps immediately amputating the leg and treating the life-threatening aspect of her injuries (and then move on to treating others)? Or, should a concern for the quality of the soldier's life also be influential in making a decision?

Certain procedures such as amputation will require less time than others, so should more time be devoted to exploring options other than amputation before performing the procedure? Adding quality of life (i.e., future quality of life after treatment) as a consideration might mean attending for a longer time to the treatment process so that the soldier will be more likely to walk rather than have to use a wheelchair. In some instances, attending to the quality of life might run contrary to the quantity of live preserved. Perhaps beyond considering these individually, the good achieved by changing the priority of which triage group to treat first in the mass-casualty/austere conditions model might be some combination of both the quantity of lives saved and quality of the life to be enjoyed by those saved. This triage procedure will not be the primary focus in this paper, but the appeal to principles of utility used to justify it will be discussed in §4.

The third level of battle conditions, what Beam calls extreme conditions, prioritizes the care of those who require only minor medical treatment, i.e., those who will live without medical care and require only minor treatment, over all others needing treatment. It is this level of military triage that is used most infrequently by the US military.[18] Beam recommends applying a triage model that is utilitarian in intent during these battle conditions, but it has a different good in view, namely, preserving the strength of the fighting force.[19] Rather than focusing on the number of lives saved (or, perhaps, on the quality of life as well), this triage procedure seeks to maximize the number of soldiers treated so that those soldiers can return to the battlefield as soon as possible. There are a number of conditions that must be met before a commander will decide that battle conditions are extreme and that these triage procedures should be used.

A condition for initiating this sort of triage reversal is that those who are most easily able to return to battle will not only live after treatment (a good) but primarily that their return to battle (as a result of the treatment) will work to the advantage of current military objectives and make a *significant* difference in winning the present

[18]Regarding this triage model and its priority on returning soldiers to duty, Beam discusses the change in priority from the 1985 Army Field Manual to the 1994 Army Field Manual. Whereas in the 1984 edition placed priority on returning soldiers to duty, this receives the lowest priority in the 1994 edition. For these guidelines, see US Department of the Army, *Planning for Health Service Support* (Washington, DC: Department of the Army, 9 September 1994), Field Manual 8–55, §§1–5, https://atiam.train.army.mil/soldierPortal/atia/adlsc/view/public/9533-1/fm/8-55/fm8_55.pdf, cited 07 June 2007.

[19] Beam, "Medical Ethics on the Battlefield: The Crucible of Military Medical Ethics," 384.

battle. For example, imagine a battalion (approximately 400 soldiers) is facing an enemy force of about 550 soldiers and that each force is equipped with comparable weaponry. After several hours of fighting, 50 soldiers in the battalion are wounded. Most of these wounds are life-threatening; in fact, imagine that 40 out of the 50 are severely wounded and that the other 10 have only superficial wounds. Although it depends on the number of physicians traveling with the battalion, in most cases this would qualify as neither an extreme nor an austere battle condition. Now imagine the same scenario, but that instead of 50 being wounded there are 300 wounded and of these only 15 have life-threatening injuries (perhaps some fit into the category of those who will die whether or not they receive treatment and others will die if they do not receive treatment). Also, assume that the battalion will be overrun in the field if the physicians are unable to quickly treat those with superficial injuries. This latter situation is one which it seems would be classified as an extreme battle condition and, all else being equal, would warrant a reversal of triage prioritization under current military recommendations.

This triage prioritization reversal during extreme battle conditions creates an ethical dilemma because it is not only the group of those who will die regardless of whether they receive care who are placed aside so that those only superficially wounded can receive care first, but it is also the group of those who will die if they do not receive medical care that is no longer given priority. In most battle conditions, this latter group receives priority for medical treatment, but during extreme battle conditions this group no longer receives priority of care, and as a result many of these soldiers who were severely wounded in battle may die. Were it not for such triage prioritization reversal, these soldiers would most likely live. This dilemma will be discussed in more detail in §4.

An example to which many refer in discussions of military triage concerns an actual application of this triage model during World War II. In this example, James Howie, the former director of the Public Health Laboratory Service in Britain, discusses a time during World War II in North Africa when British military officials were faced with a difficult decision regarding triage prioritization.[20] During the spring of 1943, while British troops in North Africa were preparing to invade Italy and Sicily, many in the ranks contracted gonorrhea after visiting local prostitutes. The debate was whether penicillin should be used to treat these soldiers who had contracted gonorrhea rather than to treat soldiers suffering from battle wounds—the goal being to return to health as many soldiers as possible so that they could resume training for the imminent invasion. Several factors heightened the tension: at this time penicillin research was still in its early stages and researchers (e.g., Cairns and Florey) were focused on learning how to treat wound victims with the medicine; the availability of penicillin was scarce and any use of the medicine was intensely scrutinized and required approval from the director of pathology at the War Office;

[20] James Howie, "Gonorrhoea—A Question of Tactics," *British Medical Journal* 6205 (1979): 1631–1632.

and, most obviously, the potential political ramifications of distributing the medicine to soldiers who had acquired gonorrhea before administering it to soldiers who had been wounded while fighting for their country.

Additionally, it was well known to researchers at the time that penicillin was highly effective in the treatment of gonorrhea, but it was uncertain how effective it would be in treating many of the wounds incurred during a battle. Howie recounts that during this debate he was working as the deputy director of army pathology and, as a result, he was involved in the deliberation process. This decision was debated by doctors and medical administrators, but it ultimately became a political issue and was passed all the way up the chain of command to Winston Churchill. In the end, the decision was made to use the available penicillin to the "best military advantage," and this meant that the soldiers who had contracted gonorrhea were treated first and allowed to return to training for the upcoming battle.[21] This decision not only stalled further research on the efficacy of penicillin for treating battle wounds (research that could have aided future injured soldiers involved in the war effort), but it also prevented presently injured soldiers from receiving it. Although this decision occurred outside of an immediate battle context, this case illustrates exactly the type of reversal of triage priorities that occurs during extreme battle conditions. This type of triage prioritization reversal employed during extreme battle conditions will dominate the remaining discussion in this paper.

At this stage, triage procedures in general as well as the current triage priorities that the US military actually uses in various battle conditions have been discussed. There has not been, however, any reflection on whether or not these procedures are the ones that *ought* to be used. This is, of course, the primary aspect that makes triage and the priorities assigned after the initial sorting interesting for ethicists. These are the procedures that military officials and field manuals recommend adopting; whether these are morally permissible, however, is a different question altogether. This will be discussed in the next section.

4 Utility, Obligations, and Triage Priorities

Since the extreme conditions triage model has been rarely employed by the US Military and since the conditions under which it should be used are limited, one might question whether it is a worthwhile area for ethics to investigate. Although the present analysis will be refined in scope (focusing primarily on those wounded from fighting and needing medical care), the argument I will make for a military commander's obligations will be broadly applicable to other areas of military bioethics. For example,

---

[21] Ibid., 1631. This case is also recounted in Henry K. Beecher, *Research and the Individual* (Boston, MA: Little, Brown, 1971), 209–210. Additionally, some question whether this case should be considered a canonical case of military triage. See, for example, the discussion in Baker and Strosberg, "Triage and Equality," 120.

whether a military physician, if asked by a commanding officer, should participate in actions such as torture or coercion by medical means would be another area to which, *mutatis mutandis*, this argument might apply. Furthermore, medical codes and ethicists alike are mostly opposed to any system of triage prioritization that appeals to any principle other than medical need. Those supporting this view often envision physicians as being required to consider only their patients' medical needs when administering care. Additionally, the Geneva Conventions (I and II) are fairly explicit on this issue: "Only urgent medical reasons will authorize priority in the order of treatment to be administered."[22] Although this principle from the Geneva Conventions aims to outline international medical care guidelines, extreme battle conditions triage models that countries in NATO recommend directly contradict it. For these reasons, I believe that the extreme battle conditions triage model should be discussed, and it will be the focus of the remainder of this paper.

Not only do the US and other NATO countries reverse triage procedures during certain battle conditions to salvage as many soldiers as possible and return them to battle, but there are also priorities about which individuals among the wounded are cared for first. The following quotation outlines these priorities and the opinion of some about them:

> [T]raditionally US combat casualty care has been directed toward US casualties first, allies second, civilians third, and enemy fourth. This is a time for reevaluation of ethical and moral principles and a reaffirmation that if the most seriously injured casualty is, in fact, an enemy soldier, he goes first.[23]

In the section that follows, I will argue that the current US (and other NATO countries) military triage guidelines that involve breaking Geneva Convention protocols with respect to treatment priorities and triage procedure reversal are both warranted and morally required on the grounds that military commanders have fiduciary obligations to win battles. In §5, I will argue that military physicians and the individuals whom they treat do not, in certain circumstances, enter into a patient-physician relationship, and that this difference warrants triage reversal should the chain of command require it.

Before arguing for these fiduciary obligations that military commanders possess, it will first be useful to address the ethical theory to which Beam appeals in his discussion of triage priorities and battle conditions, namely, utilitarianism. Beam mentions that the triage models employed during austere battle conditions as well those employed during extreme conditions would be appropriate under a utilitarian analysis. As he states regarding the latter, "The defense of the decision to treat the minimally wounded could be made on the basis of a utilitarian approach."[24] At first glance, it may seem intuitively appropriate to appeal to utilitarian calculi to justify

[22] Geneva Conventions, I, II article 12, http://www.icrc.org/, cited 30 April 2007.

[23] Kenneth G. Swan and K.G. Swan, Jr., "Triage: The Past Revisted," *Military Medicine* 161:8 (1996): 448–452.

[24] Beam, "Medical Ethics on the Battlefield: The Crucible of Military Medical Ethics," 384.

such decisions regarding triage. After all, whether or not a battle will be won may hinge on whether or not triage priorities are adequate to the needs of the chain of command. And surely, winning a battle is better than losing a battle, right?

Attempting to account for these triage prioritization decisions under a utilitarian model, however, would be a difficult task and, even if one were able to do so, the application of such triage prioritization reversal would only be acceptable for a utilitarian in a few, limited circumstances. Since for a utilitarian the "good" choice is the one which will, in the end, result in the most total aggregate happiness, to justify a triage prioritization reversal a pure utilitarian account would not only have to account for the happiness of the combatants but also for everyone who might be affected by the triage reversal. As a result, a utilitarian would be able to reverse triage only if he were sure (or at least believed it highly probable) that the decision to do so would likely effect more good than not.

Furthermore, a utilitarian view would not only have to account for the total aggregate happiness resulting from a particular decision to reverse triage but, moreover, for the happiness resulting from winning the battle at hand and, on a larger scale, for the happiness resulting from winning the war (if that were the goal). Additionally, he would have to consider the happiness of enemy belligerents and their families and all those who would be affected by the result of the battle and, ultimately, the war. Furthermore, for a utilitarian to even go to war in the first place there would have to be so great an evil that would be avoided by fighting a war that it seems doubtful that, given the overwhelming likelihood of a large amount of resulting unhappiness, a war would ever be fought. In a utilitarian framework, in fact, it is sometimes better to lose a battle if it will create more total aggregate happiness than winning. For these reasons, it seems that a utilitarian approach would not be best to defend the extreme battle conditions triage model unless one simply assumed that the army in question only fought wars that were likely to create more total aggregate happiness.[25]

Rather than attempting to analyze triage prioritization decisions through a utilitarian framework, I suggest that we view military commanders as possessing fiduciary obligations.[26] I will argue that it is the principle of "fiduciary obligations" that should guide military decisions, both on the battlefield and off. It is to this principle that a military officer or military medical commander should appeal when determining

[25] Beam seems to assume such a view. For example, regarding the extreme battle conditions model he states, "... the 'greatest good for the greatest number' would allow the decision [to reverse triage] to be made, not for the benefit of the individual patient, but for the good of the unit, the army, or the country'" ("Medical Ethics on the Battlefield: The Crucible of Military Medical Ethics," 384). Here Beam assumes that the wars in which this model would be applied would be wars in which more good would be created by winning them than not. What of the unhappiness of the enemy combatants and their countrymen? Beam does not mention this issue, but instead he seems to assume that the only happiness or good in question is the good of the army making the decision and its sponsoring country.

[26] A similar approach by Michael L. Gross ("Bioethics and Armed Conflict," *Hastings Center Report* 34.6 [2004], 22–30, esp. 25–26) makes use of the concept of "military necessity."

whether to reverse triage procedures. To support my claim that military commanders possess fiduciary obligations, I will look to business ethics literature dealing with the obligations possessed by a corporate executive. The corporate executive, then, will serve as an analogue for a particular military commander entrusted with decisions regarding triage priorities.

There has been much discussion in the business ethics literature about the duties of corporate executives and the duties of the respective businesses they manage. In business ethics there are some who believe that businesses are obliged to assist the persons living in the communities in which they operate.[27] This "assistance" might include philanthropic contributions to publicly accessible goods, such as libraries or schools. It also might take the form of scholarship programs or donations to charitable causes. Whatever the case may be, under this view a business, through the leadership of the corporate executive, is morally obliged to contribute some of its profits for the betterment of society. A second perspective regarding the obligations of a business might be that it is permissible for businesses to contribute to social causes and welfare. So, while it may not be necessary for a business to use a portion of its profits to provide such support, the business is not prohibited from doing so.

A third view on business involvement in social causes is that a business, led by a corporate executive, is permitted to contribute to social welfare only if doing so will increase the profits of her company. The justification provided for this condition is that businesses, and more specifically the corporate executives, have fiduciary obligations to their shareholders. These obligations are the result of the shareholders of a business trusting the business and the corporate executive with their money with one goal in mind, namely, generating profits for the business and a financial return for the shareholders. This view on the social obligations of business is expressed most clearly by Milton Friedman in the following quotation:

> [T]here is one and only one social responsibility of business—to use its resources and engage in activities designed to increase its profits as long as it stays within the rules of the game, which is to say, engages in open and free competition, without deception or fraud.[28]

Under this view, then, it is inappropriate for a corporate executive, acting on a corporation's behalf, to contribute to a social cause unless doing so would contribute to the corporation's profits since these funds are entrusted to him by shareholders for a specific purpose. In a sense, as Friedman argues, if an executive does this he is using someone else's money for a cause to which they did not intend to contribute. These fiduciary obligations result from the corporate executive being entrusted by the shareholders with the financial resources they have contributed.

---

[27] For example, see Gillian Brock, "Meeting Needs and Business Obligations: An Argument for the Libertarian Skeptic," *Journal of Business Ethics* 15.6 (1996): 695–702.

[28] Milton Friedman, *Capitalism and Freedom* (Chicago, IL: University of Chicago Press, 1962), 133. Also, see Milton Friedman, "The Social Responsibility of Business is to Increase Profits," *The New York Times Magazine* (13 September 1970).

This view of the obligations of business, and specifically the obligations of a corporate executive, is applicable to decisions made in a military context. Rather than being entrusted with financial resources so as to make profits, military commanders are entrusted with the duty to win wars. Thus, they possess fiduciary obligations to accomplish this goal without attending to other possible goals they as individual persons might have, unless doing so would enable them to better accomplish their primary obligation, namely winning wars.[29] In the argument that follows, I will suggest that military decisions in general should be governed by an overarching fiduciary obligation to win wars. In particular situations, this may be accomplished by triage models that are egalitarian in focus, but in others commanders must reverse triage procedures to fulfill their obligation and perform the duty with which they have been entrusted.

One question that might arise in the analogy being made between the obligations of corporations and the obligations of military commanders is related to who the shareholders might be. Are the shareholders who have entrusted military commanders to win wars the governmental officials of a particular country? Would this include just the executive of a country (for example, the president) or perhaps the larger, often more representative body such as the congress or parliament? Or further, would the shareholders include each citizen of the country that has entrusted the commander with the objective of winning the war? Rather than focus exclusively on Friedman's shareholder model, it is important at this juncture to discuss a different model for explicating the obligations businesses and corporate executive possess, namely the stakeholder model.[30] This contrast between shareholder theory and stakeholder theory will be relevant in deciding to whom military commanders are obligated and by whom they have been entrusted to win wars.

Rather than view businesses and corporate executives as having obligations only to their shareholders, stakeholder theory expands the purview of those to whom businesses have obligations. R. Edward Freeman defines a stakeholder as "any group or individual who can affect or is affected by the achievement of the firm's objectives."[31] Shareholders are, of course, also stakeholders, but stakeholder theory

---

[29] A similar argument by Brian S. Carter ("The Military Physician and Conservation of Force," *Military Medicine* 158.6 [1993]: 374–375) makes use of the principle of 'conservation' under which military commanders and military medical commanders must operate. Carter argues that "[t]he military commander uses the resources entrusted to him, men and material, to accomplish the mission assigned to him" (ibid., 374).

[30] A representative exposition of stakeholder theory is R. Edward Freeman, *Strategic Management: A Stakeholder Approach* (Marshfield, MA: Pitman Publishing, 1984). More recent discussions include the following: Anant K. Sundaram and Andrew C. Inkpen, "The Corporate Objective Revisited," *Organization Science* 15:3 (2004): 350–363; R. Edward Freeman, Andrew C. Wicks, and Bidhan Parmar, "Stakeholder Theory and 'The Corporate Objective Revisited,'" *Organization Science* 15:3 (2004): 364–369; and Max B.E. Clarkson, "A Stakeholder Framework for Analyzing and Evaluating Corporate Social Responsibility," *The Academy of Management Review* 20:1 (1995): 92–117.

[31] Freeman, *Strategic Management*, 25. Also, see Freeman's discussion on 46–47.

greatly enlarges the group of persons to whom corporate executives have duties to include the following, among others: governments, suppliers, consumer advocates. Under Friedman's view, the only group of individuals an executive must consider is the group of shareholders that have entrusted her with making profits; under Freeman's stakeholder view, however, a corporate executive must consider any stakeholder, i.e., any person who has a "stake" in the matter, who might potentially be affected by or potentially affect the attainment of corporate goals.

It should be clear from the outset that there are a number of ways to understand the phrase "any group or individual who can affect or is affected by the achievement of the firm's objectives." Does this really mean *any* group or individual? How should we understand the terms 'affect' and 'affected'? These questions and others like them that relate to where exactly the line should be drawn about who is and who is not a stakeholder have caused a great deal of debate over the applicability of stakeholder theory.[32] In fact, it certainly seems possible for almost any person or group to be included as a stakeholder under Freeman's definition,[33] perhaps even a competitor's business. The goal of this essay is, of course, not to defend a particular interpretation of stakeholder or shareholder theory but rather to make use of the insights or perhaps shortcomings of each in evaluating the decisions that must be made by military commanders.

One might object to the possibility of a coherent shareholder theory on practical grounds. That is, it would seem nearly impossible to make calculations about the effects one's decision might have on every single person or group potentially affected. Thus, there must be some (practical) limit to who is considered a stakeholder and who is not. Must the business person in Taiwan consider each and every person her choice might affect? Analogously, must the military commander consider each and every person his decision will affect? This requirement to consider all stakeholders in each decision, or at least the ones believed to be most closely affected by a particular decision (how close is close?), it seems, would create a practical impossibility.[34]

---

[32] For example of such a critique see Kenneth Goodpaster, "Business Ethics and Stakeholder Analysis," *Business Ethics Quarterly* 1:1 (1991): 53–73. R. Edward Freeman responded to this critique in the following article: "The Politics of Stakeholder Theory: Some Future Directions," *Business Ethics Quarterly* 4:4 (1994): 409–421.

[33] Ronald K. Mitchell et al. ("Toward a Theory of Stakeholder Identification and Salience: Defining the Principle of Who and What Counts," *The Academy of Management Review* 22:4 [1997]: 853–886, here 856) observe this and describe Freeman's definition as "... certainly one of the broadest definitions in the literature."

[34] Mitchell et al. surveyed the literature on stakeholder theory in 1997 and found 27 different definitions that each attempt to define who stakeholder is (ibid., 858), displaying just how difficult it is to determine with a high degree of precision who counts as a stakeholder. With this in mind, Freeman notes that rather than being a theory in the sense that we normally understand the term 'theory,' "'Stakeholder theory' is ... a genre of stories about how we could live" and also "[Stakeholder theory] is part of a narrative about how we do and could live" ("The Politics of Stakeholder Theory," 413 and 418, respectively). While interesting for discussion and perhaps useful as a heuristic, it is unclear how these views of Freeman's on stakeholder theory as a "narrative" provide definite direction as to what a business should or should not do.

The more serious objection against stakeholder views, at the least the sort of stakeholder theory for which Freeman argues, is metaphysical. It seems that giving all stakeholders equal weight in decision making fails to recognize the fundamental purpose for engaging in business activity, namely, to better one's economic position. Persons cooperate in business ventures for the purpose of creating a surplus in which they may share, a surplus that would not have existed if each individual cooperating in the venture had attempted to produce without the cooperation of others.[35] For these reasons, it seems that giving the distant individual who has a "stake" in the matter—but who has not financially or otherwise contributed to the venture—equal weight misunderstands the point.[36] Thus, I side with a shareholder view which makes a business, and analogously a military commander, required to fulfill its fiduciary obligations to their shareholders. For the corporate executive this means generating profits with the money entrusted to him by the shareholders; for the military commander this means winning wars using the means and resources entrusted to her by the shareholders.

So, this leads to the following question: who are the shareholders who have entrusted the military commander with the task of winning wars? The answer for this, it seems, would depend upon the nation who has entrusted the military commander with winning wars. For the US this would be a combination of the three branches of power, the legislative, the executive and the judicial, as each relates to the ability to engage in war. In each particular situation, those parties who have authorized the war and empowered the commanders to do what is necessary to accomplish the goal of winning the war would count as the shareholders to whom the commander has fiduciary obligations.

These fiduciary obligations that I am arguing military commanders possess oblige commanders to do what is required to accomplish the task for which they have been appointed. In most instances regarding which triage model should be chosen, it seems clear that the triage model selected would be egalitarian in design. When resources are sufficient to treat first those most needing care without breaking the obligation to win the war, it is appropriate to have medical need determine who receives priority. Furthermore, having a triage system in place which, most of the time, prioritizes individual medical need seems necessary to maintain the morale of the fighting force.[37] Thus, under the fiduciary obligations principle I am suggesting,

---

[35] Furthermore, viewing the obligations of military commander through a stakeholder theory would require him to not only consider those positively affected by the battle such as the government which has entrusted him to protect its interests but also consider the belligerents whom his decision will affect. Applying a stakeholder model to the way in which a military commander should make decisions, then, would seem to mistake the purpose of fighting a war, namely, to win and by doing so accomplish what each individual could not have done on her own.

[36] See Sundaram and Inkpen ("The Corporate Objective Revisited," 354–355) for a discussion of the difficulty and conflict that arises from having multiple goals driving a business, goals which in some cases may contradict the reason shareholders have invested in the company.

[37] Beam mentions that always having a triage model in place that gave priority only on the basis of one's ability to return to battle would have a negative effect on morale ("Medical Ethics on the Battlefield: The Crucible of Military Medical Ethics," 384).

having an extreme conditions triage model all the time would actually hamper the commander's ability to fulfill his obligation. This provides further support for the view expressed above that it seems best to have multiple options available for triage prioritization, some which are egalitarian in focus and others that are not.

Regarding the extreme battle conditions model, should a commander believe he must reverse triage to win the war,[38] then he is required to enact a triage reversal that will enable him to fulfill his obligation. This, unfortunately, may involve the deaths of those needing treatment. But reversing triage will only be done in the circumstances where it is necessary to do so. To refuse to reverse triage procedures when it is necessary to do so, perhaps by appealing to some other principle like medical need, would be for the military commander to squander the resources entrusted to her by the shareholders (the supporting nation, government, etc.) for the explicit purpose of winning a war. If a military commander refuses to reverse triage procedures and as a result loses the war, then she has violated her obligations to her shareholders.

If one grants the existence of fiduciary obligations possessed by military commanders, what remains to be discussed is physicians' participation in triage activities that seem to violate what many believe is a basic responsibility physicians possess. This responsibility is that physicians should place the well-being of their patient as the highest priority in decision making. In the section that follows, I will argue that physicians are able to support and participate in these triage procedures whether as physicians serving on the battlefield or as military medical commanders.

5 The Military Physician's Relationship with Those Needing Treatment

Many believe that physicians, both military and civilian, should always act with the goal of improving the health of those presenting themselves for medical treatment. This "duty" that physicians have for these individuals' needs is often mentioned in discussions of torture during which physicians are present (or even assisting). So, while they may support the fiduciary obligations that military commanders possess, they may not support the view that a physician should act in any other way than to help those in need of medical care. The following quotation from an article by Jerome Amir Singh is illustrative of this view:

> Military physicians should always remember that while captured terror suspects are detainees of a government they are *first and foremost patients* of the physicians and they are *owed* a

[38] Throughout the paper, I have assumed that military commanders are provided resources by the shareholders so that they may win wars. Wars are only won, of course, by winning battles, and it is in battles that triage may or may not be reversed. So, the military commander, often one who is experienced in making decisions such as these, must make a decision on a battle-by-battle basis about what to do so that the overall war will be won.

duty of care. The duty of care must supercede any blanket notion of loyalty, obligation, allegiance or patriotism that the physician may feel is owed to his or her station.[39]

Where exactly this "duty" originates is not immediately clear. Singh notes that this principle quoted above is in line with views espoused by a group called Physicians for Human rights, but this is hardly an argument for the existence of these obligations on the part of physicians. It certainly seems possible that this duty may be the result of individual rights that persons possess; perhaps this duty should be grounded in each person's right to life. It may also be possible that this duty results from medical knowledge that physicians possess. Each of these possibilities will be discussed below.

From the perspective outlined in §4, individual rights clearly play a large role in the fiduciary obligations that military commanders possess. For these fiduciary obligations to have any weight, we must presuppose that the shareholders each possess a right to their resources that they contribute, and further that they have certain rights within the relationship between them and the agent they have entrusted with their resources.[40] Although the rights of shareholders clearly play a role in that argument, in this section I will argue that in certain instances it is permissible that the rights of individuals presenting for treatment may be violated, and as a result that physicians should participate in triage reversal when a military commander commands it.

One primary reason for discussing physician participation in reverse triage procedures is that many ethicists believe that doing so fundamentally contradicts the duties a physician has to those in need of medical treatment who present themselves to him as patients.[41] Furthermore, in the opinion of the AMA *Code of Medical Ethics* physicians have "... ethical obligations to place patients' welfare above their own self-interest and above obligations to other groups."[42] It is first important to

---

[39] Jerome A. Singh, "American Physicians and dual loyalty obligations in the 'war on terror,'" *BMC Medical Ethics* 4.4 (2003): 1–10, here 8 (emphasis is mine). Note Singh's use of the term 'patients.'

[40] For another example of such a connection with individual rights being presupposed by cooperative activities such as business ventures see David Gauthier, *Morals by Agreement* (Oxford: Clarendon, 1986), esp. 221–223.

[41] For an example of theorists believing that it is a physician-soldier is a "morally unacceptable" role, see Victor W. Sidel and Barry Levy, "Physician-Soldier: A Moral Dilemma?" in *Military Medical Ethics*, vol. 1, Dave E. Lounsbury, ed., Office of the Surgeon General of the Army, http://www.bordeninstitute.army.mil/published_volumes/ethicsVol1/Ethics-ch-11.pdf, cited 17 March 2007. Also, Michael Gross discusses that decisions that take into consideration issues other than medical need may need to be done on a macro-level by policy makers and government officials so that doctors can "... fulfill their obligation to save human life when they can" (*Bioethics and Armed Conflict*, 151). My suggestion will be that military physicians may choose not to enter into a patient-physician relationship and, thus, should support such decisions by the chain of command.

[42] American Medical Association, *Code of Medical Ethics: Current Opinions with Annotations*, 2004–2005 ed. (Chicago, IL: AMA, 2004), 300. Additional references to the AMA Code will be included in the text.

note that the AMA *Code of Medical Ethics* is not intended to cover every possible ethical dilemma that a physician might face; rather, it is a collection of ethical guidelines that are open, in some areas, to various possible interpretations. Furthermore, although the annotated version contains references to legal codes and journal articles relevant to each opinion, statements in the code themselves represent the opinion of the AMA and its constituents and are not, as such, explicit moral arguments. Furthermore, while legal precedents may be important in developing an opinion on a particular issue, in certain cases legal considerations may diverge from moral considerations. With these caveats in place, it will now be useful to discuss some ambiguities regarding the patient-physician relationship that the AMA Code describes.

The AMA *Code* states that "[a] patient-physician relationship exists when a physician serves a patient's medical needs, generally by mutual consent between a patient and a physician"(300). The *Code* continues to state that "[p]hysicians must keep their professional obligations to provide care to patients in accord with their prerogative to choose whether to enter into a patient-physician relationship" (305). Furthermore, "both the patient and the physician are free to enter into or decline the relationship" (281). Given these conditions on the patient-physician relationship, there are two questions relevant to the issue of military physicians and the issue of triage. First, does a patient-physician relationship exist between a military physician and the individual needing care, and if so does it exist in only the instances where the physician agrees to consider the patients' medical needs as that which dictates triage prioritization (e.g., in non-austere battle conditions)? Second, if a physician can freely choose not to enter into a patient-physician relationship with someone requiring care is this how we should understand the situation of military physicians who must reverse triage?

It will be useful to consider the second question before the first. Since physicians are free to enter into the patient-physician relationship, it seems that we might allow for instances where a physician may use his medical knowledge for a certain purpose but not be in a patient-physician relationship while doing so.[43] In other words, it does not seem that the knowledge an individual possesses is what obligates one to consider a patients' needs above all else; rather, it is the decision to enter into a patient-physician relationship, which as the AMA *Code* notes, is a contractual decision on the part of both the physician and the patient.[44] This being the case, it seems

[43] For an example of a similar argument relating to hostile interrogation and torture, see Fritz Allhoff, "Physician Involvement in Hostile Interrogations," *Cambridge Quarterly of Healthcare Ethics* 15 (2006): 392–402.

[44] Also, see Dominick R. Rascona, "The Moral Obligation of United States Military Medical Service," in *Military Medical Ethics*, vol. 1, Dave E. Lounsbury, ed., Office of the Surgeon General of the Army, http://www.bordeninstitute.army.mil/published_volumes/ethicsVol1/Ethics-ch-11.pdf, cited 17 March 2007. Here Rascona argues that the assumption that medical ethics "... may be somehow superior to (all) ethics ... would seem to be at the heart of the problem of the legitimacy of military medical ethics." I contend that possessing medical knowledge does not imply special ethical duties any more than specialized knowledge in another field implies special ethical duties.

that since physicians affected by reverse triage procedures are aware that in certain instances, when mandated by the chain of command, medical need will not be the primary consideration for medical care, these physicians are not *de facto* entering into patient-physician relationships in these instances; rather, they are choosing to use their medical knowledge to help accomplish the goals of the chain of command (i.e., fulfilling fiduciary obligations by winning wars).

Regarding the first question, it does seem useful to describe the military physician as choosing to enter into a patient-physician relationship in the triage model recommended by non-austere battle conditions. In these situations, patient medical need is valued above all else and there is an understanding of this between the individual needing care and the physician. But, it should be noted that just as battle conditions are ever-changing and dynamic it is certainly possible that a patient-physician relationship begun during non-austere battle conditions may need to change to a non-patient-physician relationship. In this circumstance, the individual being treated may be de-prioritized, and his care may be delayed.

This should come as no surprise, though, since in civilian situations we can imagine the patient-physician relationship as dynamic as well. For example, one of the situations explicitly identified by the AMA *Code* in which a physician may decide not to enter into a patient-physician relationship with an individual is one in which the treatment requested is "known to be scientifically invalid, has no medical indication, and offers no possible benefit to the patient" (305). In such a situation, we can easily envision a physician initially choosing to enter into a patient-physician relationship and administering treatment. After assisting the patient, however, the physician discovers that the patient desires a treatment that is scientifically invalid. At this point, the physician may withdraw from the patient-physician relationship.

Having discussed these abilities that physicians have to choose not to enter into the patient-physician relationship, it is now necessary to discuss what happens to the rights of the individual soldier whose medical care is de-prioritized when triage is reversed. What of his right to life? Is this decision unfair to him? Here it is important to note and respond to a prevailing view in bioethics, the view of Michael Walzer makes most clear in the important work *Spheres of Justice*.[45] Using a principle of distributive justice as a guide, Walzer believes that elements of need in a particular situation "... generate a particular distributive sphere."[46] Since healthcare has its own particular criteria of need, Walzer argues that applying needs from other spheres to the sphere created by the needs in healthcare situations would be inappropriate. In this line of thought, Walzer notes that "... the market is ... the chief rival of the sphere of security and welfare."[47] Relating Walzer's view back to triage in military decisions, it seems he would argue that allowing any need from a different sphere to influence the medical decision would be inappropriate.

[45] Michael Walzer, *Spheres of Justice* (New York: Basic Books, 1983).

[46] Ibid., 26.

[47] Ibid., 89.

People do have rights, but how we understand these rights can widely diverge. Walzer's system is derived from a generally egalitarian standpoint, namely that each person's needs in each situation must be considered in the decision about the distribution of goods. There are certain situations, though, in which it seems appropriate for the rights of certain individuals to be violated so that a greater number of rights may be preserved. For example, imagine a situation in which the strength of a military force has been significantly decreased due to 150 soldiers being wounded. Of these 150 wounded, imagine that 140 have been wounded only superficially and, with a minor amount of medical treatment, will be able to quickly return to the battlefield. The other 10 wounded are those who will die unless they receive immediate treatment.

In this scenario, though, it seems appropriate to consider the lives of the soldiers still fighting in the battlefield as well as the soldiers needing medical attention. Imagine that there are 200 soldiers still fighting in the battlefield, and imagine that according to the military commander's judgment if the superficially wounded soldiers are not returned as soon as possible the fighting force will be overrun on the battlefield. In this situation, I argue that it is important to violate the right to medical care (and the right to life) of the lesser number of individuals, hoping to preserve the rights of the larger group. So, it's not that rights should be violated *tout court*, but rather that in certain situations it may be appropriate for rights to be violated so that the rights of a larger number may be preserved.[48]

For these reasons, it seems that military physicians and military medical commanders are morally permitted to participate in triage reversal procedures when the chain of command requires it. Rather than elevating decisions such as triage reversal to a macro-level as Gross does (see fn. 40), viewing the military physician in this way, i.e., as individuals acting with medical knowledge to preserve the strength of the fighting force, provides a realistic picture of both the medical commander's participation that occurs in military strategizing and the physician's role as one acting to serve the needs of the chain of command.

6 Conclusion

The present paper has endeavored to provide support for triage models that make use of considerations other than medical need to determine who receives priority of care. Examining these situations through the lens of the fiduciary obligations model, I have argued that commanders must consider the reason which shareholders have entrusted them with resources, namely, so that they will win the war and as a result accomplish something that each individual could not have accomplished

[48] For a similar discussion, see Fritz Allhoff, "A Defense of Torture: Separation of Cases, Ticking Time-Bombs, and Moral Justification," *International Journal of Applied Philosophy* 19.2 (2006): 243–264, esp. 249–251.

by herself. Furthermore, it is by no means clear that physicians possess special ethical obligations merely as a result of their possessing medical knowledge. Perhaps *qua* persons they do possess obligations, but holding specialized knowledge does not create special ethical obligations. Additionally, since doctors may choose when to enter into a patient-physician relationship, perhaps we should view the relationships between military physicians and those whom they treat differently.

This essay has primarily focused on the priority of care administered to soldiers returning from the battlefield. Other areas to which this view could be applied would be the case of POWs and indigenous civilians needing care who are part of the country in which a war is taking place. In each of these situations, it seems that a commander's fiduciary obligations should be the primary governing principle for decision making.

References

Allhoff, Fritz. 2006. Physician Involvement in Hostile Interrogations. *Cambridge Quarterly of Healthcare Ethics* 15: 392–402.

Allhoff, Fritz. 2006. A Defense of Torture: Separation of Cases, Ticking Time-Bombs, and Moral Justification. *International Journal of Applied Philosophy* 19.2: 243–264.

American Medical Association. 2004. Code of Medical Ethics. *Current Opinions with Annotations*, 2004–2005 ed. Chicago, IL: AMA.

Baker, Robert and Martin Strosberg. 1992. Triage and Equality: An Historical Reassessment of Utilitarian Analyses of Triage. *Kennedy Institute of Ethics Journal* 2.2: 103–123.

Beam, Thomas E. and Linette R. Sparacino, eds. 2003. *Military Medical Ethics*, vols. 1–2 (*Textbooks of Military Medicine* series; Office of the Surgeon General, Department of the Army, and Borden Institute). http://www.bordeninstitute.army.mil/. Cited 17 March 2007.

Beecher, Henry K. 1971. *Research and the Individual*. Boston, MA: Little, Brown.

Bowen, Thomas E. and Ronald F. Bellamy, eds. 1988. *Emergency War Surgery*. Second Revision of NATO Handbook, Washington, DC: Department of Defense.

Brock, Gillian. 1996. Meeting Needs and Business Obligations: An Argument for the Libertarian Skeptic. *Journal of Business Ethics* 15.6: 695–702.

Carter, Brian S. 1993. The Military Physician and Conservation of Force. *Military Medicine* 158.6: 374–375.

Childress, James F. 2003. Triage in Response to a Bioterrorist Attack. In *In the Wake of Terror*, ed. J.D. Moreno, 77–93. Cambridge, MA: MIT.

Clarkson, Max B.E. 1995. A Stakeholder Framework for Analyzing and Evaluating Corporate Social Responsibility. *The Academy of Management Review* 20.1: 92–117.

Freeman, R. Edward. 1984. *Strategic Management: A Stakeholder Approach*. Marshfield, MA: Pitman Publishing.

Freeman, R. Edward. 1994. The Politics of Stakeholder Theory: Some Future Directions. *Business Ethics Quarterly* 4.4: 409–421.

Freeman, R. Edward et al. 2004. Stakeholder Theory and 'The Corporate Objective Revisited.' *Organization Science* 15.3: 364–369.

Friedman, Milton. 1962. *Capitalism and Freedom*. Chicago, IL: University of Chicago Press.

Friedman, Milton. 1970. The Social Responsibility of Business is to Increase Profits. *The New York Times Magazine*. 13 September 1970.

Gauthier, David. 1986. *Morals by Agreement*. Oxford: Clarendon.

Geneva Conventions. I and II. http://www.icrc.org/. Cited 30 April 2007.

Goodpaster, Kenneth. 1991. Business Ethics and Stakeholder Analysis. *Business Ethics Quarterly* 1.1: 53–73.
Gross, Michael L. 2006. *Bioethics and Armed Conflict*. Cambridge, MA: MIT.
Gross, Michael. 2004. Bioethics and Armed Conflict. *Hastings Center Report* 34.6: 22–30.
Howie, James. 1979. Gonorrhoea—A Question of Tactics. *British Medical Journal* 6205: 1631–1632.
Kilner, John F. 1990. *Who Lives? Who Dies?* New Haven, CT: Yale University Press.
Mitchell, Ronald K. et al. 1997. Toward a Theory of Stakeholder Identification and Salience: Defining the Principle of Who and What Counts. *The Academy of Management Review* 22.4: 853–886.
Singh, Jerome A. 2003. American Physicians and Dual Loyalty Obligations in the 'War on Terror.' *BMC Medical Ethics* 4.4: 1–10.
Sundaram, Anant K. and Andrew C. Inkpen. 2004. The Corporate Objective Revisited. *Organization Science* 15.3: 350–363.
Swan, Kenneth G. and K.G. Swan, Jr. 1996. Triage: The Past Revisted. *Military Medicine* 161.8: 448–452.
Walzer, Michael. 1983. *Spheres of Justice*. New York: Basic Books.
Winslow, Gerald R. 1982. *Triage and Justice*. Los Angeles, CA: University of California Press.
Zimmerman, Peggy G. and Robert D. Herr. 2006. *Triage Nursing Secrets*. St. Louis, MO: Mosby/Elsevier.

Medical Neutrality and Political Activism: Physicians' Roles in Conflict Situations[1]

Justin M. List

Physicians should speak out about their values. The word 'profession' means, from the Latin, 'speaking forth.' Public avowal of values has been a distinctive feature of the professions from before medieval times.[2]

1 Introduction

Physicians in conflict situations juggle myriad duties and experience many ethical dilemmas in caring for the sick and wounded. Issues of how to triage care, allocate resources, and knowledge of injustices committed against patients by warring parties are among these concerns. Medical neutrality—care given based on criteria of medical need and urgency—has been strongly instantiated as a core value in the moral fabric of medicine and international medical ethics. Yet, physician political neutrality or activism regarding war crimes and injustices against people wartime physicians serve has been met with controversy. Medical neutrality, political neutrality, and political activism can be construed as types of moral goods in the practice of medicine. I argue that medical neutrality in the provision of care and political neutrality in conflict situations are not equivalent goods. Physicians have duties to provide care on the basis of medical neutrality, but they also have an obligation to be politically active in certain conflict situations and report allegations and abuses revealed during either the clinical encounter or in the field.

First, I review a short history of medical neutrality in medical ethics as well as offer a defense of it. Next, I discuss political neutrality, and I argue that there exists the obligation for physician political activism (e.g., reporting human rights abuses). At the same time, I argue that physicians must practice medical neutrality using ethical and public health-based arguments that combine physicians' duties to preserve equal respect for all persons (clinical role) while maximizing the protection of individuals living in communities (public health role). I conclude by examining

[1] I would like to thank Fritz Allhoff and Michael Gross for their valuable comments on earlier drafts. I also thank a fellow medical student, Saranya Kurapati, former national student coordinator for Physicians for Human Rights, for her comments. This essay is dedicated to the courageous physicians and health care workers who have paid with their lives trying to defend and restore health to the victims of armed conflicts around the world.

[2] Matthew K. Wynia et al., "Medical professionalism in society," *NEJM* 341 (1999): 1612–1616, here 1613.

F. Allhoff (ed.), *Physicians at War: The Dual-Loyalties Challenge.*

pragmatic implications of such an approach and the risks and benefits it might pose. Here I explore different ethical dilemmas military physicians and physicians working with humanitarian groups experience in wartime. Throughout the essay, I focus the discussion on physician professional duties *qua* physicians, because I argue that all physicians are bound to the same core professional principles despite differences in their affiliations.

2 Standards and Principles of Medical Neutrality

The principle of medical neutrality is in many ways an uncontroversial and relatively straightforward domain of international medical ethics. Medical neutrality has two distinct meanings: one refers to *impartiality* in providing medical care and another refers to *protections* due to health care professionals by all warring parties in armed conflict situations. Medical neutrality construed as a professional obligation requires that physicians impartially treat the wounded and injured, whether friend or foe, on the basis of medical need and urgency. Need and urgency are impartial criteria because they are not related to the non-medical affiliations of the patient. Need-based care can refer to treating those needing urgent care quickly or treating as many needy patients as possible. Thus, as a form of triaging care, these criteria represent one way of treating all persons equally and distributing medical care justly, values at the core of this version of medical neutrality. Medical neutrality understood as a protective ethical duty in conflict situations requires that warring parties not harm any medical professionals or interfere with their health care work. While the protective concept of medical neutrality in human rights, humanitarian, and professional literature is stated clearly, an understanding of medical neutrality and physician impartiality in the provision of care in armed conflict varies. This essay focuses on the impartiality notion of medical neutrality.

The Geneva Conventions serve as the benchmark for both forms of medical neutrality. The overall purpose of the four Geneva Conventions of 1949 is to protect the victims of war, especially the sick and wounded.[3] The four conventions differentiate between combatant and non-combatant status and the level of protection and medical care these persons are entitled to in conflict situations. For example, according to the 1949 Conventions, civilian non-combatants are entitled to receive physical protection from warring parties but are not guaranteed the same level of medical care to which wounded or sick combatants of either warring party are entitled. Additional Protocols I and II (1977) ended the distinction between combatants and non-combatants by expanding the definition of "wounded and sick" to include

[3] Lewis C. Vollmar, "Military medicine in war: the Geneva Conventions today," in *Military Medical Ethics Volume*, vol. 2, eds. Thomas E. Beam and Linette R. Sparacino (*Textbooks of Military Medicine* series) (Washington, DC: Office of the Surgeon General, Department of the Army, and Borden Institute, 2003), 739–771.

civilians in addition to military combatants. Additional Protocol I, Part II, Article 10 states: "In all circumstances [the wounded, sick and shipwrecked, to which ever Party they belong] shall be treated humanely and shall receive, to the fullest extent practicable and with the least possible delay, the medical care and attention required by their condition. There shall be no distinction among them founded on any grounds other than medical ones."[4]

While not as authoritative as the Geneva Conventions, other international standards include the Declaration of Tokyo and the World Medical Association Regulations in Times of Armed Conflict. In the Declaration of Tokyo, "a doctor must have complete clinical independence in deciding upon the care of a person for whom he or she is medically responsible. The doctor's fundamental role is to alleviate distress ... and no motive, whether personal, collective or political, shall prevail against this higher purpose."[5] The World Medical Association (WMA) has put forth other statements including: "[u]nder all circumstances, every person, military or civilian, must receive promptly the care he needs without consideration of sex, race, nationality, religion, political affiliation or any other similar criterion"; and "[i]n emergencies, physicians and associated medical personnel are required to render immediate service to the best of their ability. No distinction shall be made between patients except those justified by medical urgency."[6] The WMA states that "[m]edical ethics in times of armed conflict is identical to medical ethics in times of peace, as established in the International Code of Medical Ethics of the World Medical Association. The primary obligation of physicians is to their patients; in performing their professional duty, their conscience should be their guide."[7] According to the WMA statement and the concept of medical neutrality as impartiality (i.e., age, gender, religion, political affiliation, and class are completely irrelevant criteria) a decision to treat a less urgent case would be unethical.

Many understand this interpretation and application of impartiality as a type of distributive justice in medicine and a moral duty in triage situations. In this sense, medical neutrality itself is type of justice, and one argument suggests that all physicians are bound to honor it always, especially in times of armed conflict. A counterargument would posit that it is in armed conflict situations that medical neutrality may be least just in the provision of care and that other non-health-related criteria become salient, because of duties to state, political affiliations, bonds of kinship, and sympathies for a particular cause of one of the warring parties. These criteria, although relevant in parts of our lives, are not values intrinsic

[4] Protocol Additional to the Geneva Conventions of 12 August 1949, and relating to the Protection of Victims of International Armed Conflicts (Protocol 1), http://www.ohchr.org/english/law/protocol1.htm, cited 3 September 2006.

[5] World Medical Association, "Declaration of Tokyo" (1975).

[6] World Medical Association, World Medical Association Condemns Human Rights Violations in Kosovo, 16 April 1999, http://www.wma.net/e/press/1999_11.htm, cited 24 January 2005.

[7] World Medical Association, The World Medical Association Regulations in Times of Armed Conflict, http://www.wma.net/e/policy/a20.htm, cited 24 January 2005.

to the ethical duties delineated from the profession of medicine. I align with the former position based on the argument that physicians have professional moral duties *qua* physicians to protect the sick and wounded based on need and urgency alone, i.e., medical neutrality as impartiality.

The concept of medical neutrality can be defended on the basis of equal respect for persons and for treating persons as ends in and of themselves. Equal respect for human persons is best achieved through a just distribution of health care in conflict situations based on a combination of medical need and urgency. Using this as the only relevant criteria in medical decision-making, is a reflection of philosopher John Rawls' "veil of ignorance" in the sense that impartiality in triaged medical care is in the best interest for all individuals unaware of whether or not they will ever need urgent care.[8] Using this understanding, impartiality represents an egalitarian approach to justice in the provision of medical care (though philosophers debate the relationship between egalitarianism and the veil of ignorance). According to Additional Protocol I, civilians and military personnel are not separated in the needs-based pool. Therefore, depending on how need and urgency are construed, the implications of this policy means civilians could be entitled to receive a greater amount of care from military physicians than military personnel themselves. Do military physicians have a *prima facie* duty to their own soldiers? Perhaps according to military policy but not according to the Geneva Conventions and other professional statements regarding the duties of physicians. We shall return to this tension for military physicians shortly.

A right to an equal chance at health care in triage situations exists by extension of an inviolable equal respect for persons. This "right" may appear to be a charitable or unjust position when justice in other non-health related dimensions is considered, such as crime deserving punishment. For example, there may be an intuitive disconnect for some physicians in conflict situations to treat a combatant urgently needing medical attention who has perpetrated gross crimes against humanity when a civilian or combatant from a friendly warring party presents for care with less urgency. An example of this type of ethical conflict for physicians would be a humanitarian group-affiliated physician in the Darfur region of Sudan treating an injured member of the Janjaweed militia when a civilian victim of the Janjaweed presents with less urgent medical need. Based on medical neutrality as impartiality, an ethical duty of physicians, the physician should choose to care for the former first in a triage situation, despite a possible sense of repugnance in doing so. Broad deontological commitments supporting a needs-based approach to triaged medical care acknowledge that: there exists a fundamental reverence of all human life and each person has the capacity to change her or his behaviors yet remains accountable for her or his actions vis-à-vis retributive justice. These three commitments point to the idea that justice for crimes committed is not to be handed out in the clinical setting by physicians.

[8] John Rawls, *A Theory of Justice*, rev. ed. (Cambridge, MA: Belknap, 1998).

The only conceivable exception to possibly justify the incorporation of non-health-related criteria in the framework I am putting forth and still fundamentally respect persons equally would be a triage situation where people with *equally* pressing needs and medical urgency present for care. Then certain criteria such as nationality, rank, and affiliation could be argued for incorporation into triage decision-making.[9] When all things are equal, randomness in medical care allocation decisions may seem most fair on one hand and a logical extension of medical neutrality, but such randomness completely neglects human experience and relationships in an unrealistic way, both of which may offer moral guidance in this unique situation. Certainly one could make the case that non-medical criteria should always factor into the equation of need based care at the outset, but this would clearly violate the requirements of justice and equal respect for persons to which physicians should be bound to within the profession itself.

Physicians are bound to a fundamental duty to treat people equally. Depending on physician affiliation, the goals of practicing medical neutrality and triaged care will be different. The US Army's Borden Institute, which publishes the textbooks of military medicine, states that "the goal of combat medicine is to return the greatest number of soldiers to combat and preservation of life, limb, and eyesight in those who must be evacuated."[10] The language of the US military's conception of military medicine is clearly and understandably one of utility for the military's purposes. Yet Robert Baker and Martin Strosberg cite examples that they interpret military and emergency triage as egalitarian in nature, because the common good is treated secondarily to urgent individual needs.[11] Likewise, the Geneva Conventions are in effect egalitarian in nature as well. But in light of human experience and emotion, it is a tremendous duty, perhaps burden, when physicians are called to care to those who they feel least deserve it.

The American Medical Association's *Code of Medical Ethics* states in Opinion 10.05 (1): "Physicians must keep their professional obligations to provide care to patients in accord with their prerogative to choose whether to enter into a patient-physician relationship." According to this opinion, it seems physicians can then choose whether or not to enter into a relationship with the patient in the first place. In peacetime, this may be appropriate in some circumstances when the patient can be referred to another physician. But this prerogative is limited in that the *Code* states that physicians need to respond to the best of their ability in an emergency situation, cannot discriminate based on many non-health-related criteria, and must render care when operating under a contractual agreement that requires them to treat.[12] Physician refusal to provide care or a particular *treatment* that they find

---

[9] For a more thorough discussion of the calculus of triage, see Gerald R. Winslow, *Triage and Justice* (University of California Press, 1982).

[10] Borden Institute, *Emergency War Surgery* (Washington, DC: Borden Institute, 2004), 3.1.

[11] Robert Baker and Martin Strosberg, "Triage and equality: an historical reassessment of utilitarian analyses of triage," *Kennedy Institute of Ethics Journal* 2 (1992): 103–123.

[12] Council on Ethical and Judicial Affairs, *Code of Medical Ethics* (Chicago, IL: American Medical Association: 2004), Opinion 10.05.

unethical for personal or religious reasons is permissible in some situations.[13] Refusing to participate in controversial treatment, however, is ethically different than refusing to treat a person urgently needing medical care based on non-health related criteria. The former is ethically acceptable; the latter is not. Military and humanitarian groups may try to place institutional parameters on the way physicians distribute care and create contractual obligations that may compete with medical ethical duties, but physicians *qua* physicians still have fundamental professional obligations to respect all persons equally.

We now return to the implications of impartial care as defined above as a duty of physicians. If physicians are truly impartial, they may be at times aiding enemy efforts or contributing to the prolongation of war, depending on whom they treat and how treatment impacts the patient's ability to participate in conflict. Physicians may become aware of information from patients in these settings that reveals crimes committed or future conflict. Former Human Rights Watch executive director Aryeh Neier, writes, "I had discovered fairly early in my tenure that, both for better and for worse, physicians had a significant role in dealing with abuses of human rights."[14] Are there settings, such as armed conflict, where physicians have concurrent personal moral duties to act outside traditional medical professional roles through political activism? What might be at stake if they do so? If a physician treats a patient perpetrating crimes of genocide, does that physician have a moral duty to "turn in" that individual, simply report that genocide is occurring, or be silent? What relevant principles guide a moral assessment of medical treatment and political activism in armed conflict situations?

There are at least three conceptions of physician duties in armed conflict that address medical and political neutrality in the provision of care. First, physicians could be impartial in the provision of medical care and publicly politically neutral concerning geopolitical affairs that impact the populations they serve. On this account, physicians could presumably provide a maximal amount of people with need-based medical care without being perceived as taking sides by warring factions. Second, physicians could be impartial in the provision of care and, bound by a moral duty to promote health and human rights, report war crimes and abuse directly or through partnered human rights, humanitarian, or military groups. Third, physicians could be medically biased in the provision of care based on allegiances and/or personal conscience and report or not report war crimes and abuses on the same basis. I concentrate on arguing for the second position against the first one, since the third one is widely considered unethical.

[13] Council on Ethical and Judicial Affairs, *Code of Medical Ethics* (Chicago, IL: American Medical Association: 2004), Opinion 10.05.

[14] Aryeh Neier, preface to *Trust is Not Enough: Bringing Human Rights to Medicine* by David J. Rothman and Sheila M. Rothman (New York: New York Review of Books, 2006), viii.

3 Medicine Neutrality and Political Activism

The practice of medicine in an armed conflict environment presents a constellation of duties and responsibilities for physicians that they might not encounter during peacetime. That is, physicians normally politically uninvolved in peacetime may need to actively promote values in medicine during wartime, such as human rights related to health. The international declarations of physician conduct in wartime do not address these other duties, such as reporting war crimes that impact health, because reporting abuses is a related but distinctly different issue than medical neutrality. A duty to be politically active arises out of the core principle of beneficence—doing good work to foster the happiness of individuals and society. This principle does not only apply to the physician-patient encounter when physicians treat sick and wounded patients; it applies to physicians' duties to prevent further harm and maximize health through appropriate political activism in a manner which will depend on the situation at hand. For example, H. Jack Geiger et al. report, "participation of health workers in the defense of human rights now includes investigation and documentation of health effects in threatened populations as well as individual victims."[15] From this perspective of physician involvement in wartime, political activism is directly coupled with knowledge that impacts public health and patient care. Arguments for political activism are based on utility just as much as arguments for political neutrality are based on utility in the sense that physicians will want to protect the health of as many people as possible (including themselves) and treat them equally. I am arguing that the utility of political activism outweighs that of political neutrality.[16]

The argument for public political neutrality suggests that physicians as politically neutral agents maximize the amount of care they can provide to the wounded and sick. Generally speaking, this is the model the International Committee of the Red Cross follows. Political activism compromises the safety of physicians and their patients, because activism itself can incite harm from warring parties against "activist" physicians. Generally speaking, groups such as Médecins Sans Frontières (Doctors Without Borders) and Doctors of the World are more politically active. Physician political neutrality may allow physicians to better protect already vulnerable patients and themselves, a position which could potentially be jeopardized through political activism. Physicians practicing impartiality in health care delivery and political neutrality attempt to maximize health for the most people. Additionally, by providing need-based care, it may be more likely that opposing factions will view medical personnel as neutral and treat them as such (medical neutrality in the

[15] H. Jack Geiger and Robert M. Cook-Deegan, "The role of physicians in conflicts and humanitarian crises: case studies from the field missions of physicians for human rights, 1988 to 1993," *JAMA* 270 (1993): 616.

[16] For more discussion over the spectrum of professional activism see Wynia et al., "Medical professionalism in society."

protective sense). Kevin Gibson argues that, in general, medical and political neutrality in the medical field promotes trust, and that this neutrality involves distance from the substance of the dispute and the values involved.[17] He also allows that true neutrality is elusive if not undesirable in particular situations, an important point to highlight for the purposes of my defense of political activism.

For example, in an armed conflict situation it may be prudentially wise for physicians to stay political neutral. Yet, this neutrality does not necessarily aid in the prevention of health crisis in the first place where as reporting human rights abuses impacting community health might do so. The prevention of ill health should be a primary goal alongside restoring health. The decision to remain politically neutral is an assessment of the relative risks and benefits all involved parties can expect, rather than as a result of a deontological principle.[18] While there are many pragmatic reasons for remaining neutral, it is a position that fails to encompass the wider duties of physicians. Respecting persons and treating them equally entails preventing further harm to the populations being served—not just mitigating present health crises—and reporting crimes against humanity as a form of political activism serves towards this end. Preventing health crises, war being an example, is a professional and moral duty for physicians, as I will explore more shortly under the framework of a physician role as public health purveyor. Physicians should be as concerned with preventing health care emergencies as with the medically neutral provision of care in armed conflict, especially when the information they know lends to the prevention of injury.

Even though physicians themselves are not actively committing war crimes or destroying infrastructure, they are arguably morally culpable in their silence regarding human rights abuses, especially as the gravity of abuses escalates in armed conflict. The risk brought to one's own life by political activism exists in tension with a duty to do so when such activism may positively impact the lives of many. Certainly the *prima facie* obligation to help others is contingent upon risk to oneself, but professionalism in medicine requires physicians to assume greater risks in certain situations. Of course, the goal for medical professionals is to promote the health of all, including their own. If they were to jeopardize their lives through activism, their absence would leave patients even more vulnerable. The important point to highlight in this deliberation is that physicians, due to the moral nature of their profession to serve patients, take on greater risks to their own safety and health depending on the environment in which they practice medicine. Physicians should be equally concerned with preventing health care emergencies (public health role) as with the medically neutral provision of care in armed conflict (clinical role), especially when the information they know lends to the prevention of injury.

---

[17] Kevin Gibson, "Mediation in the medical field: is neutral intervention possible?" *Hastings Center Report* 29.5 (1999): 6–14.

[18] Michael L. Gross, "Bioethics and armed conflict: mapping the moral dimensions of medicine and war," *Hastings Center Report* 34.6 (2004): 22–30.

To the degree that respecting persons equally entails protecting the health of patients, political activism by physicians in armed conflict situations reflects maximizing the contribution to population health and safety *if* such activism can be expected to reduce further human rights abuses, war-related malnutrition, and structural degradation of society. For example, the MSF-France operational section board (MSF has operational section boards in 5 countries, including France, that directly control field projects and 13 non-operational sections that provide support, including the US) made a controversial call for an armed intervention to stop the Rwandan genocide, an action it had never taken before in its history.[19] The potential implications of political neutrality versus activism were also highlighted by this situation. That is, "... some MSF doctors in Rwanda defected to the ICRC, feeling that the Red Cross's discretion would offer them more safety."[20] Depending on the type of political activism expressed, the choice to become politically active or not raises salient concerns—a sense of life or death in the case just mentioned. But as I have already argued, physicians may in fact prevent more sick and wounded patients from presenting with need and urgency in the first place through strategic political activism. The sense of international silence and inaction may have been too overwhelming for the MSF physicians in Rwanda as human rights abuses continued unabated. This, in part, may have been among the arguments for MSF-France to go public and urge for intervention at great expense.

If physicians are responsible for promoting public health and war can be viewed as a public health problem, then overlapping ethical duties physicians have to populations during war bolsters a case for physician political activism as a form of justice in medicine. Joanna Santa Barbara argues:

> So compelling are the needs of people either acutely affected by an ongoing war or struggling to rehabilitate a war-torn society once hostilities have ended, that knowledge, energy, and financial resources applied to prevention are sparse. It may be useful to consider the phases of war over time, and to apply the public health concepts of primary, secondary, and tertiary prevention to these phases.[21]

War, when looked at as a public health problem, is akin to an epidemic of disease. The abuses perpetrated as a weapon of it pose health threats to individuals and society. War often brings about the degradation of infrastructure, diminished food and water supply, and an increase in crimes such as rape, all of which can cause the spread of disease, foster malnutrition, and ultimately lead to increased morbidity/mortality rates. Physicians need to conceive of war as a disease and respond accordingly in a way similar to coordinating a public health response. If war is a disease, then addressing war is a professional obligation and which could entail that physicians take on the additional personal risks that political activism in armed

---

[19] Dan Bortolotti, *Hope in Hell: Inside the World of Doctors Without Borders* (Buffalo: Firefly, 2004), 264.

[20] Ibid., 246.

[21] Joanna Santa Barbara, "Physicians and the prevention of war," *Medicine & Global Survival* (1997), http://www.ippnw.org/MGS/AllContents.html, cited 3 September 2005.

conflict may create. Reporting human rights abuses should be attempted in a manner that protects the safety of patients and health care personnel as much as possible, but the imperative to report exists nonetheless. The benefits of appropriate political activism can outweigh those of political neutrality for physician political neutrality stands no chance of preventing the ills of war when physicians withhold knowledge that could reduce harm.

4 Pragmatic Issues for Physicians in Conflict Situations

While I attempted to argue for both medical neutrality and physician political activism as part of physicians' professional duties, human experience needs to be taken into account in the assessment of what physicians do as opposed to what they should do, since idealized thought experiments are rarely instantiated in the real world. After all, I am essentially arguing for a position that likely puts physicians' lives even more at risk than they have been in the first place in light of the difficult demands of justice and beneficence placed upon them. That said, in viewing war as a public health crisis, the notion of physicians acting additionally as quasi-human rights police, in the sense that they report a variety of war crimes in the effort to protect others, is a radical but logical extension of physician duties.

Up until this point, we have concentrated on the work of physicians affiliated with humanitarian groups and military forces. Political activism through human rights agencies is another example of physicians practicing the duties of their profession. Although their work is not as clinically based as it is for physicians in humanitarian outfits, physicians affiliated with human rights groups articulate a crucial moral voice of the medical profession that promotes the health and human rights of victims of armed conflict. These physicians are oftentimes positioned to be a more effective voice for the profession than physicians who are juggling both requirements of medical neutrality and political activism in conflict situations. Two examples of such organizations include Physicians for Human Rights (PHR) and International Physicians for the Prevention of Nuclear War (IPPNW). PHR investigates and addresses human rights violations rather than participate in organized medical care. IPPNW's mission statement states that "IPPNW is committed to ending war and advancing understanding of the causes of armed conflict from a public health perspective."[22] Physicians of PHR experience a different kind of risk in conflict situations and war torn societies as they practice political activism through forensic investigations of human rights abuses in these places. For example, a recent PHR investigation team evaluated the use of rape as a weapon of war in Darfur, which brought upon the team the risks of

[22] IPPNW homepage, http://www.ippnw.org, cited 31 December 2006.

being in that region at a volatile time.[23] Although, as workers through a human rights agency, they do not practice clinical medicine in armed conflict areas, they do complete psychological and medical evaluations of survivors of torture through a political asylum network in the US.

Jennifer Leaning describes what many physicians experience as tensions between adherence to human rights standards and the humanitarian requirement to maintain access to populations in need.[24] She provides the example of human rights investigators seeking evidence about events witnessed by humanitarian workers when such information may jeopardize personal or group security in the field. It may be no surprise then that many aid workers are not able work in the field for long periods of time because of a sense of personal moral or ethical ambiguity. The difficulty seems to be greatest for humanitarian group physicians[25] compared to human rights activists in the field.

Remi Russbach and Daniel Fink suggest that the primary purpose of humanitarian groups is to protect and assist victims of conflict and alleviate their suffering in ways that differ in nature from those of *ad hoc* self-help organizations or campaigns for human rights.[26] Their definition of the duties and activities of humanitarian medicine in conflict situations, while differentiating between human rights campaigns and humanitarian efforts, does not preclude political activism. To the contrary, one of the five characteristics of humanitarian action they outline is "defending the individual [suffering physical or mental distress] in all respects, not just by saving lives and alleviating suffering, but also by safeguarding the dignity of those in need."[27] Russbach and Fink discuss humanitarian work in the context of a public health approach, and "safeguarding those in need" could include appropriate political activism that promotes both the prevention of war-related health detriments and the health of those presently suffering the ravages of armed conflict.

Military physicians are frequently in similar situations as humanitarian group physicians, but they also encounter unique dilemmas. They must honor international conventions if their country has signed onto them, e.g., Geneva Conventions. In following the Geneva Conventions, military physicians part of a warring party

[23] Physicians for Human Rights, "Rape as a Weapon of War in Darfur," http://physiciansforhumanrights.org/sudan/rape/, cited 31 December 2006. Also see PHR publications *Darfur: Assault on Survival* and *The Use of Rape as a Weapon of War in the Conflict in Darfur, Sudan*.

[24] Jennifer Leaning, "Health and human rights in times of conflict," in *Health and Human Rights in Times of Peace and Conflict* (Boston, MA: François-Xavier Bagnoud Center for Health and Human Rights, 2000), 45–49.

[25] Kenneth Roth, "Health-related aspects of international humanitarian law," in *Health and Human Rights in Times of Peace and Conflict* (Boston, MA: Francois-Xavier Bagnoud Center for Health and Human Rights, 2001), 73–80.

[26] Remi Russbach and Daniel Fink, "Humanitarian Action in Current Armed Conflicts: Opportunities and Obstacles," *Medicine & Global Survival* 1.4 (1994), http://www.ippnw.org/MGS/V1N4Russbach.html, cited 3 September 2005.

[27] Ibid.

provide medical care to their own and enemy combatants in accordance with the principle of medical neutrality. While humanitarian physicians may have qualms of treating patients that may in turn harm others in conflict situations, military physicians do not experience this dilemma in the same way. The enemy combatant patient becomes a enemy prisoner-of-war (EPW) and to the extent that one less enemy combatant on the field alleviates further war and human rights abuses, physicians in the military may have less about which to be conflicted compared to non-military physicians who provide impartial care to patients who may be future perpetrators of war crimes.[28]

At the same, time the military physician almost certainly experiences pressure to prioritize care based on non-health related criteria, such as whether or not a combatant is from a friendly warring parties or an enemy warring party. Nonetheless, the military physician has professional duties qua physician to practice impartiality in medical care. The impartial practice of medical neutrality by military physicians is a challenging ideal in reality. Victor Sidel and Barry Levy suggest,

> As long as physicians in the service of the military continue to be a part of the military, they will be susceptible to divide people into "us" and "them" rather than into categories of patients needing attention based solely upon their medical needs. It is our opinion that military physician cannot, as members of the armed forces, live up to the expectations and responsibilities of the Geneva Conventions.[29]

They conclude that it is impossible and morally unacceptable for a physician to serve both as a physician and a soldier in the US military forces and unlikely in other military forces. In a response paper to Sidel and Levy, Edmund Howe cites a report[30] that US military physicians have stated that they would violate an obligation to treat EPWs equally.[31] That military physicians "cannot" live up to international expectations and the aforementioned ethical principles seems to disrespect the autonomous will and capability of the military physicians to follow what are difficulty and lofty requirements of practicing in the medical profession. Rather than remove them from the military as Sidel and Levy would have, Howe argues that the attitude

---

[28] However, other morally problematic situations unique to military medicine, such as physician participation in torture, can arise in an EPW situation not related to medical neutrality. See M. Gregg Bloche and Jonathan Marks, "When doctors go to war," *New England Journal of Medicine* 352.1 (2005): 3–6; and Fritz Allhoff, "Physician involvement in hostile interrogations," *Cambridge Quarterly of Healthcare Ethics* 15.4 (2006): 392–402 (reprinted in this volume).

[29] Victor W. Sidel and Barry S. Levy, "Physician-soldier: a moral dilemma," in *Military Medical Ethics Volume*, vol. 2, eds. Thomas E. Beam and Linette R. Sparacino (*Textbooks of Military Medicine* series) (Washington, DC: Office of the Surgeon General, Department of the Army, and Borden Institute, 2003), 303.

[30] Brian S. Carter, "Ethical concerns for physicians deployed to Operation Desert Storm," *Military Medicine* 159 (1994): 55–59.

[31] Edmund G. Howe, "Point/counterpoint—a response to Drs. Sidel and Levy," in *Military Medical Ethics Volume*, vol. 2, eds. Thomas E. Beam and Linette R. Sparacino (*Textbooks of Military Medicine* series) (Washington, DC: Office of the Surgeon General, Department of the Army, and Borden Institute, 2003), 293–329.

present among physicians who would prioritize care using non-health related criteria requires structural change in US military policy and punishment for those who undermine need-based care.

If only urgency and need are considered in the triage of care equation, then in the hypothetical event that EPW injuries overwhelm the ability of military physicians to provide for their own soldiers, it is certainly not of utility to their military force to treat EPWs. But need-based treatment in this circumstance, while difficult, is a reflection of the type of justice demanded of physicians. This example highlights the discord between intuitive feelings and allegiances on the battlefield and transcendent moral reasoning, a tension I am not inclined to mitigate by arguing that other non-health-related criteria should in fact become relevant with the exception of the "all else being equal" case I mentioned earlier. What is in conflict for the military physician in the provision of care is a sense of competing commitments—commitments to overarching, fundamental moral norms (e.g., treat persons equally) in tension with varying commitments and obligations that originate from human experience and the unique bonding relationships found in environments such as the military.[32] An intuition that need and urgency as sole criteria are unfair in the triage situation comes from of a sense of commitment to fellow soldiers and citizens. Arguably, there exists a natural inclination to help persons based on these non-medical factors, but the professional requirements of medicine in terms of justice and beneficence as outlined in this chapter hold highest the larger moral imperative of equal respect for persons.

Physicians affiliated with humanitarian groups often have less physical protection around them that can make political activism and impartial care a more daunting experience compared to military physicians. Some groups may retaliate against physicians in humanitarian groups for treating patients impartially, e.g., when a physician treats a patient of one faction in conflict with members of another proximate faction. Humanitarian organizations tend to be less "activist" (i.e., publicly denouncing human rights abuses) than human rights organizations and the mandates of human rights groups often place humanitarian group physicians in moral quandaries as to their responsibilities in armed conflict situations.[33] Different groups have different mandates as well. The ICRC participates in the process of forming international humanitarian law[34] and making other agencies, governments, etc., aware of humanitarian crises[35] but it is purposefully neutral in other ways as

[32] For a philosophical investigation into commitment and obligation, see Margaret A. Farley, *Personal Commitments: Beginning, Keeping, Changing* (New York: HarperCollins, 1986). Also see, Gilbert C. Meilaender, *Friendship: A Study in Theological Ethics* (South Bend: University of Notre Dame Press, 1981).

[33] Bortolotti, *Hope in Hell: Inside the World of Doctors Without Borders.*

[34] International Committee of the Red Cross (ICRC), "How does humanitarian law adapt to new developments and what is the ICRC's role in the process?" http://www.icrc.org/web/eng/siteeng0.nsf/iwpList104/1F6F862CFDD6FE48C1256CF50052D2D3, cited 3 September 2005.

[35] ICRC, "Promoting International Humanitarian Law," http://www.icrc.org/Web/eng/siteeng0.nsf/htmlall/section_training_education_awareness, cited 3 September 2005.

an "impartial, neutral and independent organization whose exclusively humanitarian mission is to protect the lives and dignity of victims of war and internal violence and to provide them with assistance."[36] Due to their neutrality, they likely conceive of themselves as maximizing the amount of care that they can provide in conflict situations in ways that other groups are often unable and perhaps more likely to not be kicked out of a country than more politically-active groups.

Compared to the ICRC, MSF occasionally opts against political neutrality in hostile or conflict situations. The example of MSF in Rwanda, which I have already discussed, goes against a principal pillar of humanitarianism, but more accurately reflects the medical neutrality/political activism model for which I argue. For many MSF physicians (and indeed many other physicians in other groups), speaking out and acting out are inextricably linked so that protesting local human rights violations locally and abroad complements the provision of medically neutral care.[37] The physical costs of speaking out are often tragic for physicians in any organization that speaks out. Retaliation from different factions has resulted in the deaths of many MSF aid workers,[38] for example, including in the Darfur conflict most recently.[39] Rather than remain neutral and silent about human rights abuses, MSF has occasionally withdrawn from volatile situations (e.g., North Korea in 1998 and Ethiopia in 1985) a controversial move from a humanitarian perspective to be sure.[40] My point here is to provide an example of the complexity and risks involved when physicians execute their multiple duties in the most extreme scenarios.

5 Conclusion

In this essay, I have argued that physicians are bound to practice medical neutrality in the provision of care on the basis of core ethical values of equal respect for all persons, beneficence, and justice. I then attempted to delineate the duty for physician political activism as a commitment to patients and as a moral value intrinsic to the profession of medicine. There exists a rich debate about whether physicians and organizations should be political neutral or activist and the impacts of such a choice, but I have argued that physicians have a duty to raise their voices against

---

[36] ICRC, "The ICRC's Mission Statement," http://www.icrc.org/web/eng/siteeng0.nsf/iwpList109/9E9D6BC7913B713BC1256F8200396625, cited 3 September 2005.

[37] Bortolotti, *Hope in Hell: Inside the World of Doctors Without Borders*, 242.

[38] See Bortolotti, *Hope in Hell: Inside the World of Doctors Without Borders*; and François Jean, ed., *Life, Death and Aid: The Médecins Sans Frontiéres Report on World Crisis Intervention* (New York: Routledge, 1993).

[39] Integrated Regional Information Networks, "Chad: MSF Worker Killed, Clinic Looted," http://www.alertnet.org/thenews/newsdesk/IRIN/6ccd91c15556f99c4632c54d9a54bed4.htm, cited 31 December 2006.

[40] Bortolotti, *Hope in Hell: Inside the World of Doctors Without Borders*, 243.

the disease of war in the most strategic and appropriate manner given their role as healers and public health professionals. Although different contracts impinge on the practice of medicine either through military, humanitarian, or human rights agency affiliation, I have attempted to make clear the universal ethical duties of physicians in armed conflict situations regarding medical neutrality and political activism.

MSF is an example of one group among others that, while juggling medical neutrality and political action, seems to model the moral argument of dual responsibilities to medical neutrality and political activism that I want to make for physicians practicing in armed conflict situations. In trying to connect ethical theory with public policy, I have sought to argue that the moral duty to provide medically neutral care may require calling upon other professional duties, such as political activism, in armed conflict. Speaking and acting out are inextricably linked and morally imperative when the overarching norms of respecting persons as equals in the medical setting and protecting populations from further harms can complement one another despite the risks in doing so.

Some argue that "the proper purpose of government may be served by dealing with rogues, liar, and cruel tyrants. That of medical organizations cannot be advanced on the same basis."[41] Prudentially, I agree that having different agents working simultaneously for a just distribution of goods—health, human rights, punishment, etc.—is ideal. Physicians, like many other health care professionals, often have a multitude of ethical dilemmas to mediate in medical settings even without armed conflict—they alone cannot stop genocide by their silence or in speaking out. They pay a price for doing so when other agents that could end war do not. Yet, my final conclusion is that physicians have *prima facie* professional obligations to provide impartial care and speak out against or report human rights abuses in order to promote public health and the reverence of life for each person in communities suffering the ravishes of armed conflict.

References

Allhoff, Fritz. 2006. Physician involvement in hostile interrogations. *Cambridge Quarterly of Healthcare Ethics* 15.4: 392–402 (reprinted in this volume).

Baker, Robert and Martin Strosberg. 1992. Triage and equality: an historical reassessment of utilitarian analyses of triage. *Kennedy Institute of Ethics Journal* 2: 103–123.

Beam, Thomas E. and Linette R. Sparacino, eds. 2003. *Military Medical Ethics* vols. 1–2 (*Textbooks of Military Medicine* series). Washington, DC: Office of the Surgeon General, Department of the Army, and Borden Institute.

Bloche, M. Gregg and Jonathan Marks. 2005. When doctors go to war. *New England Journal of Medicine* 352.1: 3–6.

[41] Harold Merskey, "Political neutrality and international cooperation in medicine," *Journal of Medical Ethics* 4.2 (1978): 74–77, here 76.

Borden Institute. 2004. *Emergency War Surgery*. Washington, DC: Borden Institute.
Bortolotti, Dan. 2004. *Hope in Hell: Inside the World of Doctors Without Borders*. Buffalo: Firefly.
Carter, Brian S. 1994. Ethical concerns for physicians deployed to Operation Desert Storm. *Military Medicine* 159: 55–59.
Council on Ethical and Judicial Affairs. 2004. *Code of Medical Ethics*. Chicago, IL: American Medical Association.
Farley, Margaret A. 1986. *Personal Commitments: Beginning, Keeping, Changing*. New York: HarperCollins.
Geiger, H. Jack and Robert M. Cook-Deegan. 1993. The role of physicians in conflicts and humanitarian crises: case studies from the field missions of physicians for human rights, 1988 to 1993. *JAMA* 270: 616–620.
Gibson, Kevin. 1999. Mediation in the medical field. *Hastings Center Report* 29.5: 6–14.
Gross, Michael L. 2004. Bioethics and armed conflict: mapping the moral dimensions of medicine and war. *Hastings Center Report* 34.6: 22–30.
International Committee of the Red Cross. How does Humanitarian Law Adapt to New Developments and What is the ICRC's Role in the Process? http://www.icrc.org/web/eng/siteeng0.nsf/iwpList104/1F6F862CFDD6FE48C1256CF50052D2D3. Cited 3 September 2005.
International Committee of the Red Cross. The ICRC's Mission Statement. http://www.icrc.org/web/eng/siteeng0.nsf/iwpList109/9E9D6BC7913B713BC1256F8200396625. Cited 3 September 2005.
International Committee of the Red Cross. Promoting International Humanitarian Law. http://www.icrc.org/Web/eng/siteeng0.nsf/htmlall/section_training_education_awareness. Cited 3 September 2005.
International Physicians for the Prevention of Nuclear War. IPPNW Homepage. http://www.ippnw.org. Cited 31 December 2006.
Integrated Regional Information Networks. Chad: MSF Worker Killed, Clinic Looted. http://www.alertnet.org/thenews/newsdesk/IRIN/6ccd91c15556f99c4632c54d9a54bed4.htm. Cited 31 December 2006.
Jean, François ed. 1993. *Life, Death and Aid: The Médecins Sans Frontiéres Report on World Crisis Intervention*. New York: Routledge.
Leaning, Jennifer. 2000. Health and human rights in times of conflict. In *Health and Human Rights in Times of Peace and Conflict*, 45–49. Boston, MA: Francois-Xavier Bagnoud Center for Health and Human Rights.
Meilaender, Gilbert C. 1981. *Friendship: A Study in Theological Ethics*. South Bend: University of Notre Dame Press.
Merskey, Harold. 1978. Political neutrality and international cooperation in medicine. *Journal of Medical Ethics* 4.2 (1978): 74–77.
Neier, Aryeh. 2006. Preface to *Trust is Not Enough: Bringing Human Rights to Medicine* by David J. Rothman and Sheila M. Rothman, vii–xiv. New York: New York Review of Books.
Office of the United Nations High Commissioner of Human Rights. Protocol Additional to the Geneva Conventions of 12 August 1949, and relating to the Protection of Victims of International Armed Conflicts (Protocol 1). http://www.ohchr.org/english/law/protocol1.htm. Cited 3 September 2005.
Physicians for Human Rights. Rape as a Weapon of War in Darfur. http://physiciansforhumanrights.org/sudan/rape/. Cited 31 December 2006.
Rawls, John. 1998. *A Theory of Justice*, rev. ed. Cambridge, MA: Belknap.
Roth, Kenneth. 2001. Health-related aspects of international humanitarian law. In *Health and Human Rights in Times of Peace and Conflict*, 73–80. Boston, MA: Francois-Xavier Bagnoud Center for Health and Human Rights.
Russbach, Remi and Daniel Fink. 1994. Humanitarian action in current armed conflicts: opportunities and obstacles. *Medicine & Global Survival* 1.4: http://www.ippnw.org/MGS/V1N4Russbach.html. Cited 3 September 2005.
Santa Barbara, Joanna. 1997. Physicians and the prevention of war. *Medicine & Global Survival*. http://www.ippnw.org/MGS/AllContents.html. Cited 3 September 2005.

Winslow, Gerald R. 1982. *Triage and Justice*. Berkeley, CA: University of California Press.
World Medical Association. 1975. Declaration of Tokyo.
World Medical Association. The World Medical Association Regulations in Times of Armed Conflict. http://www.wma.net/e/policy/a20.htm. Cited 24 January 2005.
World Medical Association. World Medical Association Condemns Human Rights Violations in Kosovo. http://www.wma.net/e/press/1999_11.htm. Cited 24 January 2005.
Wynia, Matthew K. et al. 1999. Medical Professionalism in Society. *New England Journal of Medicine* 341: 1612–1616.

Appendix 1
Regulations in Time of Armed Conflict[1]

World Medical Association

1. Medical ethics in times of armed conflict is identical to medical ethics in times of peace, as stated in the *International Code of Medical Ethics* of the WMA. If, in performing their professional duty, physicians have conflicting loyalties, their primary obligation is to their patients; in all their professional activities, physicians should adhere to international conventions on human rights, international humanitarian law and WMA declarations on medical ethics.
2. The primary task of the medical profession is to preserve health and save life. Hence it is deemed unethical for physicians to:

   (a) Give advice or perform prophylactic, diagnostic or therapeutic procedures that are not justifiable for the patient's health care.
   (b) Weaken the physical or mental strength of a human being without therapeutic justification.
   (c) Employ scientific knowledge to imperil health or destroy life.
   (d) Employ personal health information to facilitate interrogation.
   (e) Condone, facilitate or participate in the practice of torture or any form of cruel, inhuman or degrading treatment.

3. During times of armed conflict, standard ethical norms apply, not only in regard to treatment but also to all other interventions, such as research. Research involving experimentation on human subjects is strictly forbidden on all persons deprived of their liberty, especially civilian and military prisoners and the population of occupied countries.
4. The medical duty to treat people with humanity and respect applies to all patients. The physician must always give the required care impartially and without discrimination on the basis of age, disease or disability, creed, ethnic origin, gender, nationality, political affiliation, race, sexual orientation, or social standing or any other similar criterion.

[1] Adopted by the 10th World Medical Assembly, Havana, Cuba, October 1956, and Edited by the 11th World Medical Assembly, Istanbul, Turkey, October 1957, and Amended by the 35th World Medical Assembly, Venice, Italy, October 1983 and The WMA General Assembly, Tokyo 2004, and editorially revised at the 173rd Council Session, Divonne-les-Bains, France, May 2006.

5. Governments, armed forces and others in positions of power should comply with the Geneva Conventions to ensure that physicians and other health care professionals can provide care to everyone in need in situations of armed conflict. This obligation includes a requirement to protect health care personnel.
6. As in peacetime, medical confidentiality must be preserved by the physician. Also as in peacetime, however, there may be circumstances in which a patient poses a significant risk to other people and physicians will need to weigh their obligation to the patient against their obligation to other individuals threatened.
7. Privileges and facilities afforded to physicians and other health care professionals in times of armed conflict must never be used for other than health care purposes.
8. Physicians have a clear duty to care for the sick and injured. Provision of such care should not be impeded or regarded as any kind of offence. Physicians must never be prosecuted or punished for complying with any of their ethical obligations.
9. Physicians have a duty to press governments and other authorities for the provision of the infrastructure that is a prerequisite to health, including potable water, adequate food and shelter.
10. Where conflict appears to be imminent and inevitable, physicians should, as far as they are able, ensure that authorities are planning for the repair of the public health infrastructure in the immediate post-conflict period.
11. In emergencies, physicians are required to render immediate attention to the best of their ability. Whether civilian or combatant, the sick and wounded must receive promptly the care they need. No distinction shall be made between patients except those based upon clinical need.
12. Physicians must be granted access to patients, medical facilities and equipment and the protection needed to carry out their professional activities freely. Necessary assistance, including unimpeded passage and complete professional independence, must be granted.
13. In fulfilling their duties, physicians and other health care professionals shall usually be identified by internationally recognized symbols such as the Red Cross and Red Crescent.
14. Hospitals and health care facilities situated in war regions must be respected by combatants and media personnel. Health care given to the sick and wounded, civilians or combatants, cannot be used for morbid publicity or propaganda. The privacy of the sick, wounded and dead must always be respected.

Appendix 2
Statement on Torture, Cruel, Inhuman or Degrading Treatment[1]

World Medical Association

The World Medical Association,

1. Considering the Preamble to the United Nations Charter of 26 June 1945 solemnly proclaiming the faith of the people of the United Nations in the fundamental human rights, in the dignity and value of the human person
2. Considering the Preamble to the Universal Declaration of Human Rights of 10 December 1948 which states that disregard and contempt for human rights have resulted in barbarous acts which have outraged the conscience of mankind
3. Considering Article 5 of that Declaration which proclaims that no one shall be subjected to torture or cruel, inhuman or degrading treatment
4. Considering the American Convention on Human Rights adopted by the Organization of American States on 22 November 1969 and which entered into force on 18 July 1978 and the Inter-American Convention to Prevent and Punish Torture, which entered into force on 28 February 1987
5. Considering the Declaration of Tokyo, adopted by the WMA in 1975, which reaffirms the prohibition of any form of medical involvement or presence of a physician during torture or inhuman or degrading treatment
6. Considering the Declaration of Hawaii (World Psychiatric Association), adopted in 1977
7. Considering the Declaration of Kuwait (International Conference of Islamic Medical Associations), adopted in 1981
8. Considering the Principles of Medical Ethics Relevant to the Role of Health Personnel, Particularly Physicians, in the Protection of Prisoners and Detainees Against Torture and Other Cruel, Inhuman or Degrading Treatment or Punishment, adopted by the United Nations General Assembly on 18 December 1982, and particularly Principle 2, which states: "*It is a gross contravention of medical ethics ... for health personnel, particularly physicians, to engage, actively or passively, in acts which constitute participation in, complicity in, incitement to or attempts to commit torture or other cruel, inhuman or degrading treatment...*"

[1] Full title: "The World Medical Association Resolution on the Responsibility of Physicians in the Denunciation of Acts of Torture or Cruel or Inhuman or Degrading Treatment of Which They Are Aware."

9. Considering the Convention Against Torture and Other Cruel, Inhuman or Degrading Treatment or Punishment, adopted by the United Nations General Assembly on December 1984
10. Considering the European Convention for the Prevention of Torture and Inhuman or Degrading Treatment or Punishment, which was adopted by the Council of Europe on 26 June 1987 and entered into force on 1 February 1989
11. Considering the Resolution on Human Rights adopted by the WMA in Rancho Mirage, in October 1990 during the 42nd General Assembly and amended by the 45th, 46th and 47th General Assemblies
12. Considering the Declaration of Hamburg, adopted by the WMA in November 1997 during the 49th General Assembly and calling on physicians to protest individually against ill-treatment and on national and international medical organizations to support physicians in such actions
13. Considering the Istanbul Protocol (Manual on the Effective Investigation and Documentation of Torture and Other Cruel, Inhuman or Degrading Treatment or Punishment), adopted by the United Nations General Assembly on 4 December 2000

Recognizing

14. That careful and consistent denunciation by physicians of cases of torture and of those responsible contributes to the protection of the physical and mental integrity of victims and in a general way to the struggle against a major affront to human dignity
15. That physicians, by ascertaining the sequelae and treating the victims of torture, either early or late after the event, are privileged witnesses of this violation of human rights
16. That the victims, because of the psychological sequelae from which they suffer or the pressures brought on them, are often unable to formulate by themselves complaints against those responsible for the ill-treatment they have undergone
17. That the non-denunciation of acts of torture may be considered as a form of tolerance thereof and of non-assistance to the victims
18. That nevertheless there is no consistent and explicit reference in the professional codes of medical ethics and legislative texts of the obligation upon physicians to report or denounce acts of torture or inhuman or degrading treatment of which they are aware

Recommends that National Medical Associations

19. Support the adoption in their country of ethical rules and legislative provisions:
    19.1 Aimed at affirming the ethical obligation on physicians to report or denounce acts of torture or cruel, inhuman or degrading treatment of

which they are aware; depending on the circumstances, the report or denunciation would be addressed to medical, legal, national or international authorities, to non-governmental organizations or to the International Criminal Court. Doctors should use their discretion in this matter, bearing in mind paragraph 68 of the Istanbul Protocol.[2]

19.2 Establishing, to that effect, an ethical and legislative exception to professional confidentiality that allows the physician to report abuses, where possible with the subject's consent, but in certain circumstances where the victim is unable to express him/herself freely, without explicit consent.

19.3 Cautioning physicians to avoid putting individuals in danger by reporting on a named basis a victim who is deprived of freedom, subjected to constraint or threat or in a compromised psychological situation.

20. Disseminate to physicians the Istanbul Protocol
21. Promote their training on the identification of different modes of torture and their sequelae
22. Place at their disposal all useful information on reporting procedures, particularly to the national authorities, nongovernmental organisations and the International Criminal Court

[2] Istanbul Protocol, paragraph 68: "In some cases, two ethical obligations are in conflict. International codes and ethical principles require the reporting of information concerning torture or maltreatment to a responsible body. In some jurisdictions, this is also a legal requirement. In some cases, however, patients may refuse to give consent to being examined for such purposes or to having the information gained from examination disclosed to others. They may be fearful of the risks of reprisals for themselves or their families. In such situations, health professionals have dual responsibilities: to the patient and to society at large, which has an interest in ensuring that justice is done and perpetrators of abuse are brought to justice. The fundamental principle of avoiding harm must feature prominently in consideration of such dilemmas. Health professionals should seek solutions that promote justice without breaking the individual's right to confidentiality. Advice should be sought from reliable agencies; in some cases this may be the national medical association or non-governmental agencies. Alternatively, with supportive encouragement, some reluctant patients may agree to disclosure within agreed parameters."

Appendix 3
Physician Participation in Interrogation (Res. 1, I-05)[1,2,3,4]

Council on Ethical and Judicial Affairs, American Medical Association

1 Introduction

At the 2005 Interim Meeting, the House of Delegates adopted amended Resolution 1, I-05, "Physician Participation in the Interrogation of Prisoners and Detainees," which directed the Council on Ethical and Judicial Affairs to delineate the boundaries

---

[1] This report has been reformatted to accord with this volume. Use with permission. Copyright American Medical Association, 2006.

[2] The Council gratefully acknowledges the following individuals and organizations for reviewing an earlier draft of this Report. (This acknowledgement does not represent endorsement of the final report nor its recommendations): American Academy of Child and Adolescent Psychiatry (David Fassler, M.D.); American Academy of Pediatrics (Eileen M. Ouellette, M.D., JD, FAAP, Tomas J. Silber, M.D., MASS, Chairperson, Executive Committee on Bioethics); American Academy of Psychiatry & the Law (Howard Zonana, M.D., Robert Phillips, M.D., Ph.D.); American Psychiatric Association (Steven Sharfstein, M.D., Paul Appelbaum, M.D.); Office of the Army Surgeon General (Col Elspeth Ritchey, M.D.); Physicians for Human Rights (Leonard S. Rubenstein, JD); Uniformed Services University (Edmund Howe, Ph.D.; Thomas A. Grieger, M.D.); United States Air Force Medical Service (Brig Gen David Young, M.D.; Col Arnyce Pock, M.D.; Lt Col Paul Friedrichs, M.D.; Maj Val Finnell, M.D., Joe Procaccino, JD); Vice Admiral Donald C. Arthur, M.D., US Navy Surgeon General; Lieutenant General Kevin C. Kiley, M.D., FACOG, US Army Surgeon General; Lieutenant General George "Peach" Taylor, M.D., US Air Force Surgeon General; Scott A. Allen, M.D., Clinical Assistant Professor of Medicine, Brown Medical School; George J. Annas, JD, MPH, Edward R. Utley Professor, Boston University School of Public Health; M. Gregg Bloche, M.D., JD, Professor of Law, Georgetown University; Burton J. Lee, M.D.; Steven Miles, M.D.; William Winkewerder, Jr., M.D., Assistant Secretary of Defense, Health Affairs; Stephen N. Xenakis, M.D., Brigadier General (Retired) US Army.

[3] Reports of the Council on Ethical and Judicial Affairs are assigned to the reference committee on Constitution and Bylaws. They may be adopted, not adopted, or referred. A report may not be amended, except to clarify the meaning of the report and only with the concurrence of the Council.

[4] Note: The Council on Ethical and Judicial Affairs presents CEJA Report 10, A-06, "Physician Participation in Interrogation," as a Late Report, acknowledging that this limits the time during which Delegates can review the full report. However, the Council sought input from a large number of interested organizations and individuals by sharing an early draft of the Report. Because this topic has been the focus of considerable ongoing public debate, the Council believes it is in the best interest of the AMA and particularly of colleagues currently serving in the military to present the Report to the House at this time, as a Late Report.

of ethical practice with respect to physicians' participation in the interrogation of prisoners and detainees.

The resolution arose from concerns in recent years regarding the role of physicians in interrogation practices, including involvement as Behavioral Science Consultants to advise interrogators.[5] This report focuses on the role of physicians in the interrogation process in the specific contexts of domestic law enforcement and military or national security intelligence gathering.

2 Elements of the Debate

2.1 Interrogation: Definition and Description

For the purpose of this Report, we define a "detainee" as a criminal suspect, prisoner of war, or any other individual who is detained and is potentially subject to interrogation. An individual who undergoes interrogation is referred to as an "interrogatee." Most broadly, interrogation has been defined as formal and systematic questioning.[6] However, in this Report, we define interrogation more narrowly, as questioning related to law enforcement or to military and national security intelligence gathering designed to prevent the occurrence or recurrence of harm or danger to individuals, the public, or national security. The interrogation aims to elicit information from a detainee that is useful to the purposes of the interrogators. Interrogations are also distinct from questioning used to assess the medical condition of an individual or to determine mental status. Accordingly, forensic medicine practices that include assessing competence to stand trial or criminal responsibility, and pre-sentencing evaluations are excluded from this report. Appropriate interrogations should be carefully distinguished from those coupled with coercive acts that are intended to intimidate and that may cause harm through physical injury or mental suffering. In general, this Report does not address participation of physicians in developing strategies to deal with individuals who are not in detention, such as negotiations

---

The Council considers that the time required to process the wide range of comments that were solicited, which resulted in the delay in submitting this Report to the House, was time well spent. After thorough reflection and deliberation on the broad spectrum of sharply conflicting opinions of reviewers, the Report now strongly and clearly describes the ethics of physicians as they relate to interrogations. The Council members are deeply grateful to all those who participated in this process.

[5] Michael Wilks, "A Stain on Medical Ethics," *Lancet* 366 (2005): 429–431; Peter Slevin and Joe Stephens, "Detainees' medical files shared," *Washington Post* (20 June 2004): A1; Robert Jay Lifton, "Doctors and Torture," *New England Journal of Medicine* 351 (2004): 415–416; M. Gregg Bloche and Jonathan H. Marks, "When Doctors Go to War," *New England Journal of Medicine* 352 (2005): 3–6; Neil A. Lewis, "Interrogators Cite Doctors' Aid at Guantanamo," *New York Times* (24 June 2004): A1.

[6] Bryan A. Garner, ed., *Black's Law Dictionary*, 8th ed. (St. Paul, MN: Thomson West, 2004).

with hostage takers and profiling of criminal suspects. From the physician's perspective, an interrogation is distinct from questioning conducted for purposes of making a diagnosis, assessing physical capacity, or determining mental capacity related to legal status.

The military and related government agencies refer to interrogations, debriefings and tactical questioning as means to gain intelligence from captured or detained personnel.[7] The Army Field Manual further defines interrogation as "the process of questioning a source to obtain the maximum amount of usable information. The goal is to obtain reliable information in a lawful manner, in a minimum amount of time, and to satisfy intelligence requirements of any echelon of command."[8]

2.2 Interrogation Techniques

The Army Field Manual provides detailed guidance on interrogations and describes methods to establish rapport with or exert control over a detainee. Specific psychological strategies that rely primarily on incentives, emotions, fear, pride and ego are generally considered acceptable, although it is recognized that approaches that rely on fear presents "the greatest potential to violate the law of war."[9]

Significant concerns regarding interrogations arise from the risk of abuse. Domestic and international law prohibit the use of coercive interrogations that might involve the application of mild to severe physical or mental force.[10]

In criminal law, coercion or undue intimidation violates the rights of individuals being interrogated. Moreover, such abuses can undermine the veracity of information derived from an interrogation and can jeopardize subsequent legal proceedings intended to establish true facts about a crime.[11] Therefore, safeguards of due process have been placed on interrogatory powers in order to protect against coercive techniques.[12] Actions by law enforcement agents may be legally reviewed, and information gathered by coercive means may be rejected from court proceedings.

---

[7] United States Department of Defense, *Intelligence Interrogations, Detainee Debriefings and Tactical Questioning*, DOD Directive 3115.09 (3 November 2005).

[8] United States Department of Defense, *Army Field Manual 34–52* (Washington, DC: 1992), P. 1–6.

[9] Ibid.

[10] Robert Galvin, "The Complex World of Military Medicine: A Conversation with William Winkenwerder," *Health Affairs* 2005: W5-353–360; Alan Elsner, "Experts See Medical Ethics Violations at Guantanamo," *Reuters* (24 February 2006).

[11] American courts recognize that confessions elicited by physical intimidation are involuntary and may not be admitted against the confessor at trial. Additionally, under certain circumstances threats, deception, and trickery may render a confession involuntary and inadmissible. 29 Am. Jur. 2d Evidence §731.

[12] The Fifth and Fourteenth Amendments to the Constitution protect individuals against involuntary self-incriminating statements. *Dickerson v. United States*, 530 US 428 (2000); *Miranda v. Arizona*, 384 US 436 (1966).

may be difficult, but when the obligations seem approximately equal, the weight should shift toward individuals.

The principles of respect for autonomy, beneficence, non-maleficence and protection of confidentiality are at risk of being violated during interrogations. Therefore, it is essential that the ethical role of physicians in interrogations be clearly defined.

3.1.1 Physicians' Dual Loyalties

In the clinical setting, physicians' obligations are first to their patients. However, in many other settings, physicians confront dual loyalties, which place the medical interests of the individuals with whom they interact in tension or conflict with those of third parties to whom the physicians are accountable. For example, when a physician assesses an employee's health for an employer, the physician has certain ethical responsibilities to the examinee as well as contractual responsibilities to the employer. However, the AMA's *Code of Medical Ethics* makes clear that the physician must not fulfill responsibilities to the employer in a manner that is detrimental to the employee's medical condition,[21] nor disclose medical information without the consent of the employee.[22]

Physicians who provide medical care in detention or correctional facilities face divided loyalties: to the medical interests of the detainees and respect for their (legally limited) autonomy, and to the correctional facility's control over detainees and need for information. Concerns are heightened when interrogations are conducted.[23] Some, including military and government officials,[24] have suggested that physicians who do not provide medical care to interrogatees are not bound by physicians' ethical obligations to patients because they act outside of the patient-physician relationship. However, various Opinions in the AMA's *Code of Medical Ethics* suggest that physician interactions under the authority of third parties are governed by the same ethical principles as interactions involving patients.[25] Physicians must apply medical knowledge and skills within the profession's ethical standards, which are distinct from and often more stringent than those of the law.

---

[21] Council on Ethical and Judicial Affairs of the American Medical Association, "Opinion E-10.03, Patient-Physician Relationship in the Context of Work-Related and Independent Medical Examinations," Code of Medical Ethics (Chicago: AMA, 2004).

[22] Council on Ethical and Judicial Affairs of the American Medical Association, "Opinion E-5.09, Confidentiality: Industry-Employed Physicians and Independent Medical Examiners," Code of Medical Ethics (Chicago: AMA, 2004).

[23] M. Gregg Bloche, "Caretakers and Collaborators," Cambridge Quarterly of Healthcare Ethics 10 (2001): 275–284.

[24] United States Department of Defense, Medical Program Principles and Procedures for the Protection and Treatment of Detainees in the Custody of the Armed Forces of the United States, HA Policy 05–006 (3 June 2005); United States Department of Defense, Medical Program Support for Detainee Operations, Instruction 2310.08E (6 June 2006).

[25] Council on Ethical and Judicial Affairs of the American Medical Association, "Opinion E-2.06, Capital Punishment" and "Opinion E-2.065, Court-Initiated Medical Treatments in Criminal Cases," Code of Medical Ethics (Chicago: AMA, 2004).

3.1.2 Confidentiality of Detainee Information

Confidentiality is of particular concern when physicians provide medical care in settings where interrogations might occur. Interrogators might believe that interrogation will be more effective if informed by medical information, and might pressure physicians to share information obtained in the course of a patient-physician encounter. Opinion E-5.05, "Confidentiality," places great emphasis on the confidentiality of personal information that patients provide to physicians. The Opinion recognizes limited circumstances in which breaching confidentiality may be justifiable, for example, disclosures related to foreseeable and preventable harm to identifiable third parties. It is otherwise unethical to divulge personal information without the authorization of the patient. When medical records belong to the detention facility, physicians should warn detainee-patients that the information they provide for the medical record is accessible to facility authorities.

Moreover, in the context of physician employment by third parties, information should not be communicated to the third party without prior notification of the interrogatee that any information they provide may be passed on to a third party.[26] The fact that interrogation may be legally mandated or protected does not ethically justify communication of confidential information by a physician without notification and the individual's approval.

3.2 *Specific Roles*

To assess the ethics of physician involvement in interrogations, it is useful to distinguish various activities in which physicians may be involved.

Physicians are ethically justified in acting to prevent harm to individuals. In this regard, the suggestion that physicians should observe or monitor interrogations to prevent harm requires careful scrutiny. As defined in this report, appropriate interrogations present no reason for medical monitoring, because interrogators ought to abstain from coercive questioning. Physicians can determine that harm has been inflicted but, in many instances, cannot predict whether an interrogation practice will or will not cause harm.

Physicians may be asked to determine the overall medical fitness of detainees or their mental capacity, and to use their knowledge and skills to assess the health of detainees; questioning to elicit medical information of this kind is distinct from interrogations and is appropriate. The presence of a physician at an interrogation, particularly an appropriately trained psychiatrist, may actually benefit the interrogatee because of the belief held by many psychiatrists that kind

[26] Council on Ethical and Judicial Affairs of the American Medical Association, "Opinion E-5.09, Confidentiality: Industry-Employed Physicians and Independent Medical Examiners," Code of Medical Ethics (Chicago: AMA, 2004).

Printed in the United States
107667LV00002BA/277-300/P

9 781402 069116